W0043060

Springer

Tokyo
Berlin
Heidelberg
New York
Barcelona
Budapest
Hong Kong
London
Milan
Paris
Singapore

Takashi Tokoro

Atlas of Posterior Fundus Changes in Pathologic Myopia

With 564 Figures, Including 333 in Color

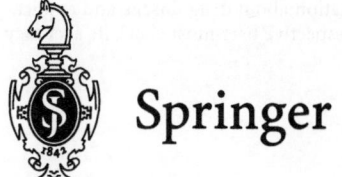 Springer

TAKASHI TOKORO, M.D.
Professor and Chairman
Department of Ophthalmology
Tokyo Medical and Dental University School of Medicine
1-5-45 Yushima, Bunkyo-ku
Tokyo 113-8519, Japan

This publication was supported by the Ministry of Education, Science, Sports and Culture of Japan, Grant-in-Aid for Scientific Research, Grant-in-Aid for Publication of Scientific Research Result

ISBN-13: 978-4-431-68018-5   e-ISBN-13: 978-4-431-67951-6
DOI: 10.1007/978-4-431-67951-6

Library of Congress Cataloging-in-Publication Data

Tokoro, Takashi, 1932–
      Atlas of posterior fundus changes in pathologic myopia/Takashi Tokoro.
         p.   cm.
      Includes bibliographical references and index.

      1. Fundus oculi—Diseases—Atlases.   2. Myopia—Complications—Atlases.   I. Title.
      [DNLM: 1. Choroid Diseases—pathology atlases.   2. Retinal Degeneration—pathology atlases.   3. Myopia—complications atlases.   4. Fundus Oculi atlases.   5. Atrophy atlases.   WW 17 T646a   1998]
      RE545.T65   1998
      617.7′2—dc21
      DNLM/DLC
      for Library of Congress   98-3242

Printed on acid-free paper

©Springer-Verlag Tokyo 1998

Softcover reprint of the hardcover 1st edition 1998

This work is subject to copyright. All rights are reserved, whether the whole or part of the material is concerned, specifically the rights of translation, reprinting, reuse of illustrations, recitation, broadcasting, reproduction on microfilms or in other ways, and storage in data banks.
The use of registered names, trademarks, etc. in this publication does not imply, even in the absence of a specific statement, that such names are exempt from the relevant protective laws and regulations and therefore free for general use.
Product liability: The publisher can give no guarantee for information about drug dosage and application thereof contained in this book. In every individual case the respective user must check its accuracy by consulting other pharmaceutical literature.

Typesetting: Best-set Typesetter Ltd., Hong Kong

SPIN: 10670522

Preface

Pathological myopia due to axial elongation results in thinning of the retina, particularly in cases of posterior staphyloma. As a result of this myopia, various kinds of chorioretinal atrophy develop in the posterior pole, especially in the macula. These atrophic changes are characterized by gradual progression during a chronic course that usually extends over several decades. Throughout this degenerative process, many complications can occur, producing multiple manifestations. Until now, however, studies of atrophic lesions and their clinical course have been incomplete, and diagnostic standards and classifications of chorioretinopathy have been unclear.

In 1987, the High Myopia Branch of the Research Committee on Chorioretinal Degenerations, which was established by the Ministry of Health and Welfare of Japan for serious diseases, published *The Manual for the Diagnosis of Pathologic Myopia*. This manual describes the classification, degenerative process, and stages of atrophic lesions, primarily based on ophthalmoscopic findings in the posterior pole.

The Department of Ophthalmology at the Tokyo Medical and Dental University established a special clinic on high myopia in 1974. Since then, we have observed progressive changes in chorioretinal atrophy in patients with high myopia. Through these observations, we have been able to differentiate various types of this disease and their modes of progression. From fundus records and accompanying photographs, we have determined that the degeneration of pathologic myopia commonly progresses slowly over a period of more than 20 years. Visual acuity, however, decreases rapidly if macular hemorrhage develops in association with posterior staphyloma. Conversely, some patients retain normal visual acuity for a long period. Although experiments using animal models of myopia and associated research to clarify the mechanism of axial elongation continue to be carried out, no effective methods for inhibiting axial elongation in pathologic myopia have been found. It is important, therefore, to forecast an effective prognosis of visual acuity in routine clinical situations according to an understanding of the progression of chorioretinal atrophy.

In this volume, we describe a classification of disease types, a classification of disease stages, and a course of disease progression based on long-term observations. All of the patients described here were examined in our clinic and include those who could be observed over a long period and whose conditions represented different types of chorioretinal atrophy.

TAKASHI TOKORO
March 1998

Acknowledgments

Many individuals have contributed to the completion of this book. In 1974, I started a special clinic on high myopia with Dr. K. Hayashi. Since the opening of the clinic many doctors have cooperated with us and have aided in our studies of the changes in the fundus of pathologic myopia. I would like to thank the members of the special high myopia clinic for their assistance.

A number of people were involved in the preparation of this book, especially Dr. Y. Akazawa, who very kindly spent many hours working with me. I appreciate his careful study and review, which has contributed greatly to this book. Certainly, without Dr. Y. Akazawa's help, this book would not have been possible.

I would like to express my appreciation to the following people: Dr. M. Kiyosawa and Dr. H. Pang, for their translation of Chapters 1 to 7 into English; Dr. K. Ohno-Matsui and others for their translation into English of additional case reports; and Mr. T. Yanagida, who photographed the fundus of the high myopia patients.

I am deeply grateful to Ms. M. A. Gere for her splendid English editing. Also, I am greatly indebted to my office staff member Miss Y. Arai, for her dedication in completing this task.

Last, I would like to thank the staff of Springer-Verlag Tokyo for their support and advice in publishing this book.

TAKASHI TOKORO

Table of Contents

1 Criteria for Diagnosis of Pathologic Myopia

Myopia is commonly classified into three groups: mild (≤3.0 diopters, D), moderate) >3.0 D), and high (>6.0 D). The limits of these types vary with each investigator. Many researchers have designated values such as >4.0 D, >6.0 D, or >8.0 D as high myopia [1]. On the basis of this information, Duke-Elder had suggested that high myopia, which is primarily caused by retinal degeneration in the posterior pole, should be named pathologic myopia. The pathological form can be distinguished from simple myopia, which is defined as variations within normal limits of the optical system of the eye [2]. However, it is sometimes difficult to define pathologic myopia as the eye with retinal degeneration in the posterior pole. Another definition states that high myopia accompanied by visual dysfunction is pathologic myopia and that this is distinguishable from simple myopia [3]. Although theoretically acceptable, this definition is not suitable for clinical practice and mass screening because it must be confirmed by various examinations.

To determine pathologic myopia, a simple standard classification is necessary. There is no doubt that axial elongation of the eyeball is the primary cause of high myopia. Therefore, if axial length exceeds three times the standard deviation from a normal distribution of the emmetropic axis, it is possible to define this condition as pathologic myopia. When the refractive degree of the eye is calculated from the long axial length outside its normal distribution, pathologic myopia is determined when the measurement of refraction exceeds −4.0 D in patients less than 5 years of age, −6.0 D between the ages of 6 and 8 years, and −8.0 D in those older than 9 years [4,5].

Using this definition, we examined 246 eyes in a population ranging in age from 5 to 72 years. Our results showed that the corrected visual acuity was less than 0.7 in 157 eyes (63.8%). The other 89 eyes had good corrected visual acuity, but 88.8% of these 89 eyes had abnormalities in visual field or in the fundus or both. Among all 246 eyes, 96% had abnormalities in visual acuity, visual field, or the fundus. Accordingly, we think that using this diagnostic criteria for pathologic myopia is reasonable [6]. Based on these criteria, the frequency of pathologic myopia is 0.1% in Japanese elementary school children, 0.5% in junior high school students, and 1.5% in senior high school students [7]. Also, according to a prospective investigation among 61 025 outpatients in 67 hospitals affiliated with medical schools in Japan, the frequency of pathologic myopia was 2.16% in the whole country [8]. Although the frequency of affected patients in the general Japanese population is not clear, it is estimated at approximately 1%.

This diagnostic criterion, based on refractive error, is enhanced if we also consider corrected vision, which is regarded as representative of visual function (Table 1.1) [9,10].

Table 1.1. Criteria for the diagnosis of pathologic myopia

Age (years)	Degree of refraction	Corrected vision
<5	>4.0 D	<0.4 D
6–8	>6.0 D	<0.6 D
>9	>8.0 D	<0.6 D

2 Methods of Examining the Posterior Pole of the Fundus

Several methods have been used to examine the fundus: direct ophthalmoscopy, indirect ophthalmoscopy, and slit lamp biomicroscopy. To examine the posterior pole in patients with pathologic myopia, indirect binocular ophthalmoscopy and slit lamp microscopy with an accessory lens are useful. Photographs taken with a fundus camera are used to record fundus changes.

2.1 Indirect Binocular Microscopy

The indirect binocular microscope allows a wide view of the fundus. The relationship between the extent and depth of posterior staphyloma and the relationship between posterior staphyloma and chorioretinal atrophy can be established by this method and with the use of a +20.0 D lens. It is necessary to look carefully at cupping of the optic disc because of complications of glaucoma in pathologic myopia. Because the frequency of complicated retinal detachment in pathologic myopia is relatively high, we have performed indirect ophthalmoscopy to examine details of the peripheral retina. On occasion, scleral depression may be used to examine the peripheral fundus as well.

2.2 Slit Lamp Biomicroscopy

To observe the fundus with a slit lamp microscope, an accessory lens, such as a contact type, for example, Goldmann's three-mirror contact lens, or a noncontact type, for example, a +90 D lens, is needed, The +90 D noncontact type of lens works best in the routine clinical setting, because it produces a three-dimensional view that can be used to confirm the findings of indirect ophthalmoscopy.

2.3 Fundus Photography

In eyes with posterior staphyloma, a fundus camera that has a picture angle greater than 45° is needed. Occasionally, it is difficult to focus the fundus lesion because of posterior staphyloma. It is very important, however, to know the chorioretinal changes and to record them with fundus photographs. A stereoscopic camera is not suitable to analyze posterior staphyloma because its picture angle is not wide enough. Also, a method that obtains the stereoscopic image using two photographs by achieving slight parallel shifting of the camera to the right and left is not suitable in quantitative analysis because the stereoscopic image differs with the distance moved.

2.4 Fundus Angiography

Fundus angiography is used to identify chorioretinal lesions or Fuchs' spot in eyes with pathologic myopia. Both fluorescein angiography (FAG) and indocyanine green angiography (IA) can be used. IA carried out by angiography after intravenous injection of indocyanine green (ICG) is best suited for observing choroidal vessels. High myopia manifests in a tessellated fundus, and the choroidal vessels can be shown clearly with this method. Scanning laser ophthalmoscopy (Rodenstock, München, Germany), which scans the fundus with a laser using a confocal scanning method, can achieve a clear picture in the early phase following ICG intravenous injection. On the other hand, the ICG infrared fundus angiography device 50 IA (Topcon, Tokyo, Japan) is excellent in obtaining the late-stage image.

3 Types of Fundus Changes in the Posterior Pole

Ophthalmoscopic findings observed in chorioretinal atrophy in eyes with pathologic myopia include four kinds of changes (Table 3.1):

1. Tessellated fundus, in which the choroidal vessels can be seen through the retina and the optic disc appears crescent shaped
2. Yellowish-white and ill-defined diffuse chorioretinal atrophy
3. Grayish-white and well-defined patchy chorioretinal atrophy
4. Macular hemorrhage

Although these changes associated with posterior staphyloma are common, some eyes with pathologic myopia exhibit no such changes.

3.1 Tessellated Fundus and Crescent

Hypoplasia of the retinal pigment epithelium (RPE) following axial elongation reduces the pigment, allowing the choroidal vessels to be seen. Sometimes a mild degree of this change can also be observed in aging or in a normal fundus that has a decreased amount of pigment:

a. Slight degree (T_1): well-defined choroidal vessels can be observed clearly (Fig. 3.1)

Table 3.1. Classification of chorioretinal atrophy in the posterior pole in pathologic myopia [10]

1. Tessellated fundus (T)
   a. Slight degree (T_1)
   b. Advanced degree (T_2)
2. Diffuse chorioretinal atrophy (D)
   a. Spotty or linear lesion of diffuse atrophy (D_1) (Lacquer crack lesion (Lc))
   b. Enlarged lesion of diffuse atrophy (D_2)
   c. Chorioretinal atrophy of the macula (MA)
3. Small patchy atrophy (P)
   a. Spotty lesion of patchy atrophy (P_1)
   b. Patchy lesion of patchy atrophy (P_2)
   c. Chorioretinal atrophy of the macula (MA)
4. Small macular hemorrhage (H)
   a. Neovascular macular hemorrhage (HN) (active stage, HN_1; scar stage, HN_2; atrophic stage, MA)
   b. Simple macular hemorrhage (HS) (active stage, HS_1; scar stage, HS_2)

b. Advanced degree (T_2): the choroidal blood vessel appears in relief (Fig. 3.2)

Tessellated fundus is usually associated with a crescent. The exposed sclera comes in contact with the papillary edge following axial elongation and forms a semilunar or annular white surface. Temporal and annular crescents are very common in the myopic fundus

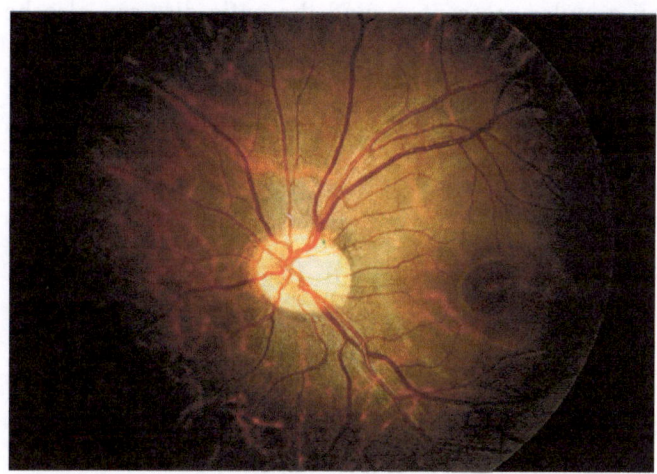

Fig. 3.1. Tessellated fundus (T_1), 17-year-old girl, left eye; refraction, $-10.0\,D$; axial length, 25.4 mm. A small temporal crescent and large choroidal vessels can be seen through the retina

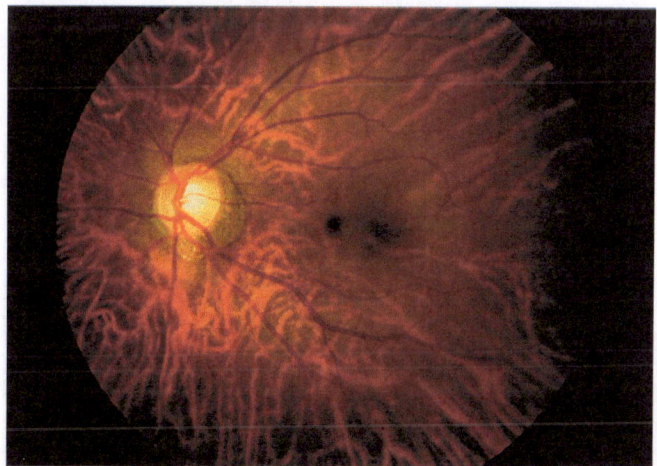

Fig. 3.2. Tessellated fundus (T_2), 37-year-old woman, left eye; refraction, $-14.5\,D$; axial length, 29.7 mm. The choroidal vessels appear as in relief

and are called myopic crescents. The other parts of the crescent are called atypical crescent. The characteristic change of crescent formation is the displacement of the edge of the lamina vitrea with its associated choriocapillaris and retinal pigment epithelium from the margin of the nerve. By degree of displacement, crescents are designated choroidal, scleral, and pigmentary. In high grades of myopia, the lamina vitrea, choroid, and sclera are superimposed over the nasal half of the optic nerve surface. (Fig. 3.3).

1. Choroidal crescent: the atrophied choroid is visible because the retinal pigment epithelium (RPE) is hypoplastic or broken down at the papillary edge. Although most crescents appear semilunar in the temporal region, an annular crescent around the optic disc can also be found.

2. Scleral crescent: in high myopia, semilunar or annular white patches can be seen because of scleral exposure.

3. Pigmentary crescent: a black ring of pigment at the optic disc edge or outer edge of the choroidal crescent.

4. Crescent by supertraction: axial elongation causes the nasal sclera and choroid to protrude at the optic disc, forming a light semilunar pigmentary ring.

Along with axial elongation, cupping of the optic disc contracts temporally; its center is easily found in the temporal region. Eyes with glaucoma and high myopia show greater cupping of the optic disc, which may be plate shaped in most cases and is different from the typical picture seen in glaucoma [11].

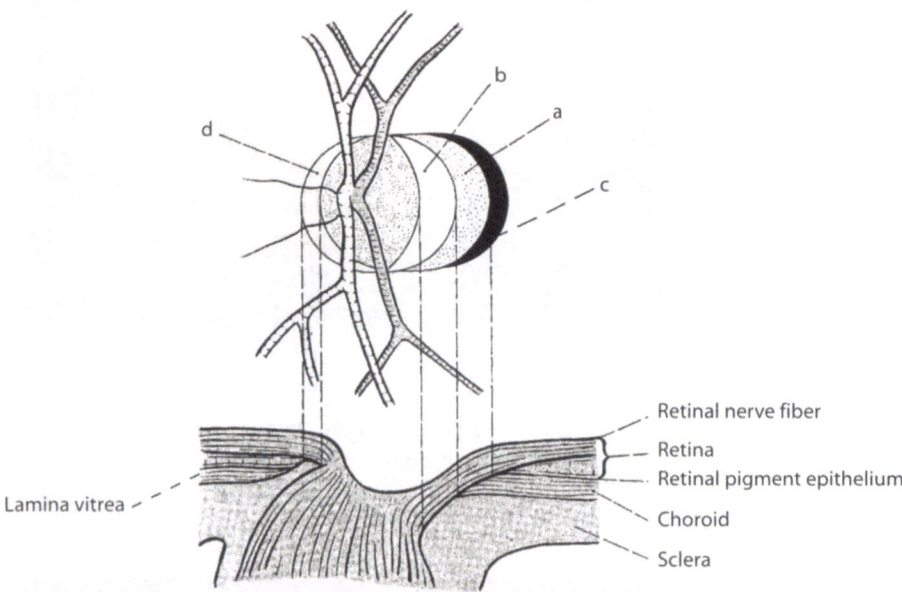

Fig. 3.3. Various types of crescent: *a*, choroidal crescent; *b*, scleral crescent; *c*, pigmentary crescent; *d*, crescent by supertraction

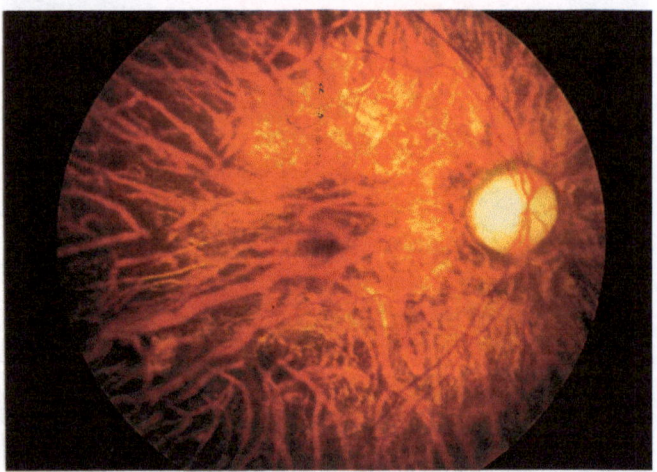

Fig. 3.4. Spotty or linear lesion of diffuse atrophy (D_1), 17-year-old girl, right eye; −12.5 D; axial length, 28.4 mm. In an obviously tessellated fundus, the choroidal vessels can be seen through the retina. A yellowish-white tessellated lesion lies along the choroidal vessels

3.2 Diffuse Chorioretinal Atrophy (D)

Characteristic diffuse chorioretinal atrophy appears as a yellowish-white fundus in the posterior pole. Spotty and linear lesions of the enlarged area of diffuse atrophy can be observed mainly in the macula and around the optic disc [10,12].

3.2.1 Spotty or Linear Lesions of Diffuse Atrophy (D₁)

Spotty or linear lesions of diffuse atrophy can be classified into two subtypes according to their location: with the choroidal blood vessels or across the choroidal blood vessels.

3.2.1.1 Lesion with the Choroidal Vessels

The spotty or linear yellowish-white lesion appears with the choroidal vessels. It exists in the macular area or around the optic disc and contacts the medium- or large-sized vessel walls in the choroid. Sometimes the choroidal vessels also appear yellowish white (Fig. 3.4). During fluorescein angiography (FAG), no abnormality can be observed from the early stage to the middle stage, but fluorescence corresponding to this lesion gradually appears at the late stage. This hyperfluorescent area is thought to be produced by staining of the connective tissue around the choroidal vessels. Therefore, this lesion may represent damage to the choroidal vessels or to the surrounding tissues. In indocyanine green angiography (IA), no abnormality is detected.

3.2.1.2 Lesion Across Choroidal Vessels

Called a lacquer crack (Lc), this lesion exists in most cases in the macular area [13]. The lesion is linear and usually is seen at almost a right angle, with straight lines that form by connecting the center of the optic disc and the fovea (Figs. 3.5, 3.6, 3.7a, 3.8, 3.9a). A lesion parallel to this straight line can also be found. In the earliest stage of the choroidal flush that occurs during FAG, spotty hyperfluorescence can be observed along with medium- or large-sized vessels in the choroid that cross the lesion (Fig. 3.7b). Later, the lesion becomes hyperfluorescent, forming a window defect following the filling of the surrounding choroidal capillary (Fig. 3.7c). Next, the fluorescence gradually increases and appears hyperfluorescent until the late stage [14]. The hyperfluorescence is considered tissue staining of the repaired RPE–Bruch's membrane–choroidal capillary after the breakdown of Bruch's membrane [12,13]. However, no leakage from the lesion can be observed (Fig. 3.7d).

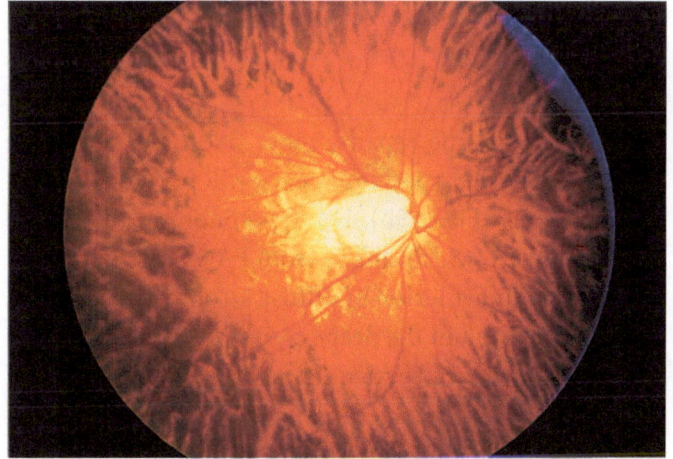

Fig. 3.5. Spotty or linear lesion of diffuse atrophy (D₁), 33-year-old man, right eye; refraction, −15.0 D; axial length, 28.8 mm. A yellowish-white spotty or linear lesion can be observed between the optic disc and fovea

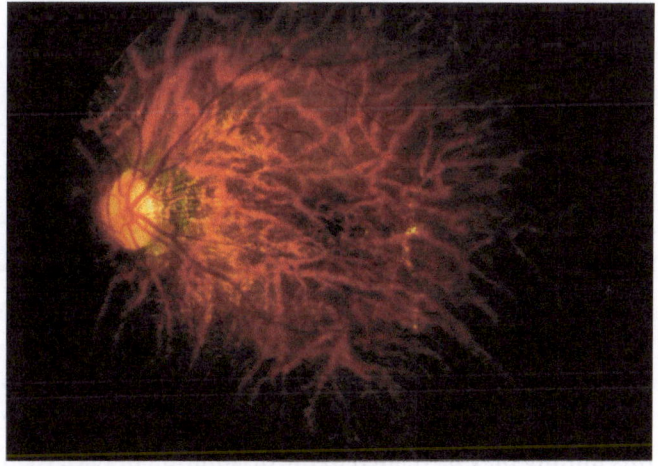

Fig. 3.6. Lacquer crack (Lc) lesion, 23-year-old woman, left eye; refraction, −20.0 D; axial length, 30.7 mm. A linear lesion, crossing the choroidal vessels, is observed in the temporal part of the fovea

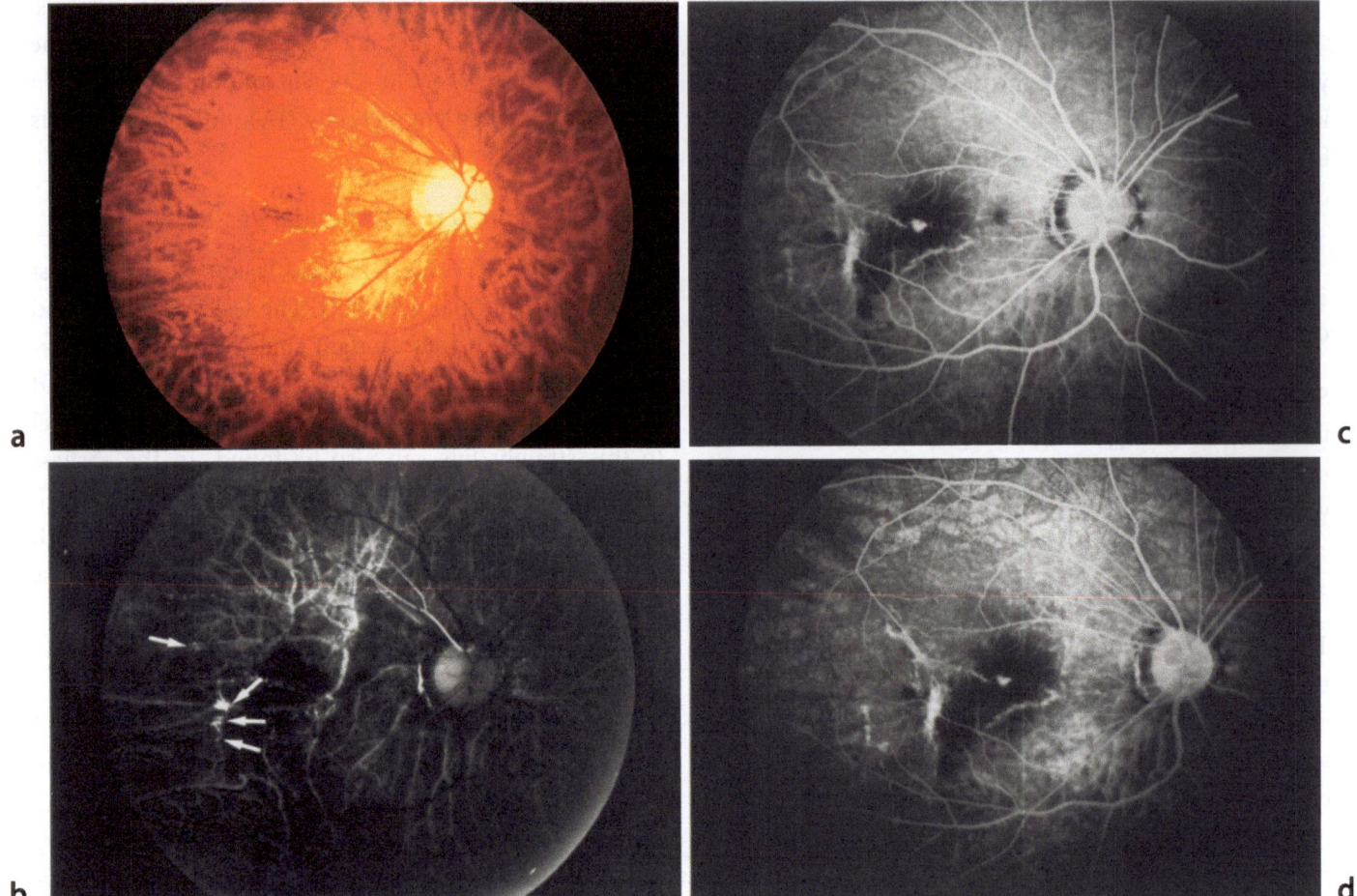

Fig. 3.7. a Spotty or linear lesion of diffuse atrophy (Lc), 24-year-old woman, right eye; refraction, −18.5 D; axial length, 30.8 mm. A yellowish-white atrophic lesion can be observed temporal to the optic disc. If a straight line were drawn between the fovea and the optic disc, the linear lesion would be at a right angle or parallel to this line. It would also be at an oblique angle to this line. **b** Photograph of fluorescein angiography (FAG) in **a**. At 10 sec, FAG shows limited area of retinal arteries filling in the choroidal phase. The Lc crossing the medium- and large-sized choroidal vessels is hyperfluorescent (*arrows*). **c** At 1 min, FAG reveals that all Lc show linear hyperfluorescence. **d** In the late phase of FAG, Lc continues in silhouette, with a comparatively strong fluorescence, even after the fluorescein has washed out of the choroidal vessels. This strong fluorescence may be derived from staining of the repaired tissue

In IA, the most common type of lesion appears as a clear hypofluorescent area in the late stage (Fig. 3.8b,c). It is thought that this hypofluorescence reflects both the filling defect of the choroidal capillary and the repaired tissue. Furthermore, the longer the time after the formation of the Lc, the stronger is the blockage. Even when abnormal fluorescence can be detected in IA, its length is usually shorter than that of the Lc in FAG. The reason for this finding may be related to the dissolution of ICG. Also in IA, as the tissue repairs, more fluorescence will be blocked, and the hypofluorescence will become increasingly obvious (Fig. 3.9b). No hyperfluorescence can be observed in IA, which differs from FAG [15].

Spotty or linear lesion of diffuse atrophy can be interpreted as a lesion in the deep layer of the choroid, which mainly involves connective tissue around the choroidal vessel and a lesion in the superficial layer of the choroid, which mainly involves Bruch's membrane.

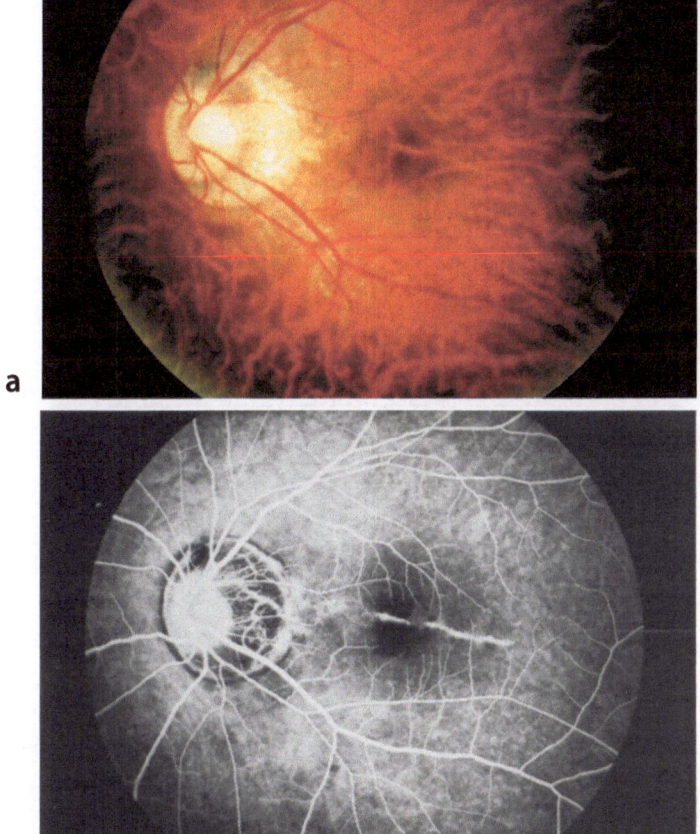

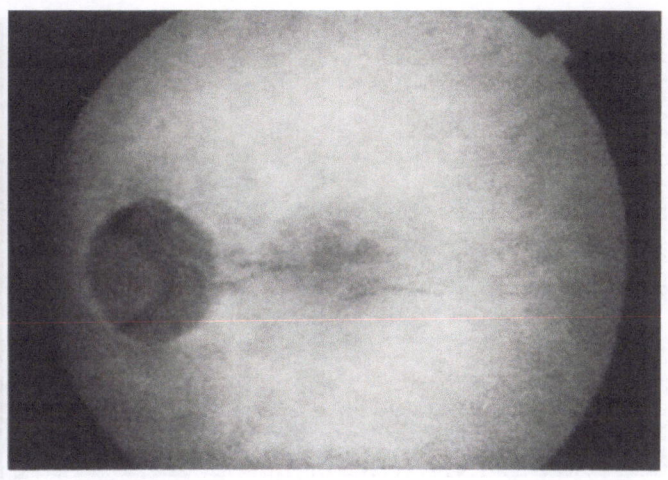

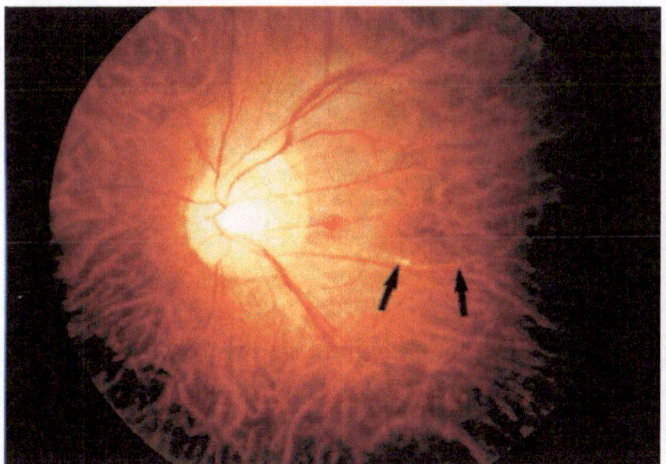

Fig. 3.8. a Lacquer crack (Lc) lesion, 30-year-old woman, left eye; refraction, −7.5 D; axial length, 28.3 mm. The linear lesion is visible crossing the fovea. **b** Photograph of FAG in **a**. Lc shows a clearer hyperfluorescence in FAG than in the fundus color photograph. **c** Photograph in late phase of indocyanine green angiography (IA). Lc is gradually becoming hypofluorescent. Extent of hypofluorescence continues to the optic disc, past that seen in the fundus color photograph or FAG.

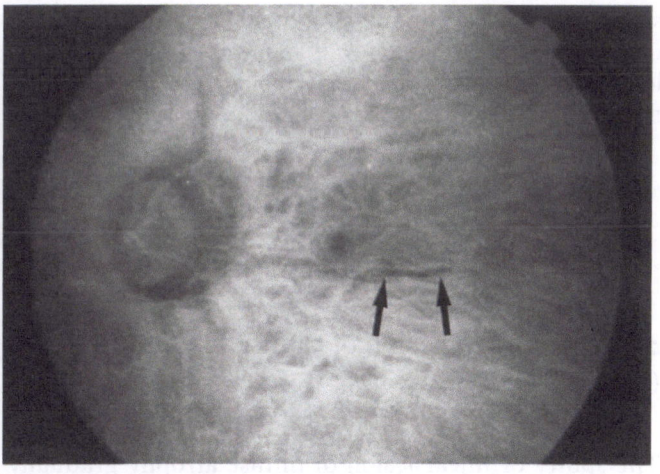

Fig. 3.9. a Lacquer crack (Lc) lesion, 27-year-old man, left eye; −15.0 D; axial length, 31.8 mm. Linear lesion (*arrows*) can be seen in the inferior part of the fovea. **b** Photograph of late phase of IA in **a** shows strong hypofluorescence in the temporal part of the Lc (*arrows*)

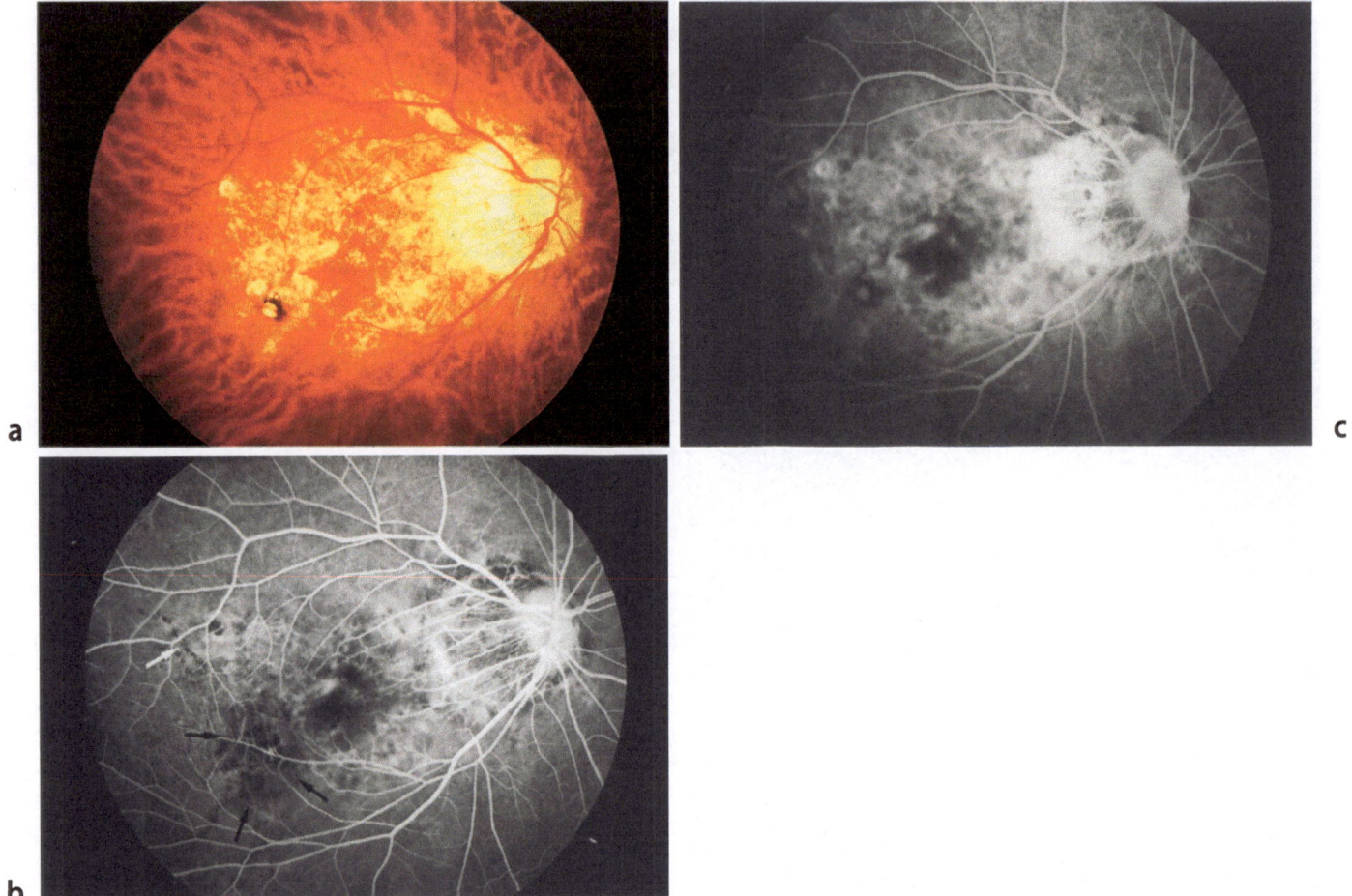

Fig. 3.10. a Enlarged lesion of diffuse atrophy (D₂), 44-year-old woman, right eye; refraction, −10.0 D; axial length, 29.2 mm. Although the yellowish-white lesion covers the entire macula, the normal orange fundus can still be observed. Two small patches of patchy atrophy appear in the temporal part of the macula, and one lesion with pigmentation is seen in the lower part of the macula. **b** Photograph of FAG in **a**. D₂ lesion manifests a mixture of hyperfluorescence and hypofluo- rescence, demonstrating an irregular fluorescent view. An obvious filling defect of the choriocapillaris appears around the pigmentation in the temporal part of the macula (*black arrows*). Also, the area without abnormal findings reveals a linear hypofluorescence caused by some unknown blockage (*white arrow*). **c** Photograph of same patient in late phase of FAG. D₂ lesion shows hyperfluorescence from tissue staining

3.2.2 Enlarged Lesion of Diffuse Atrophy (D₂)
(Figs. 3.10a, 3.11a)

The spotty or linear lesion of diffuse atrophy gradually increases in number with the years and appears yellowish white. Although the diffuse enlargement of the spotty or linear lesion is discolored, the fundus between lesions remains normal in color. The extent of this enlargement varies, from the restricted area in the optic disc and a part of the macula to the whole posterior pole. The tessellated change within the lesion disappears, and any choroidal vessels smaller than medium size also become unclear.

In FAG, the enlarged area of diffuse atrophy that is restricted to the posterior pole shows hypofluorescence by a delayed filling of the choroid in the late stage (Fig. 3.10b). After that, the area of hypofluorescence decreases because of gradual extravasation from the surrounding choroidal vessels. Hyperfluorescence can be observed in the late stage, caused by tissue staining that corresponds to the enlarged lesion of diffuse atrophy (Fig. 3.10c). Meanwhile, irregular linear hypofluorescence can also be seen in the late stage (Fig. 3.12). (Accumulated pigment in the hypofluorescent area corresponding to this blockage is not seen by ophthalmoscopy.) In the late stage of FAG, the medium- or large-sized choroidal vessels running through the enlarged lesion of diffuse atrophy often appear in silhouette, and hyperfluorescence is observed in part of the connective tissue around the blood vessels [12]. Therefore, it is conceivable that the tissue staining derives from the connective tissue (Fig. 3.11b). These findings show that the atrophy has reached the RPE, Bruch's membrane, choroidal capillary, and extensive tissues of the choroid.

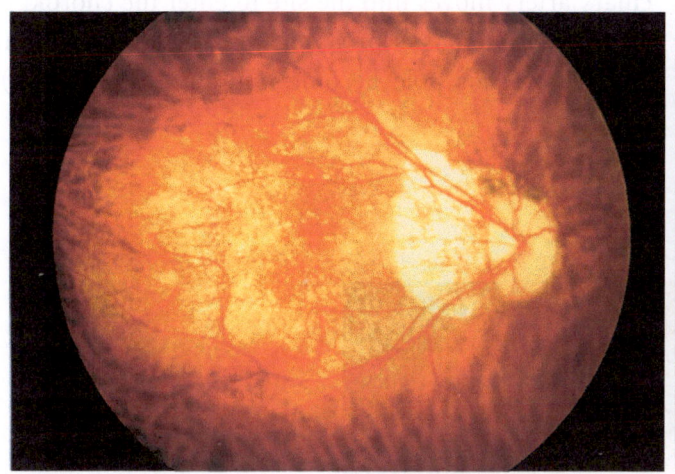

a

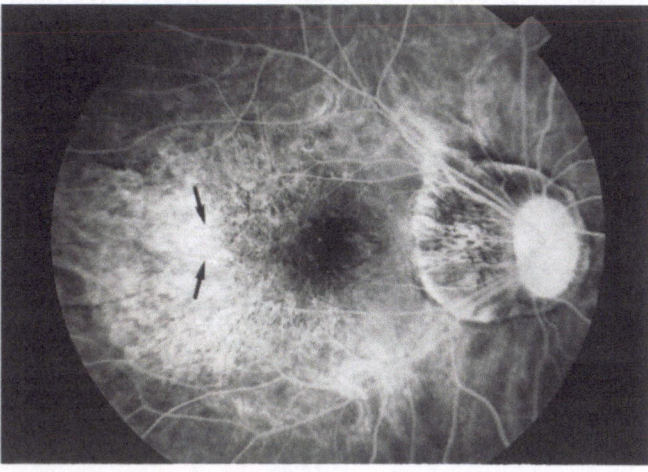

b

Fig. 3.11. a Enlarged lesion of diffuse atrophy (D$_2$), 32-year-old woman, right eye; refraction, −22.0 D; axial length, 32.1 mm. The lower part of a posterior staphyloma has an enlarged lesion, through which large choroidal vessels are visible. **b** Photograph in late phase of FAG in **a**. Granular hypofluorescent tissue staining is obvious within a D$_2$ lesion in the temporal part of the macula. Choroidal vessels within the lesion appear in silhouette against the linear hypofluorescence (*arrows*)

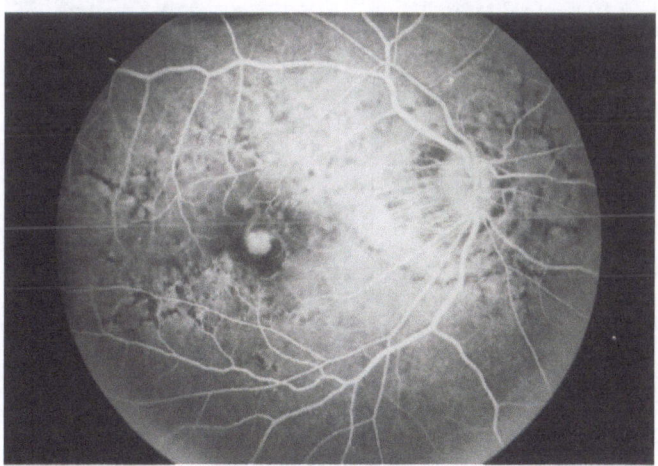

Fig. 3.12. A 64-year-old woman, right eye; refraction, −18.0 D; axial length, 29.3 mm. Photograph of D$_2$ lesion in late phase of FAG. Lesion is complicated by a macular hole. Exten-sive linear hypofluorescence can be observed within the D$_2$ lesion and around the optic disc

3.2.3 Diffuse Chorioretinal Atrophy of the Macula

The posterior pole of the fundus, including the macula, appears yellowish white and has a sunset appearance (Figs. 3.13a, 3.14). Granular hyperfluorescence produced by tissue staining can be found in the late stage of FAG (Fig. 3.11b). The filling of the background fluorescence in the choroid is delayed sporadically from the early stage to the late stage. There is also reduced fluorescence in this lesion. Although these findings do not show com-

plete blockage of the choroidal capillary, it is conceivable that an advanced obstacle in the choroidal circulation has involved the whole lesion. With IA, the enlarged lesion of diffuse atrophy not only involves the choroidal capillary, but the medium- and large-sized vessels in the choroid have also obviously decreased, and the blood vessels in the back of the eyeball may be seen through the sclera in the posterior pole. Because the short posterior ciliary artery moves into the site to enter the choroid at the edge of the posterior staphyloma, the blood vessels in the posterior pole become less dense (Fig. 3.13b).

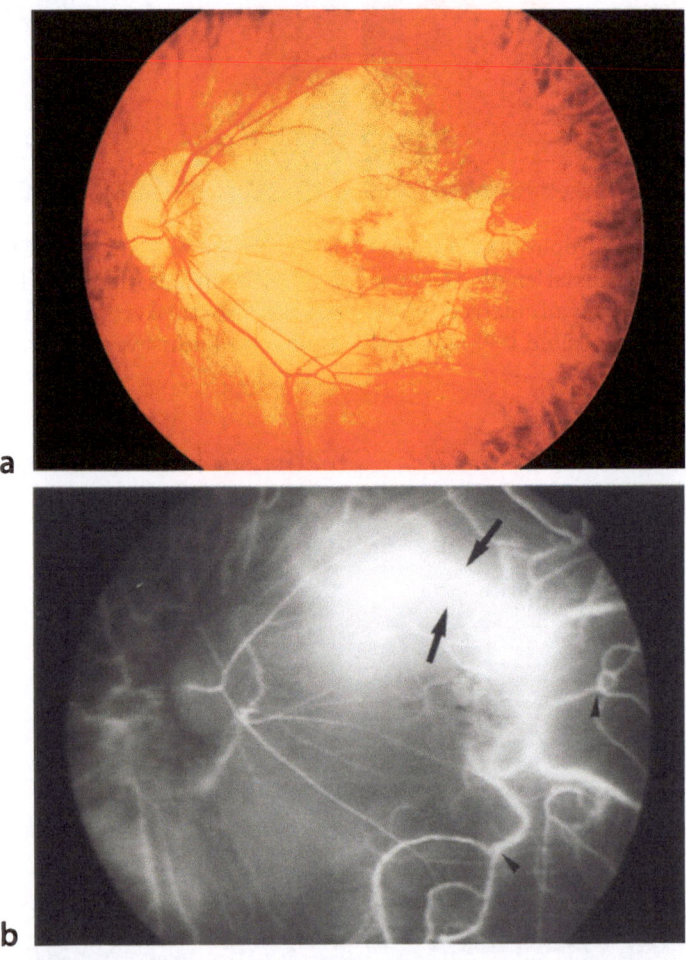

Fig. 3.13. a Diffuse chorioretinal atrophy of the macula (MA), 47-year-old man, left eye; refraction, −16.0 D; axial length, 29.4 mm. The area from optic disc to macula is yellowish-white; no normal fundus color can be observed within this area. **b** Photograph in early phase of IA (**a**). The choroidal vessels lose density in the posterior pole, clearly revealing the retrobulbar artery (*arrows*) through the sclera. The site where the short posterior ciliary artery enters the choroid has shifted closer to the edge of the posterior staphyloma (*arrowheads*)

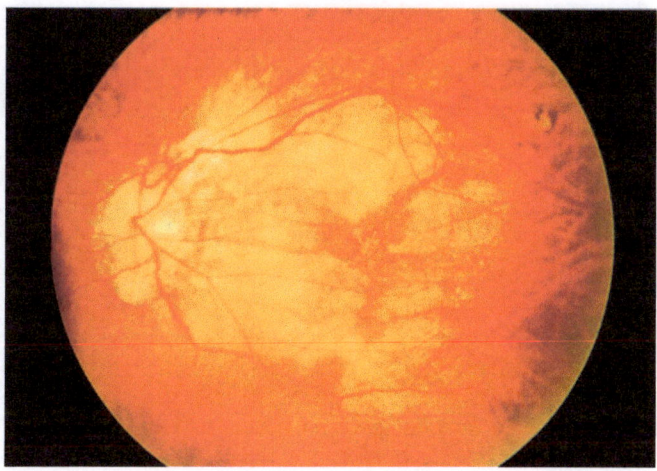

Fig. 3.14. Diffuse chorioretinal atrophy of the macula (MA), 64-year-old woman, left eye, −25.0 D; axial length, 31.8 mm. Yellowish-white color appears in the macular area, in which the fovea is centered

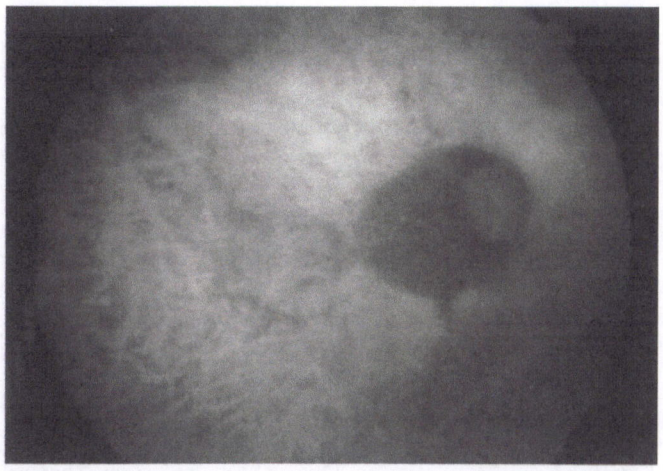

Fig. 3.15. A 61-year-old woman, right eye; refraction −17.5 D; axial length, 28.1 mm. Photograph in late phase of IA. A fairly wide linear hypofluorescence appears very clearly in the lesion and gains in clarity in the later phase of IA. These hypofluorescence of this lesion is similar to that of Lc, although it is slightly wider than is seen in the Lc. These differ in that the hypofluorescence is almost a curved lesion, while the Lc is a linear lesion. It is conceivable that the blockage could be caused by something unknown

Also, the number of hypofluorescent lines that cross the lesion are seen more clearly in the late stage, compared with FAG. The linear hypofluorescence in the late stage of IA is very similar to that of the Lc lesion (Fig. 3.15).

Histological specimens of eyes with high myopia often exhibit multiple layers of RPE. Sometimes, hypofluorescence can also be detected in the late stage of FAG. It has been speculated, therefore, that linear hypofluorescence in the late stage of IA is the reflection of blocked fluorescence. Diffuse chorioretinal atrophy includes a lesion from RPE to choroidal vessels. The ophthalmoscopic characteristic of this lesion is that it looks more yellowish, as compared with the white scleral conus, and ill defined, which is important to differentiate it from patchy atrophy.

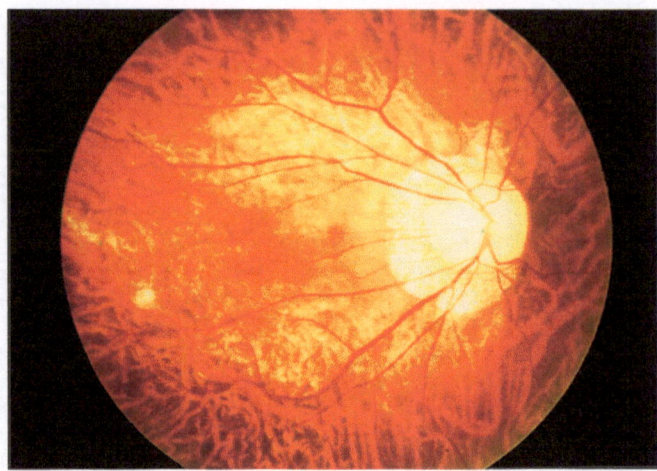

Fig. 3.16. Spotty lesion of patchy atrophy (P_1), 34-year-old man, right eye; refraction, -14.5 D; axial length, 29.2 mm. D_2 can be seen in the posterior pole of the fundus. A small well-defined area of patchy atrophy is observed in the inferotemporal area of the fundus

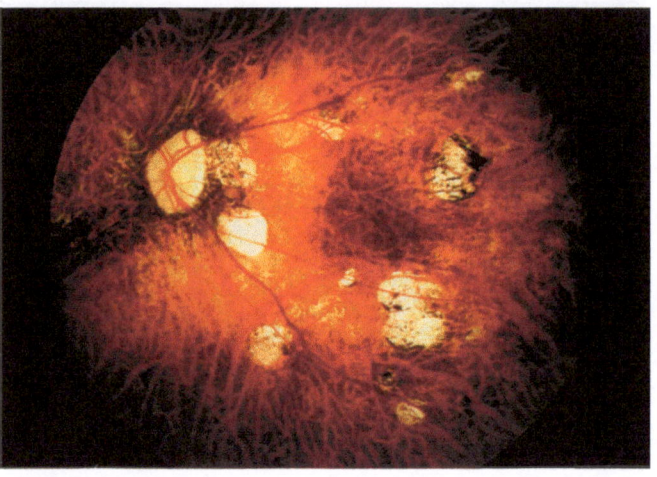

Fig. 3.17. Spotty and patchy lesions of patchy atrophy (P_1, P_2), 63-year-old woman, left eye; refraction, -3.75 D (aphakia); axial length, 32.3 mm. Spotty (P_1) and patchy (P_2) lesions of patchy atrophy coexist in the posterior pole. Although both lesions are well defined and grayish white, some lesions are associated with pigmentation. Also, an enlarged lesion of diffuse atrophy is visible

3.3 Patchy Chorioretinal Atrophy (P)

The ophthalmoscopic finding of patchy atrophy is a grayish-white, well-defined lesion [10,12].

3.3.1 Spotty Lesion of Patchy Atrophy (P_1)

Spotty lesions are from one to several choroidal lobules in diameter (0.6–0.8 mm; less than 0.5 optic disc diameter) and appear in the macular area or around the optic disc. This small lesion looks somewhat brighter than its surroundings, or it may appear grayish white (Fig. 3.16). Occasionally slight pigmentation can be found around the lesion (Fig. 3.17). If no detailed examination is done, it is difficult to find this small lesion. When the lesion coexists with diffuse atrophy, it is difficult to differentiate the two (Fig. 3.18a). In the early stage of FAG, hypofluorescence caused by delayed filling of choroidal fluorescence can be observed in a small zone that includes the spotty atrophy. After that, as the fluorescein leakage progresses from its surrounding choriocapillaris, spotty hyperfluorescence (window defect) appears. Alternatively, no hyperfluorescence may be observed, even in the late stage of FAG (Fig. 3.18b–e). It is difficult to detect spotty atrophy in this stage of IA because of poor resolution.

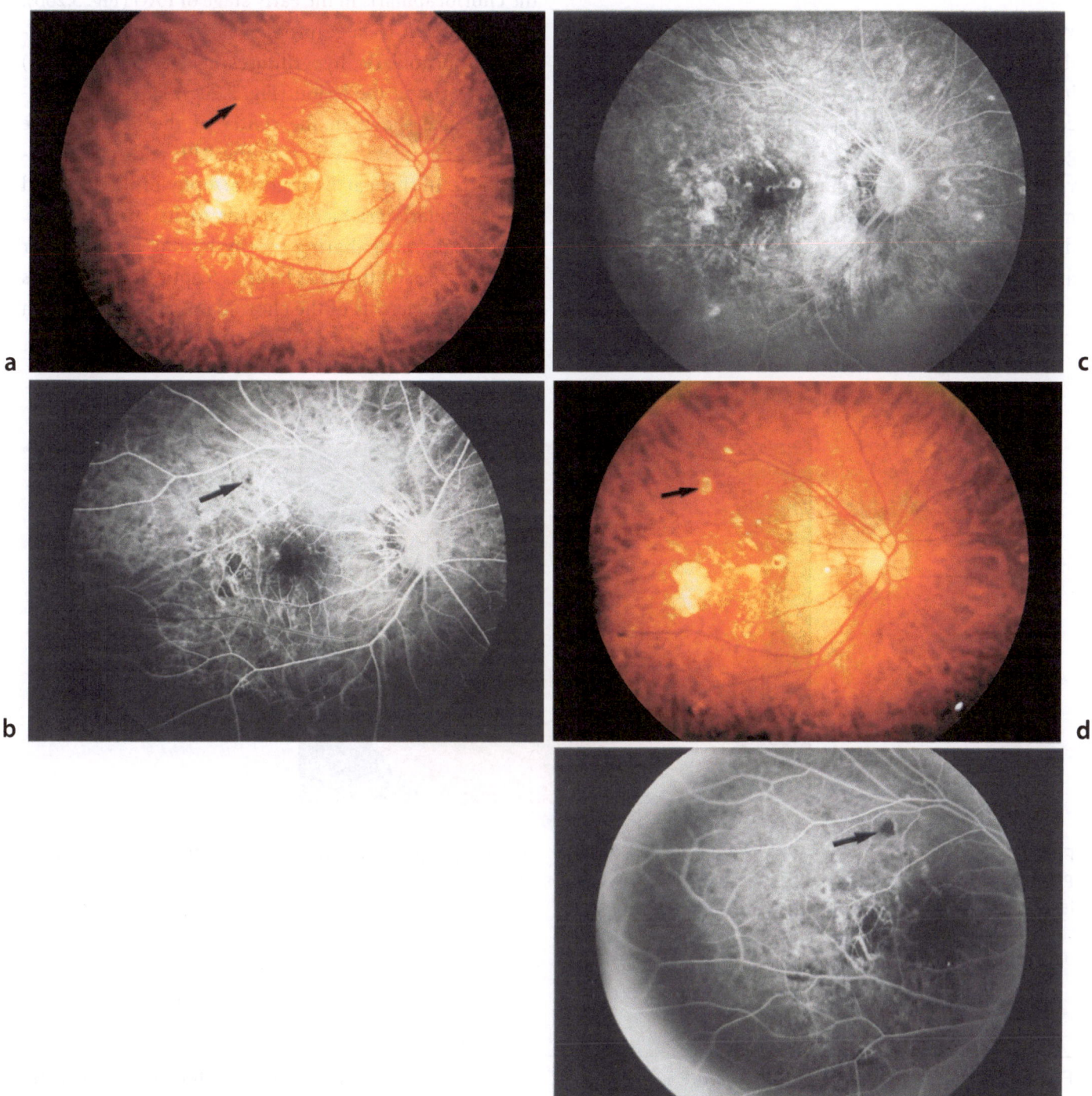

Fig. 3.18. a Spotty and patchy lesions of patchy atrophy (P_1, P_2), 24-year-old man, right eye; refraction, -21.0 D; axial length, 30.5 mm. Spotty (P_1) and patchy (P_2) lesions with diffuse atrophy. A small undefined area is seen (*arrow*). A simple hemorrhage occurs in the macular area. **b** Photograph of FAG in **a**. At 42 sec after intravenous injection, the hypofluorescence produced by delayed filling of the choroid is observed in the position P_1 (*arrow*). **c** Photograph in late phase of FAG in **a**. As

fluorescein leaks from the surrounding choriocapillaris, the hypofluorescence in the position of P_1 disappears. Also, no hyperfluorescence appears in this position during the angiography. Atrophy of the retinal pigment epithelial cell (RPE) may not occur in the same position. **d** Photograph of the same patient as in **a** after 1 year. A spotty lesion is enlarged (*arrow*). **e** In the position of an enlarged P_1, very clear, delayed choroidal filling is shown (*arrow*)

3.3.2 Patchy Lesion of Patchy Atrophy (P₂)

When individual areas of spotty atrophy become larger than 0.5 optic disc diameter after many years of spreading, a well-defined round or oval lesion will form. The color of the patchy lesion of patchy atrophy is mainly grayish white (Fig. 3.19). The medium- or large-sized vessels of the choroid within the lesion can be observed more clearly, as compared with those in tessellated fundus. Sometimes, the atrophy is dark green and is associated with pigmentation (Fig. 3.20a)

P_2 shows the typical choroidal filling defect in FAG, which is hypofluorescence produced by delayed filling of the choriocapillaris in the early stage of FAG (Fig. 3.20b). As fluorescein leakage progresses from the surrounding choriocapillaris, hyperfluorescence (tissue staining) appears around the lesion (Fig. 3.20c). However, hypofluorescence shows in the center of the lesion as the result of complete atrophy in the RPE and the choriocapillaris. In this patchy lesion, atrophy of the RPE and choriocapillaris gradually spreads to its surroundings. Occasionally, neighboring patchy lesions fuse together and form a lesion that is as large as 5 optic disc diameters (Fig. 3.22). Sclerosis of the choroidal vessels can be seen

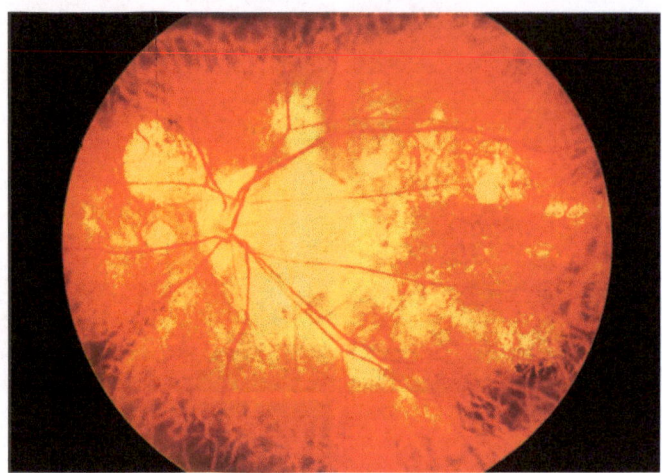

Fig. 3.19. Spotty and patchy lesions of patchy atrophy (P_1, P_2), 69-year-old woman, left eye; refraction, −21.0 D; axial length, 30.2 mm. Spotty (P_1) and patchy (P_2) lesions of patchy atrophy coexist around the optic disc. Posterior staphyloma (type 1) is also present

Fig. 3.20. a Patchy lesion of patchy atrophy (P_2), 40-year-old man, left eye; refraction, −22.0 D; axial length, 32.1 mm. A patchy lesion of 2 disc diameters is observed in the inferotemporal part of the fovea. Pigmentation is seen in the center of this lesion. Visual acuity is 0.8 because the fovea is not involved. **b** Photograph in early phase of FAG. Within the P_2 lesion, medium- or large-sized choroidal vessels behind the atrophied RPE can be seen clearly. Because the choriocapillaris has disappeared, hypofluorescence within the lesion contrasts with the surrounding area. **c** Photograph in late phase of FAG in the same patient (**a**). As fluorescein leaks from normal capillaris around the lesion, the fibrous tissue within the lesion stains and turns hyperfluorescent. **d** Photograph in early phase of IA in the same patient (**a**). Typical of most cases complicated with the P_2 lesion, the area surrounding the choroidal circulation has decreased in the area surrounding the P_2 lesion. The number of medium- or large-sized vessels in the choroid is obviously decreasing. Sometimes the retrobulbar artery is visible through the lesion (*arrows*). **e** Photograph in late phase of IA in the same patient (**a**). Because indocyanine green dye leaking from the choriocapillaris around the lesion is reduced, no hyperfluorescence is shown as P_2. Hypofluorescence appears in the late phase of IA, reflecting the disappearance of the choriocapillaris behind the lesion (*arrowheads*). P_2 is, however, often complicated with severe D_2, which decreases the choroidal circulation surrounding the lesion, and the hypofluorescence is less conspicuous, as compared with the surrounding areas. Therefore, it is thought that FAG is useful in detecting the range of P_2

within such a big patchy lesion, and it is also obvious that the number of vessels is decreasing.

In the early stage of IA, retrobulbar arteries behind the posterior pole of the globe can be seen clearly through the decreasing vessels in the choroid (Fig. 3.20d). When the choriocapillaris fills with fluorescein, the surroundings show a veil-like hyperfluorescence. Mean-while, hypofluorescence exists only within the lesion because no filling occurs. Even in the late stage of IA, the lesion does not fill with fluorescein, although diffuse hyperfluorescence appears around the lesion. Subsequently, the boundary of the patchy atrophy becomes gradually more delineated in the late stage (Fig. 3.20e). However, FAG is a better choice for determining the ex-

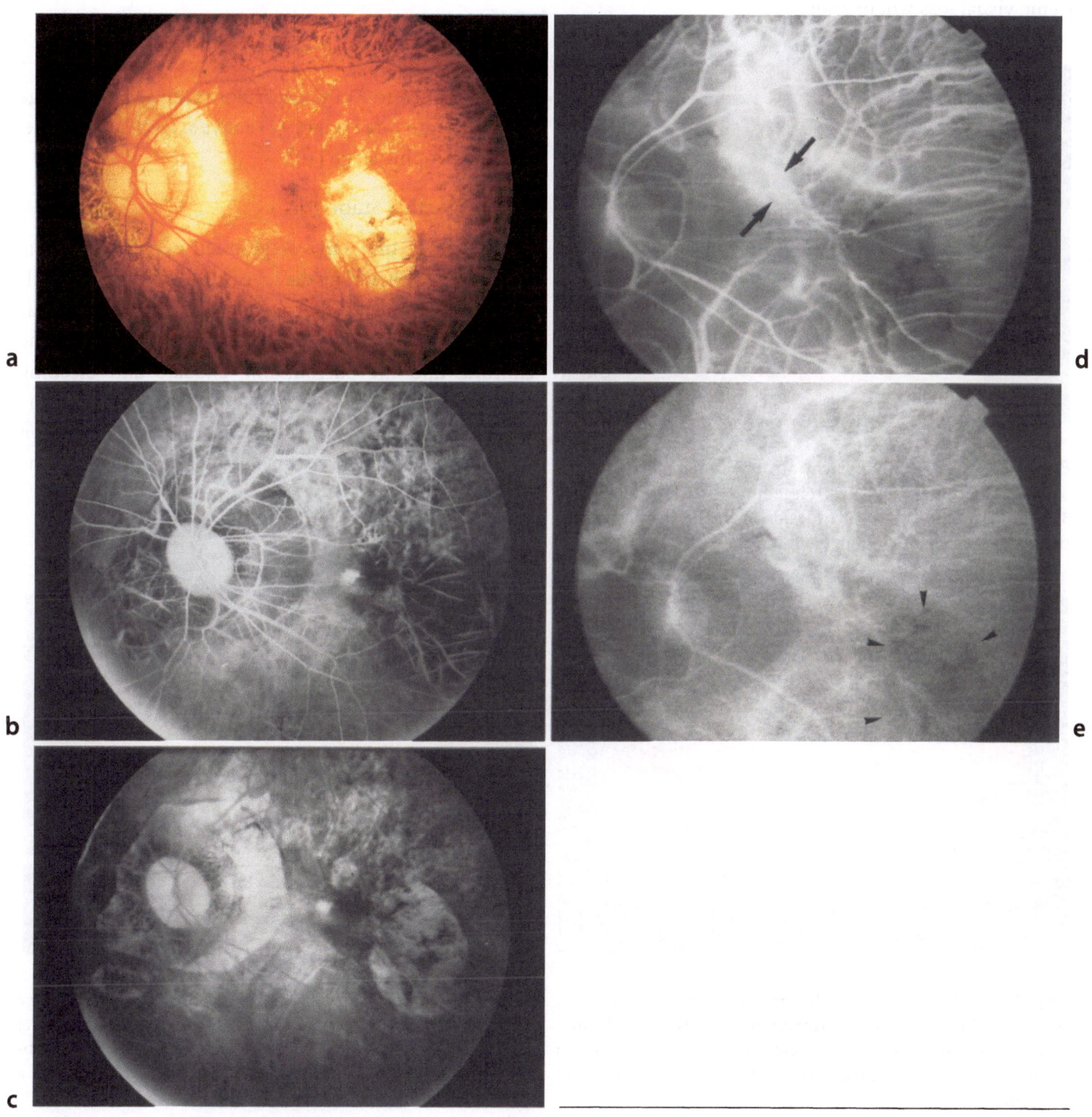

tent of the lesion, because the hypofluorescence seen in IA that corresponds to the patchy lesion is too weak.

Patchy atrophy is characterized by complete atrophy in a restricted area of RPE and choriocapillaris. The similar grayish-white color of the scleral conus and the well-defined morphological features are important ophthalmoscopic findings to make the diagnosis.

3.3.3 Chorioretinal Atrophy of the Macula
(Figs. 3.21, 3.22)

If chorioretinal atrophy occupies the macular area, extreme visual loss will develop.

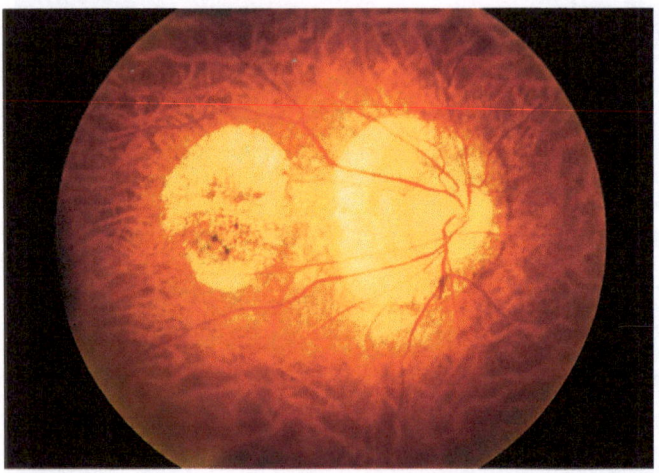

Fig. 3.21. Chorioretinal patchy atrophy of the macula (MA), 50-year-old woman, right eye; refraction, −18.0 D; axial length, 31.1 mm. A well-defined patchy lesion of patchy atrophy covers the entire macula, including the fovea

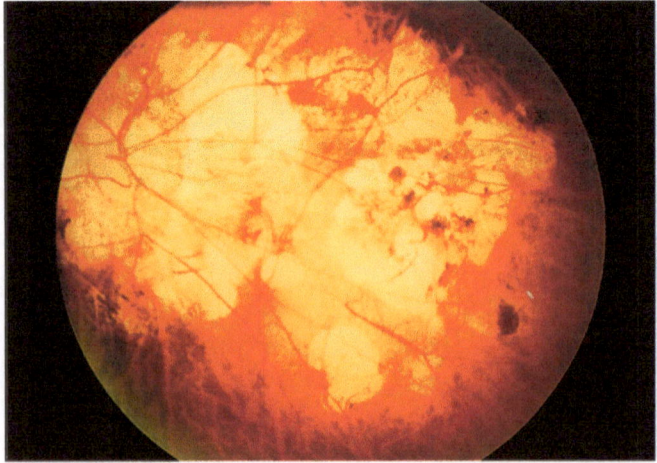

Fig. 3.22. Chorioretinal patchy atrophy of the macula (MA), 59-year-old woman, left eye; refraction, −28.0 D; axial length, 30.2 mm. A large temporal crescent and a large patchy lesion cover the macula. The lesions are fused and are associated with a pigmented spot

3.4 Macular Hemorrhage (H)

Macular hemorrhage can be classified as two types: neovascular macular hemorrhage, which may originate from the choroidal neovascularization, and simple macular hemorrhage, which is considered idiopathic choroidal hemorrhage [16,17]. The morphological features, which form after absorption of the hemorrhage, are different from the two types of macular hemorrhage. The prognoses also differ. Therefore, it is clinically very important to identify the type of macular hemorrhage at the onset of disease.

3.4.1 Neovascular Macular Hemorrhage (HN)

The clinical course of neovascular macular hemorrhage is divided into three stages: (1) active stage, (2) scar stage, and (3) atrophic stage [10].

3.4.1.1 Active Stage (HN₁)

The lesion of the active stage often occurs within the macular area, including the fovea [16]. A typical ophthalmoscopic finding is the proliferation of fibrovascular membrane, which includes neovascularization from the choroid, and the surrounding exudate and bleeding (Figs. 3.23, 2.24, 2.25a). In general, most of the hemorrhage and exudate of the lesion are mild in comparison with those of senile disciform macular degeneration. The

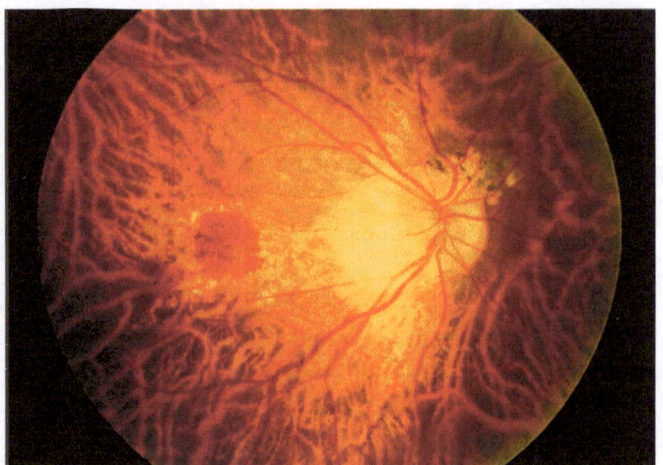

Fig. 3.23. Neovascular macular hemorrhage, active stage (HN₁), 55-year-old woman, right eye; refraction, −16.0 D; axial length, 30.0 mm. A hemorrhage 1 disc diameter in size is observed over the fovea. In the center of the hemorrhage is a proliferation of fibrovascular membrane

Fig. 3.24. Neovascular macular hemorrhage, active stage (HN$_1$), 54-year-old man, right eye; refraction, -12.0 D; axial length, 30.2 mm. A proliferating dark-colored fibrovascular membrane is observed over the fovea. A hemorrhage of about 1 disc diameter surrounds the lesion

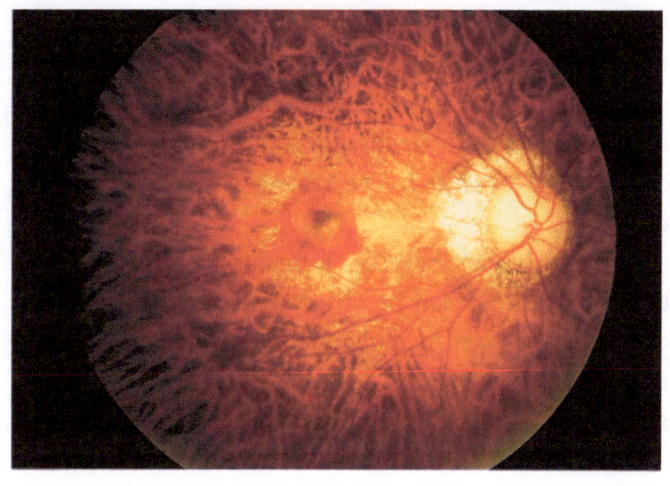

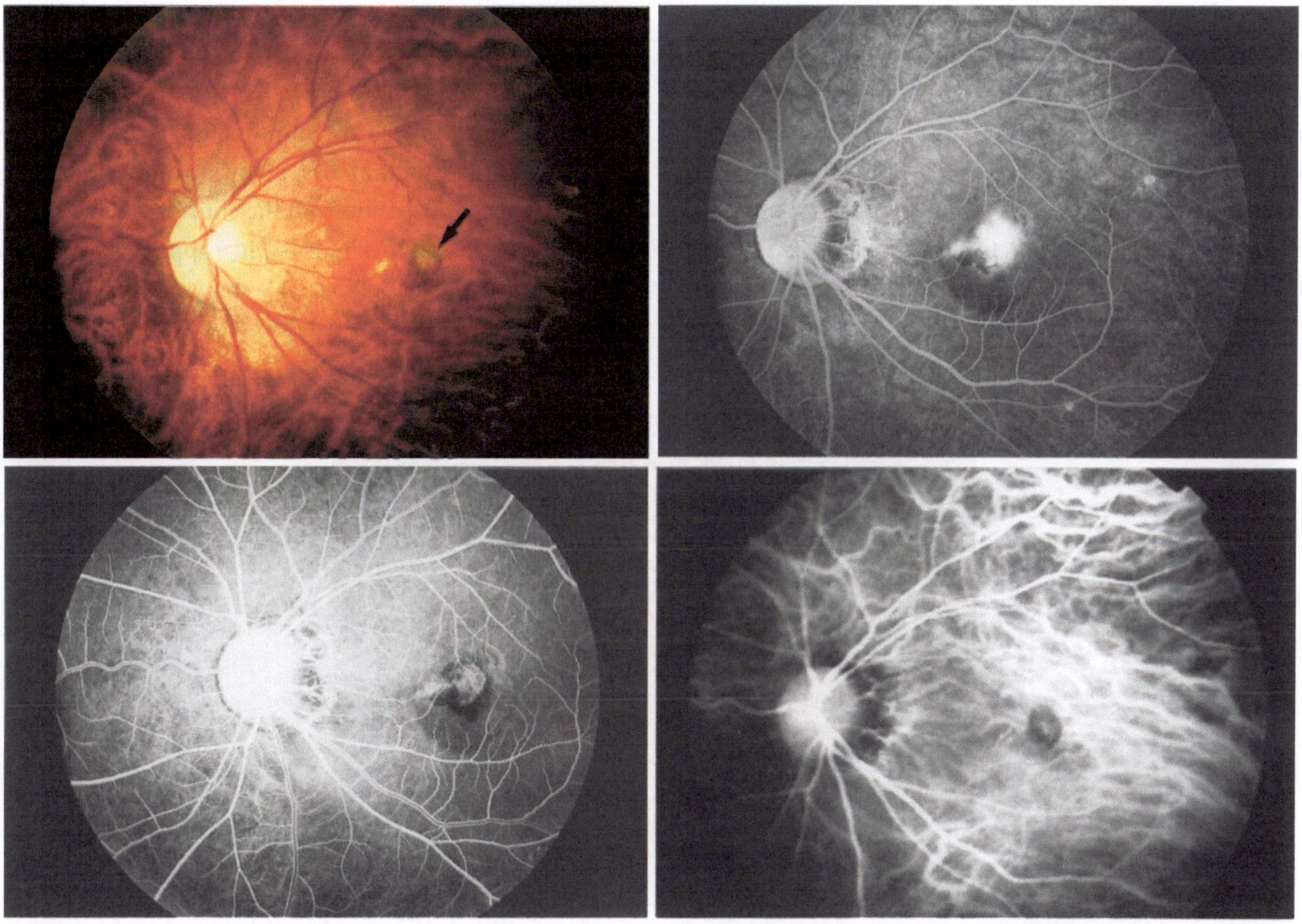

Fig. 3.25. a Neovascular macular hemorrhage, active stage (HN$_1$), 39-year-old man, left eye; refraction, -15.0 D; axial length, 30.7 mm. A dark-colored fibrovascular membrane with a hemorrhage is observed over the fovea (*arrow*). **b** Photograph in early phase of FAG in **a**. Reticular choroidal neovascular membrane can be observed within the lesion. **c** Photograph in late phase of FAG in **a**. Although fluorescein leaks from Fuchs' spot, generally it is mild, as compared with that in other diseases that are associated with choroidal neovascular membrane. **d** Photograph in late phase of IA in the same patient (**a**). Fuchs' spot shows only mild hypofluorescence, and almost no fluorescein is leaking. Annular hypofluorescence (called a dark rim) appears around the Fuchs' spot more clearly than that seen by FAG. It is suspected that this blockage is produced by the proliferation of RPE around the choroidal neovascular membrane

size of each lesion is approximately 1 optic disc diameter. Occasionally, the fibrovascular membrane that mainly consists of severe exudate and subretinal hemorrhage, similar to that of senile disciform macular degeneration, can also be observed. The reason why this occurs is unknown.

In the early stage of FAG, a reticular neovascular membrane of choroid can be observed (Fig. 3.25b). Next is observed leakage of fluorescein from the abnormal neovascular vessel. This leakage, which is usually very slight (Fig. 3.25c), is called Fuchs' spot [18].

Proliferation of fibrovascular membrane and exudate in addition to hemorrhage are the key factors for the ophthalmoscopic diagnosis. FAG is necessary, however, to diagnose the location, size, and shape of the neovascular membrane correctly.

In IA, almost no leakage of fluorescein occurs because the activity of the choriocapillaris in pathologic myopia is usually very low. Even in the active stage of neovascular macular hemorrhage, there is only slight hyperfluorescence from the middle to the late stage of IA. The blocked fluorescence produced by proliferation of the RPE around the lesion (dark rim) will sometimes occur from a more active stage (Fig. 3.25d). IA can determine the range of the dark rim more clearly than FAG.

3.4.1.2 Scar Stage (HN$_2$)

The hemorrhage and exudate surrounding the fibrovascular membrane will be gradually absorbed from 3 to 6 months after the onset. The lesion will become drier, and even the fibrovascular membrane itself will reduce its size and form a grayish-white scar lesion, which sometimes is associated with pigmentation (Fig. 3.26). The FAG finding of blocked fluorescence by pigmentation and tissue staining, which corresponds to scar tissue, is observed. No fluorescein leakage can be observed.

3.4.1.3 Atrophic Stage (MA)

The scar tissue of fibrovascular membrane will reduce 2–3 years after its formation. In some cases, a well-defined round chorioretinal atrophic lesion, which is dark green or grayish white and 2–4 optic disc diameters in size, appears from the regressed fibrovascular membrane [19] (Figs. 3.27, 3.28a). The filling defect of the choriocapillaris is observed by FAG. The filling defect corresponds to the area surrounding the atrophic lesion, which is similar to that of patchy atrophy. Following the leakage of fluorescein from the choriocapillaris in the late phase of FAG, hyperfluorescence appears around the atrophic lesion (Fig. 3.28b,c). IA shows similar findings with the patchy lesion of patchy atrophy (Fig. 3.28d).

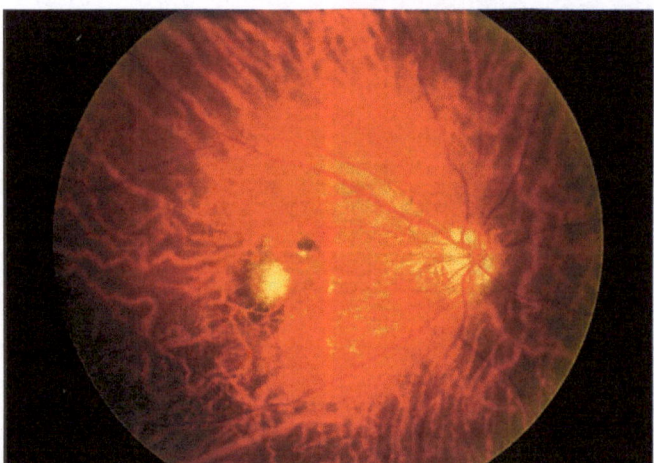

Fig. 3.26. Neovascular macular hemorrhage, scar stage (HN$_2$), 64-year-old man, right eye; refraction, −17.25 D; axial length, 29.9 mm. Grayish-white scar tissue about 1 disc in diameter is observed over the fovea. In the superonasal part of the lesion are pigmented spots and a small spot of bleeding undergoing absorption

Fig. 3.27. Neovascular macular hemorrhage, scar stage (MA), 76-year-old woman, left eye; refraction, −11.0 D; axial length, 29.9 mm. Ten years after a neovascular macular hemorrhage, the lesion is becoming an atrophic lesion covering the entire macula. Pigmentation can be observed where the Fuchs' spot has been

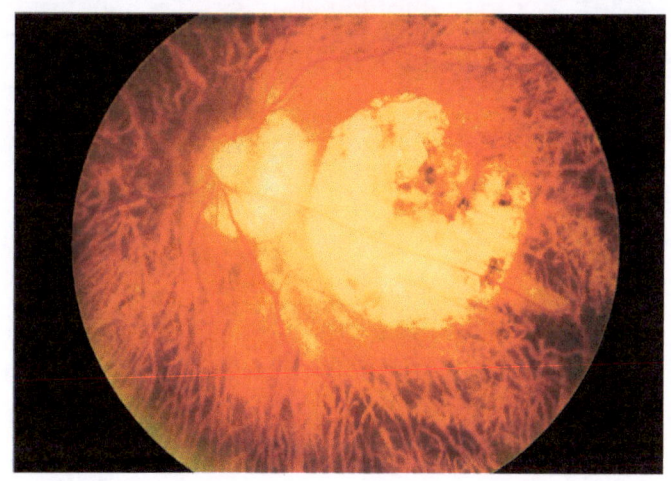

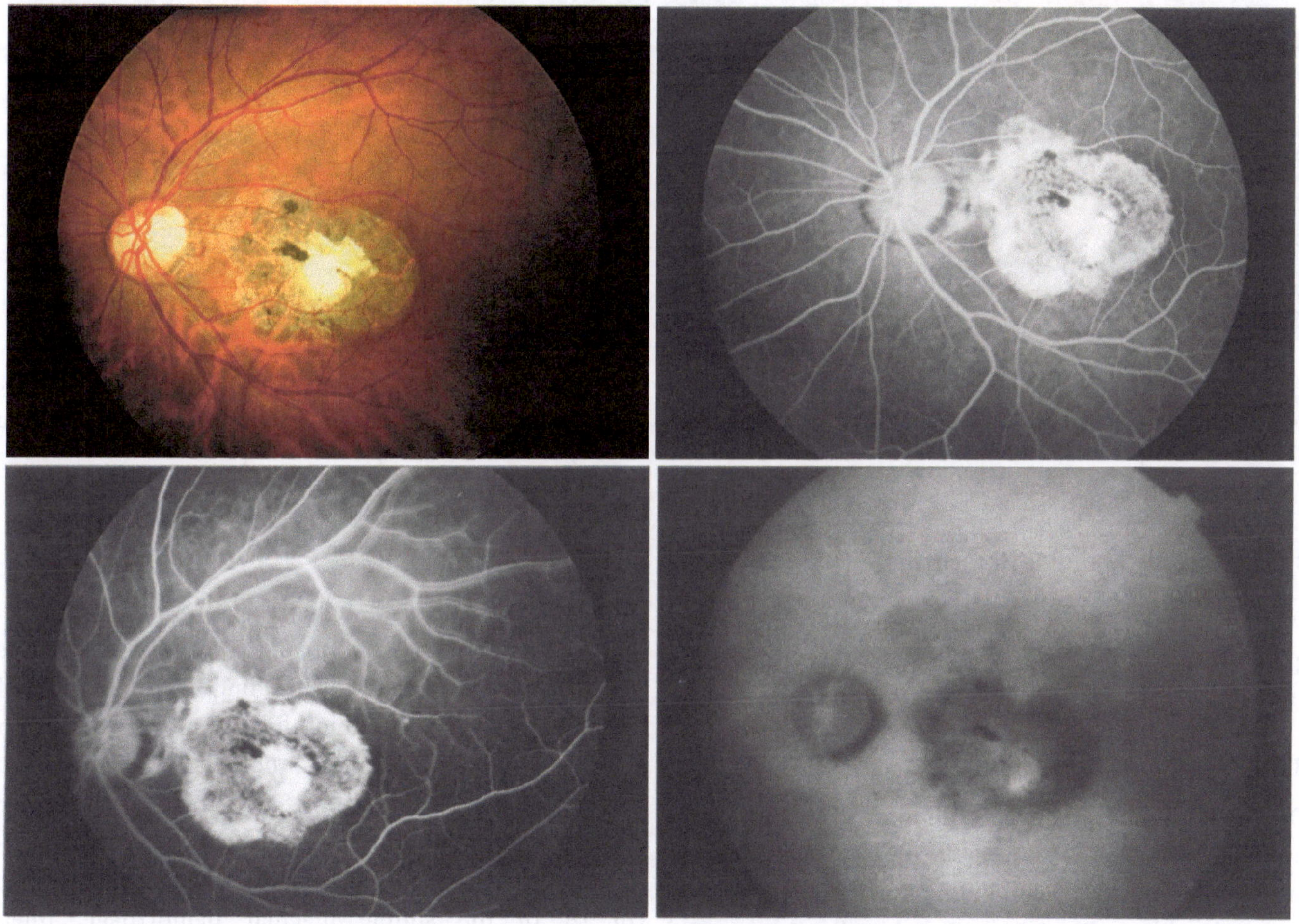

a

b

c

d

Fig. 3.28. **a** Neovascular macular hemorrhage, atrophic stage (MA), 39-year-old man, left eye; refraction, −7.0 D; axial length, 27.8 mm. Five years after a neovascular macular hemorrhage, the grayish-white fibrovascular membrane has proliferated in the center of the lesion. The atrophic lesion exceeds 3 discs in diameter. Pigment can be observed within the lesion. **b** Photograph in early phase of FAG in **a**. Picture is similar to that of P_2. A filling defect of the choroid appears hypo-

fluorescent. **c** Photograph in late phase of IA in the same patient (**a**). The fluorescein leaking from the surrounding choriocapillaris turns the hypofluorescence into hyperfluorescence gradually, by staining tissue within the lesion. **d** Photograph in late phase of IA in the same patient (**a**). Similar to the P_2 lesion, a clear hypofluorescence appears, reflecting the disappearance of the choriocapillaris within the lesion

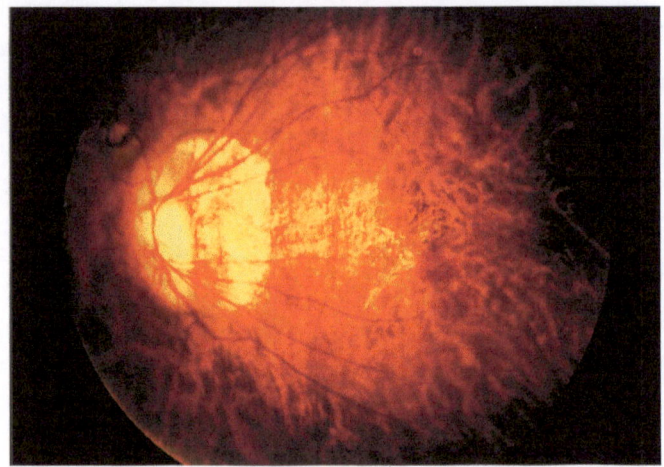

Fig. 3.29. Simple macular hemorrhage, active stage (HS₁), 16-year-old girl, left eye; refraction, −11.0 D; axial length, 28.5 mm. Two bleeding spots as large as 0.5 disc diameter are observed in the inferotemporal part of the fovea. This simple macular hemorrhage occurs without a neovascular membrane

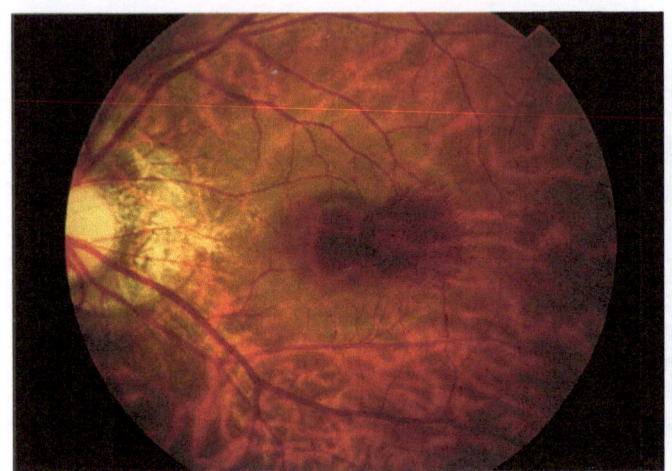

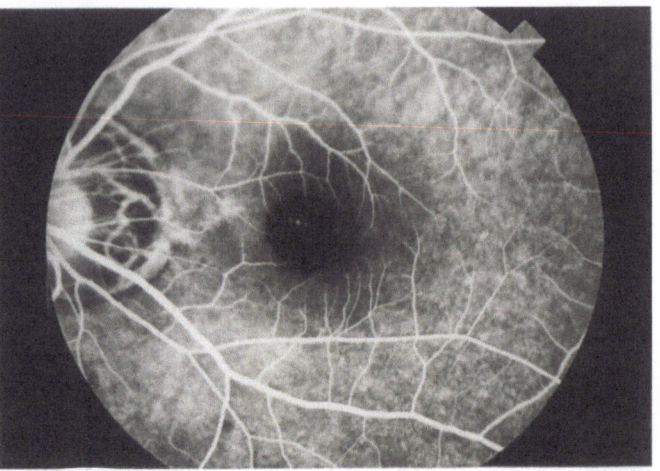

a   b

Fig. 3.30. a Simple macular hemorrhage, active stage (HS₁), 24-year-old woman, left eye; refraction, −27.75 D; axial length, 31.4 mm. A simple macular hemorrhage is observed near the fovea. **b** Photograph in late phase of FAG in **a** after 3 months. The simple macular hemorrhage seen in **a** has been absorbed. A lacquer crack lesion appears in its place

3.4.2 Simple Macular Hemorrhage (HS)

The clinical course of simple macular hemorrhage is divided into two stages: (1) active stage and (2) scar stage [17].

3.4.2.1 Active Stage (HS₁)

One or more bleeding spots, round or oval, and 0.25–1 optic disc diameter in size, can be observed in the macular area (Fig. 3.29). The lesion that involves the fovea will cause visual loss (Fig. 3.30a). Only bleeding is observed in this type of lesion. It does not accompany proliferation of the fibrovascular membrane, serous retinal detachment, or exudate. Blocked fluorescence caused by the bleeding spots is the only abnormal finding seen by FAG (see Fig. 3.18b).

3.4.2.2 Scar Stage (HS₂)

Most simple macular hemorrhage can be absorbed within 1–2 months. It is difficult to recognize the original lesion, which has caused the bleeding, even with ophthalmoscopic and FAG examination. In some cases, spotty or linear atrophy of the RPE can occur after absorption of the hemorrhage (see Fig. 3.18d,e). In FAG, the hyperfluorescence of the window defect, which corresponds to a spotty or linear lesion, can be observed. Sometimes, in IA of the simple macular hemorrhage, linear hypofluorescence (lacquer crack lesion) that crosses the bleeding area can be detected immediately after the bleeding [20].

By observing the progression of the lesion, which has developed to scar stage, the progressive changes of diffuse atrophy and the lacquer crack (Lc) lesion occasionally appear (Fig. 3.30b).

4 Explanatory Factors of Chorioretinal Atrophy

Chorioretinal atrophy includes diffuse atrophy, patchy atrophy, and atrophy after macular hemorrhage. It also can manifest as peripapillary atrophy, which includes the optic disc crescent.

4.1 Percentage of Chorioretinal Atrophy in Each Age Group

The incidence of chorioretinal atrophy in high myopia increases with aging [1,3,21–26]. It is also understood that various chorioretinal atrophies in high myopia will occur following long-term observation. These changes are very slow. Usually, the incidence of this atrophy increases in high myopia after middle age [3,22,27–29].

In this chapter, chorioretinal atrophy is divided into diffuse atrophy, lacquer crack (Lc) lesion, patchy atrophy, and macular hemorrhage. These incidences are shown in each age group and gender and in eyes with or without staphyloma. The cases that are used here include eyes with high myopia from −8.50 D to −37.0 D. Monocular high myopia and bilateral high myopia associated with cataract or other eye disease have been excluded (because of the complication of amblyopia in monocular high myopia). The number of affected male subjects is 258 (447 eyes), and the number of affected female subjects is 395 (695 eyes). The total number of affected patients is 653 (1106 eyes). The distributions of age, refractive error, and axial length are shown in Fig. 4.1.

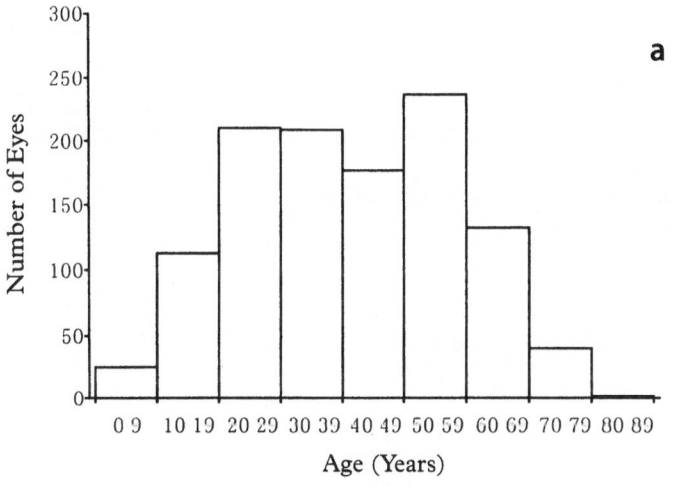

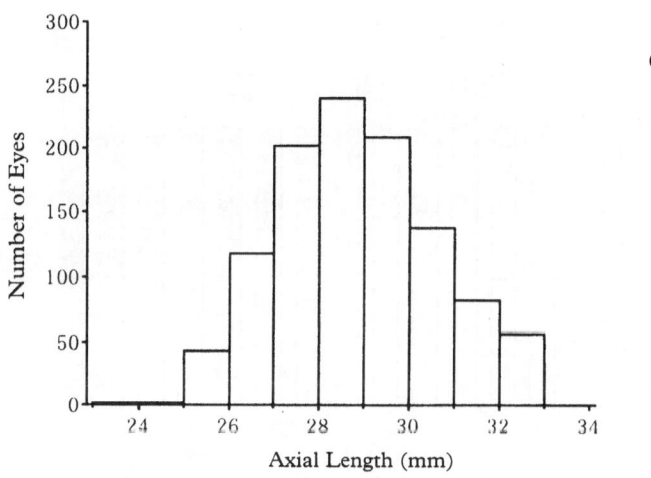

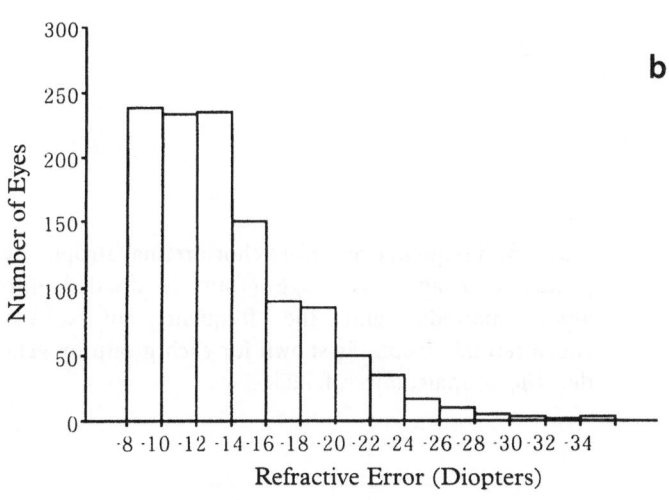

Fig. 4.1a–c. Distribution by age (**a**), refraction (**b**), and axial length (**c**) in all high myopic eyes observed in this study

4.1.1 Frequency of Diffuse Chorioretinal Atrophy in Each Age Group

Diffuse chorioretinal atrophy in total high myopia occurs in 62.8% (696 eyes), D_1 in 33.8% (375 eyes), D_2 in 24.6% (273 eyes), and MA in 4.4% (48 eyes). The remainder manifest tessellated fundus only.

From the percentages in each age group (Fig. 4.2), it is clear that the frequency of atrophic lesions increases with aging. Tessellated fundus appears in about 80% of those

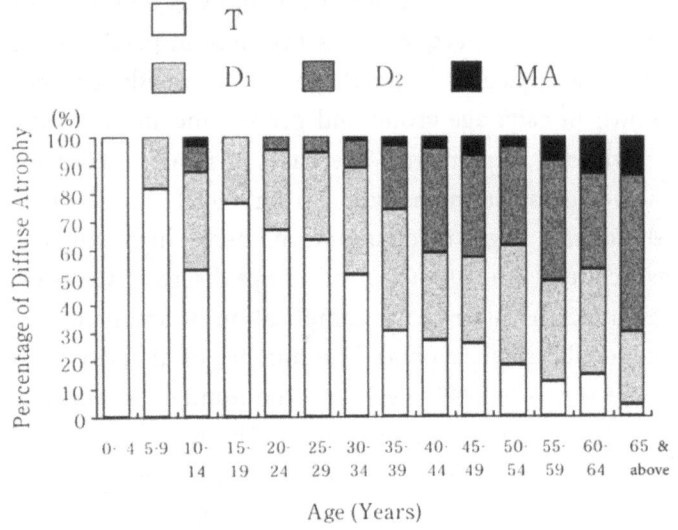

Fig. 4.2. Frequency of diffuse chorioretinal atrophy in all high myopic eyes by age group. Ages are divided into 5-year periods, and the frequency of diffuse chorioretinal atrophy is shown for each group. *T*, tessellated fundus; D_1, spotty or linear lesion of diffuse chorioretinal atrophy; D_2, enlarged lesion of diffuse chorioretinal atrophy lesion; *MA*, chorioretinal atrophy of the macula

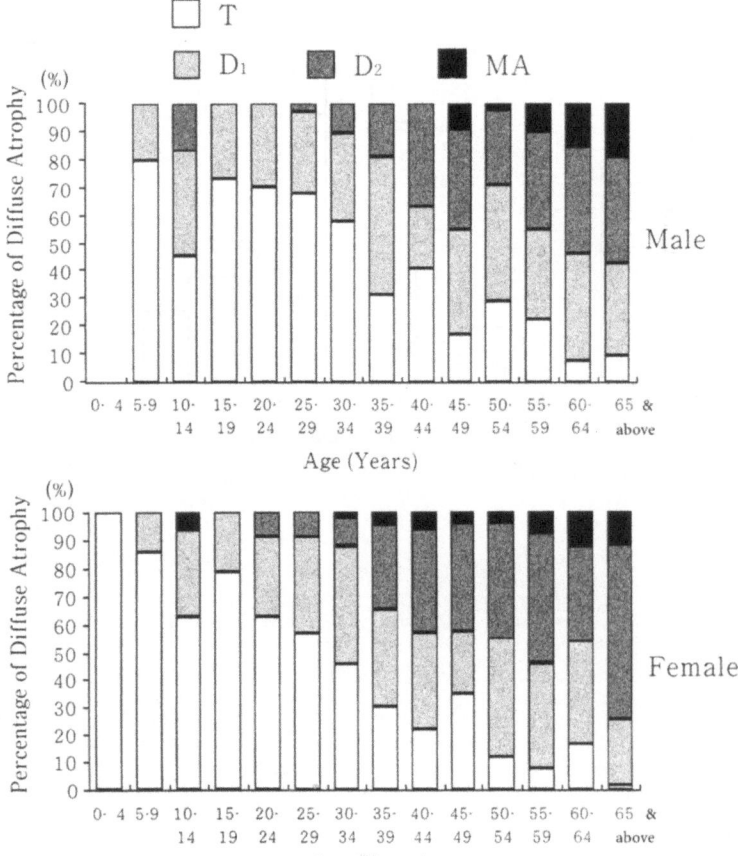

Fig. 4.3. Frequency of diffuse chorioretinal atrophy by gender and age. Each age group is divided into 5-year periods, and the frequency of diffuse chorioretinal atrophy is shown for each group by gender. *Upper*, male; *lower*, female

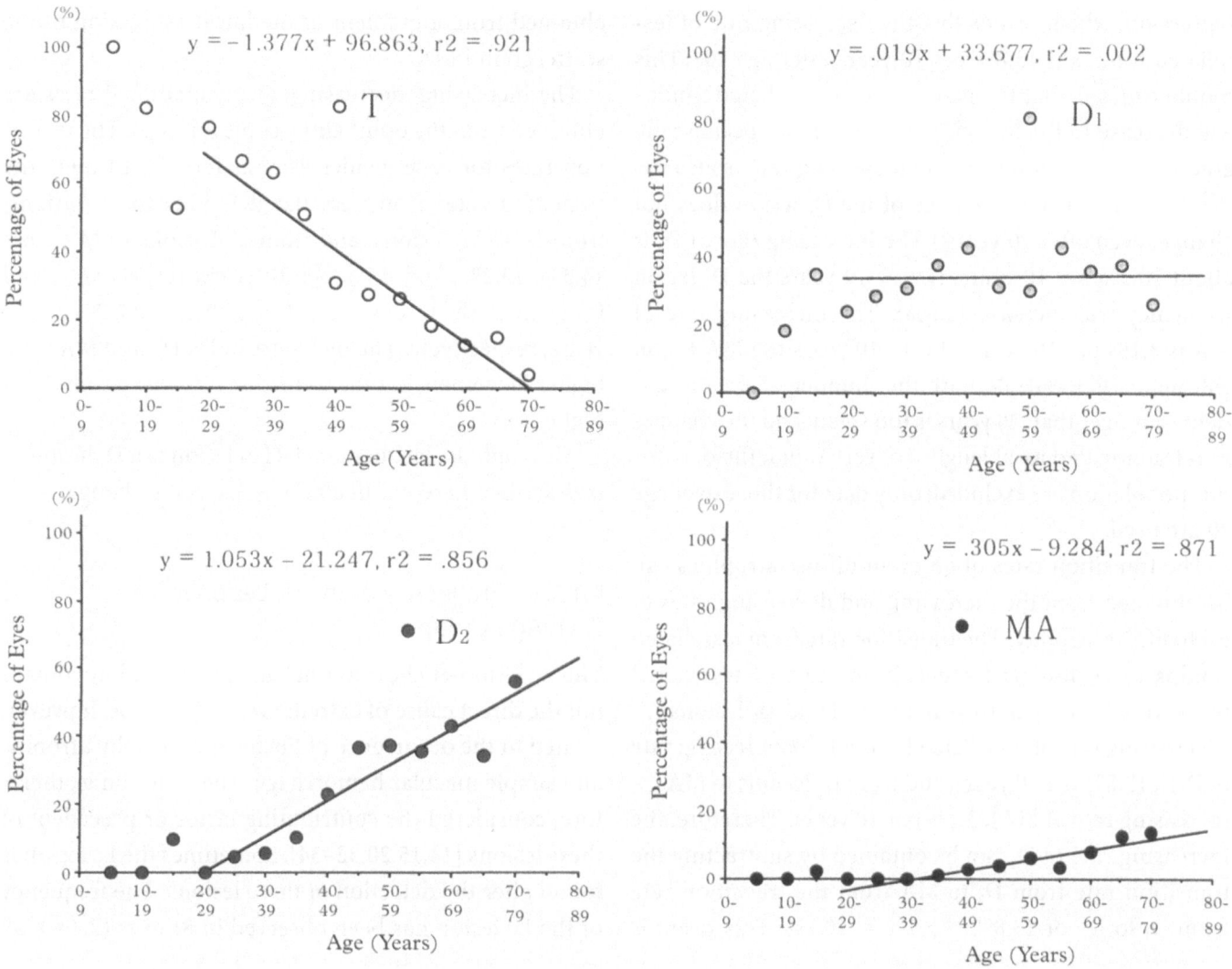

Fig. 4.4. Scattergrams of diffuse chorioretinal atrophy by age. For patients more than 20 years of age, the frequency distribution of diffuse chorioretinal atrophy by age groups is shown with linear regression. Data from patients less than 20 years of age were excluded from these calculations

younger than age 10 years, and decreases with aging. Tessellated fundus is seen in about 10% of those older than 60 years. The percentage of D_1 lesions in diffuse atrophy increases before age 40, and is about 30%–40% after age 40. No D_2 lesions exist in diffuse atrophy under the age of 10 years. From age 20 years, D_2 lesions increase. More than 50% of the patients older than age 55 have D_2 lesions. The progression to diffuse chorioretinal atrophy in the macula (MA) does not occur in those younger than age 30, and will increase gradually after age 30. There is no predilection for gender in any age group of patients with diffuse atrophy (Fig. 4.3).

The results shown in Fig. 4.2 indicate that with aging tessellated fundus will change to D_1 lesions, D_1 lesions will change to D_2 lesions, and D_2 lesions will progress to

MA [10,30,31]. Therefore, the percentage of tessellated fundus that develops to D_1 lesions with aging will decrease by linear regression. Because the transition of tessellated fundus to D_1 lesions is consistent with that of D_1 to D_2 lesions, the percentage of D_1 lesions remains almost constant. It is thought that the percentages of D_2 and MA will increase linearly after age 30 because D_1 lesions will develop into D_2 lesions and D_2 lesions will develop into MA.

To illustrate this process, the high myopic patients were divided into groups by age, with a difference of 5 years between groups. Using a scattergram of percentages of diffuse atrophy for each age group, a linear regression was calculated. A gradient of the linear regression is shown in Fig. 4.4. The percentage of tessellated fundus shows a negative gradient of the linear regression, which means that the decreasing rate of tessellated fundus is 13.8% per 10 years after age 20. (This number means that the percentage of tessellated fundus will decrease 13.8% in each 10 year interval.) Because the gradient of D_1 is almost 0, the increasing rate is also 0% per 10 years. (The percentage of the D_1 lesion does not change, even after 10 years.) The increasing rate of D_2 is about 10.5% per 10 years. (Every 10 years the D_2 lesion frequency will increase 10.5%). The increasing rate of MA is 3.1% per 10 years. (Every 10 years the MA lesion will increase 3.1%). Because the number of eyes in patients younger than 20 years is too small, and the changes in refraction and axial length are very rapid, the data for this population are excluded; only data for those over age 20 are used.

The transition rates of different diffuse atrophies can be obtained from the increasing and decreasing rates of each diffuse atrophy. The transition rate from tessellated fundus to D_1 lesions (= decreasing rate of tessellated fundus) is 13.8% per 10 years; from D_1 to D_2 lesions [= (decreasing rate of tessellated fundus) − (increasing rate of D_1)], 13.8% per 10 years; and from D_2 lesions to MA (= increasing rate of MA), 3.1% per 10 years. Therefore, the increasing rate of D_2 can be obtained by subtracting the transition rate from D_2 to MA from the transition rate from D_1 to D_2, or 13.8% − 3.1% = 10.7%. This result is almost the same as that of 10.5% per 10 years, which is obtained from a gradient of the linear regression of the scattergram in D_2.

The increasing, decreasing, and transitional rates are obtained from the ophthalmoscopic findings. The transition rates for each gender were as follows. In men, the transition rates from tessellated fundus to D_1 lesions, from D_1 to D_2 lesions, and from D_2 Lesions to MA were 14.3%, 13.2%, and 4.1% per 10 years, respectively, and for women, the rates were 13.0%, 13.0%, and 2.7% per 10 years, respectively. The incidence of D_1, D_2, and MA were higher in women, but the transition rates were somewhat higher in men.

Although the lacquer crack (Lc) lesion is a D_1 lesion, it is described here, particularly as a specific change.

4.1.1.1 Frequency of the Lc Lesion in Each Age Group

The Lc lesion of chorioretinal atrophy in high myopia is not the direct cause of extreme visual loss. It is, however, related to the occurrence of Fuchs' spot, patchy atrophy, and simple macular hemorrhage. The Lc lesion is, therefore, considered the contributing factor or precedent of these lesions [14,15,20,32–34]. Sometimes the Lc lesion is found after the detection of these lesions. The frequency of the Lc lesion has been observed in 81 eyes (7.4%), all

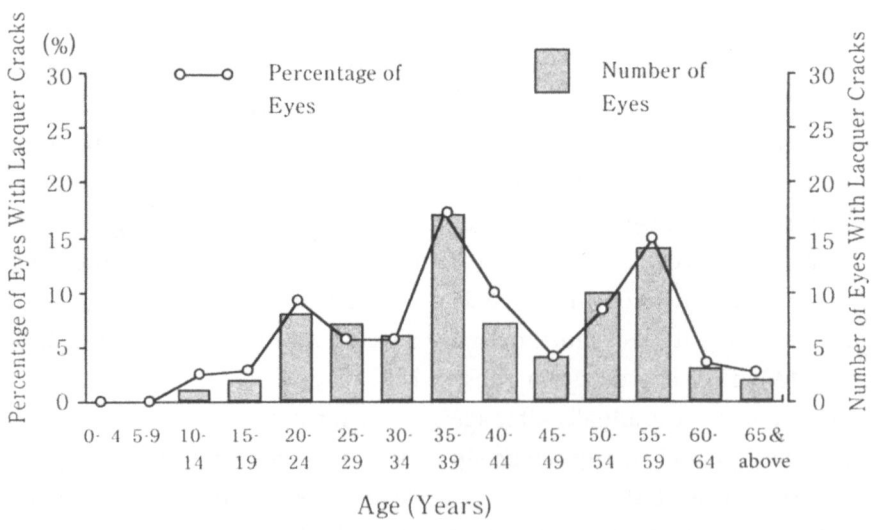

Fig. 4.5. Number of eyes (*bars*) and frequency of lacquer crack lesions (*circles*) by age group, divided into 5-year periods

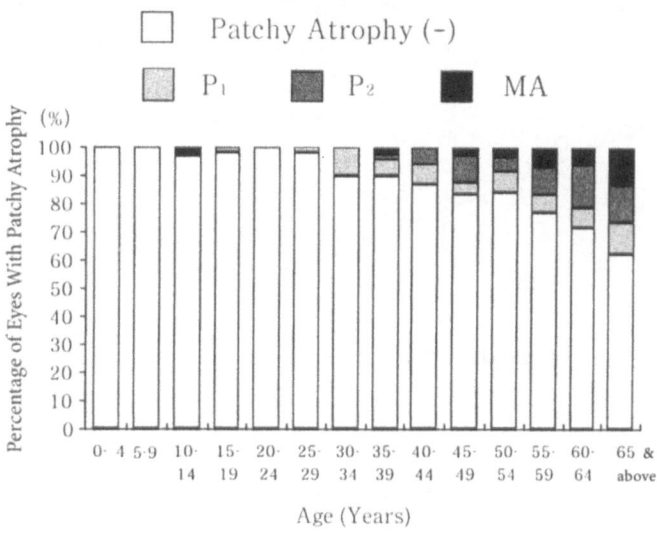

Fig. 4.6. Percentage of eyes with patchy atrophy (P) by age group, divided into 5-year periods. P_1, spotty lesion; P_2, patchy lesion

with high myopia. The incidence in our findings is nearly the same as that reported previously [28].

The frequency of the Lc lesion in each age group is shown in Fig. 4.5. It is lower in those younger than age 20 years and in the elderly, but increases around ages 40 and 60 years (35–39 years old, 17%; 55–59 years old, 15%). The frequency distribution of the Lc lesion shows two peaks. No difference by gender is observed in this type of frequency distribution.

4.1.2 Frequency of Patchy Atrophy in Each Age Group

Patchy atrophy exists in 144 eyes, or 13.1% of all high myopic eyes (P_1, 58 eyes, 5.3% P_2, 57 eyes, 5.2%; MA, 29 eyes, 2.6%). This frequency is lower, as compared with the 23% obtained by Curtin and Karlin [28] and the 28.5% obtained from a national investigation conducted by a research committee established by the Ministry of Health and Welfare of Japan [8]. It is conceivable that the many subjects under age 30 which are included in our investigation may have influenced the results (see Fig. 4.1). In all high myopic eyes, P_1 appears in those aged 25–29 years; P_2 and MA begin to increase after ages 35–39

years. The frequency of all patchy atrophy increases with aging and reaches 32.5% after age 60 years (Fig. 4.6).

Eyes without patchy atrophy decrease 7.4% per 10 years after 20 years of age. The rates of increase are 1.5% per 10 years in P_1, 3.6% in P_2, and 2.3% in MA (Fig. 4.7). Therefore, using a method of calculation similar to that for the transition rate of diffuse atrophy after age 20 years, the transition rates of patchy atrophy (from no patchy atrophy to P_1, P_1 to P_2, and P_2 to MA) obtained were 7.4%, 5.9%, and 2.3%, respectively, per 10 years. When the transition rates of patchy atrophy were compared with the transition rates of diffuse atrophy (tessellated fundus to D_1 is 13.8%, D_1 to D_2 is 13.8%, and D_2 to MA is 3.1% per 10 years), the progression of patchy atrophy is about half that of diffuse atrophy.

The transition rate of patchy atrophy has been investigated by gender. The transition rate from no patchy atrophy to P_1, from P_1 to P_2, and from P_2 to MA is 4.9%, 2.4%, and 2.2% per 10 years, respectively, in men and 8.1%, 7.1%, and 2.5% per 10 years in women. These findings indicate that patchy atrophy has a predilection for women. The rate of progression from P_1 to P_2 to MA is also faster in women than in men. In addition, many cases of patchy atrophy are associated with diffuse atrophy.

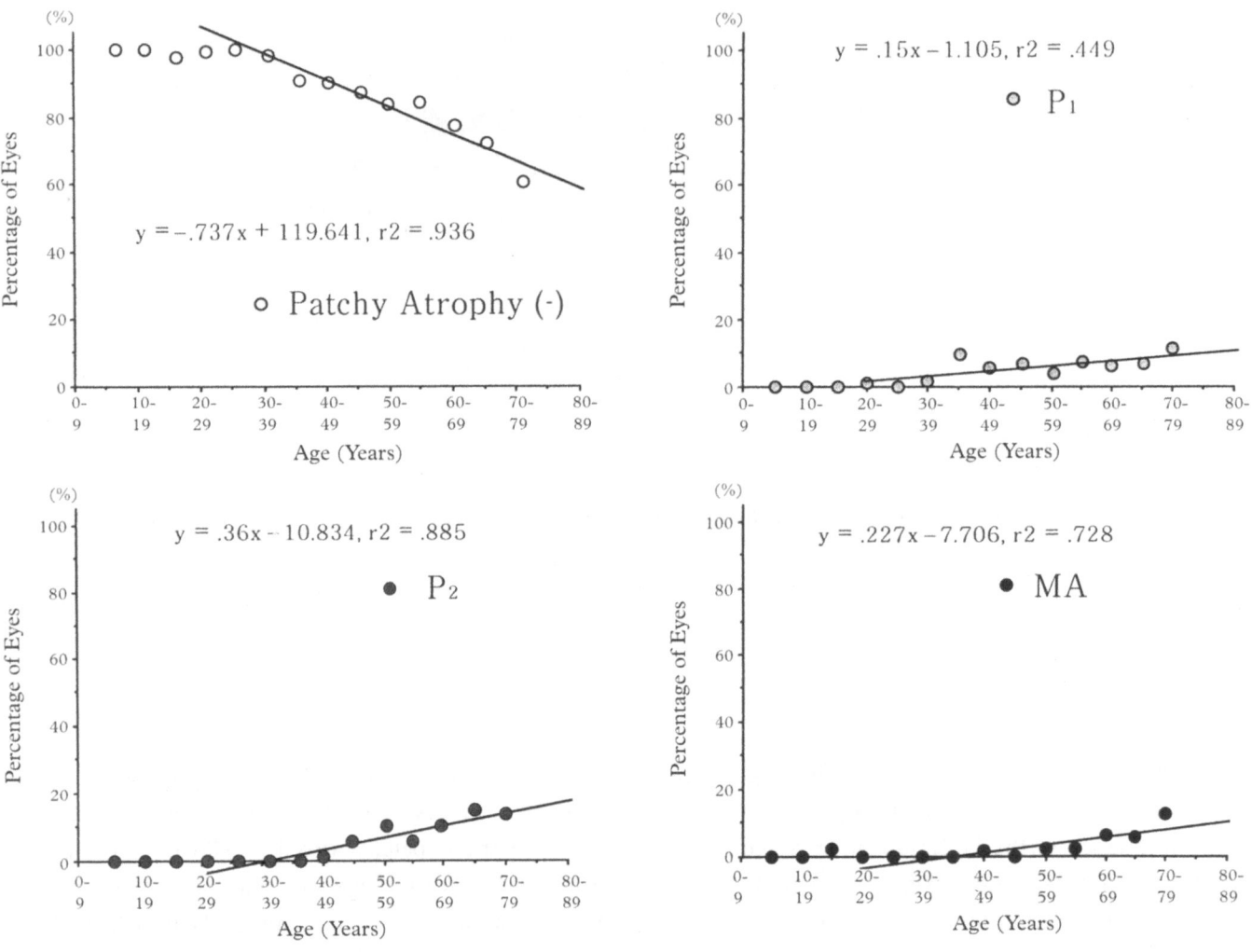

Fig. 4.7. Scattergrams of patchy atrophy by age. The frequency distribution of patchy atrophy by age group is shown with linear regression

4.1.3 Frequency of Eyes with Macular Hemorrhage by Age

4.1.3.1 Neovascular Macular Hemorrhage (Choroidal Neovascular Membrane)

Choroidal neovascular membrane is an important factor in determining the prognosis of visual acuity in pathologic myopia [35,36]. We calculated the percentage of eyes with choroidal neovascular membrane in those with pathologic myopia to be 11.6% in 128 eyes. Of these 128 eyes, 46 (4.2%) had HN_1, 51 eyes (4.6%) had HN_2, and 31 eyes (2.8%) had MA. No choroidal vascular membrane was seen in 974 eyes (88.4% of all pathologic myopic eyes). This percentage of eyes with choroidal neovascular membrane is somewhat higher than the 5.2% reported by Curtin [28] and the 3.7% reported in the national survey conducted by a research group

from the Ministry of Health and Welfare of Japan [8]. The difference in percentages may be because most of the patients we describe have severe complications and were referred to our high myopia clinic by other physicians.

The percentage of choroidal vascular membrane tends to increase gradually with aging after 20 years, although no choroidal vascular membrane is observed in those under age 20 (Fig. 4.8). A linear regression can be determined from the percentage of cases of choroidal vascular membrane in each age group greater than 20 years (Fig. 4.9). The incidence of choroidal vascular membrane can then be obtained from the gradient of the linear regression, that is, 5.2% per 10 years. Therefore, about 30% of the patients between ages 70 and 80 years will have involvement of the choroidal vascular membrane, which is considered the main cause of visual loss. The mean

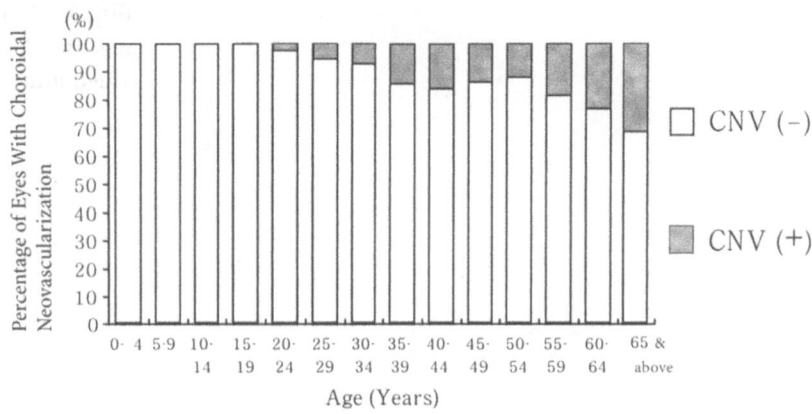

Fig. 4.8. Percentage of eyes with neovascular macular hemorrhage (choroidal neovascular membrane, *CNV*) by age group, divided into 5-year periods

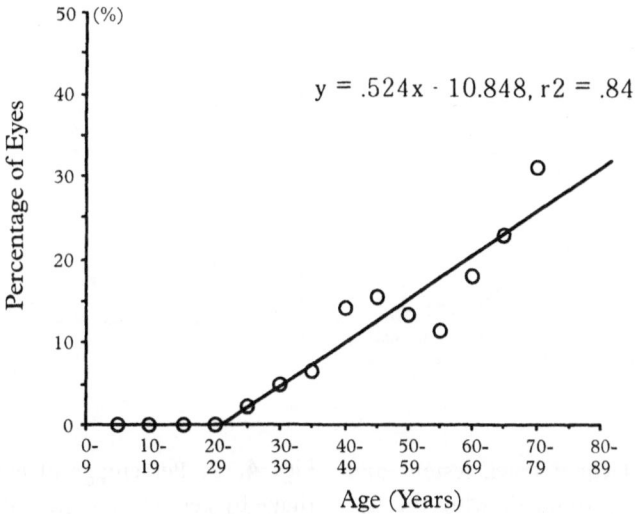

$$y = .524x - 10.848, r2 = .842$$

Fig. 4.9. Scattergram of choroidal neovascular membrane by age shows frequency distribution with linear regression in patients more than 20 years of age

value of visual acuity in 128 eyes with choroidal vascular membrane is 0.13, which is considerably lower than 0.62 in the other 974 eyes without choroidal neovascular membrane.

Choroidal vascular membrane was found in 24 eyes in men (5.4% in the total number of male eyes) and in 104 eyes in women (15.8% of the total number of female eyes). The incidence of choroidal neovascular membrane was investigated in men and women older than 20 years of age. In men, choroidal neovascular membrane occurred in 2.5% per 10 years; in women, it was 5.7% per 10 years. On the basis of these findings, the incidence of choroidal vascular membrane in women is two times higher than in men. Between ages 70 and 80 years, the rate increases to about 15% in men and to about 30% in women. From the previous data, we know

that the transition rate of patchy atrophy in women is about two times that in men. This dominance holds true for the incidence of choroidal vascular membrane as well.

4.1.3.2 Simple Macular Hemorrhage

To evaluate visual loss, a fundus examination is usually performed, and sometimes simple macular hemorrhage near the fovea can be found. In many cases, however, the hemorrhage has formed far from the fovea and cannot be found without periodic examination, because the hemorrhage absorbs after several months. Therefore, the incidence of simple macular hemorrhage is the lowest among chorioretinal lesions found in pathologic myopia [16,17]. Our data also show a low incidence: 3.1% in only 34 eyes.

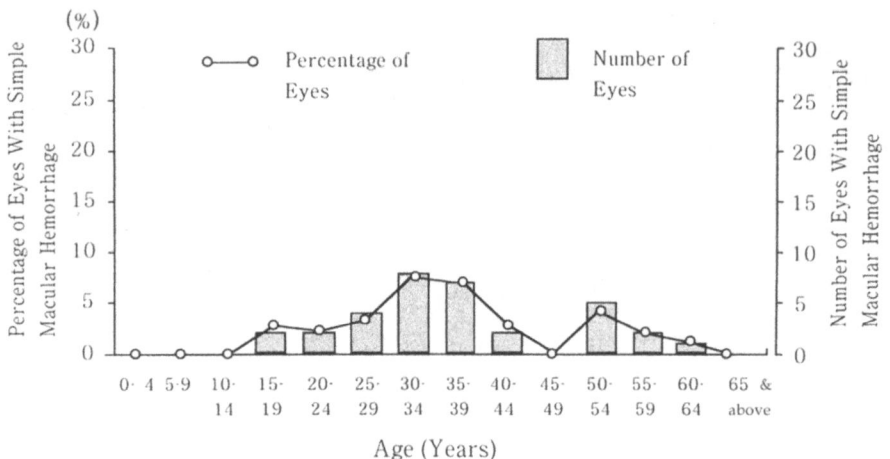

Fig. 4.10. Percentage of eyes with simple macular hemorrhage by age group, divided into 5-year periods

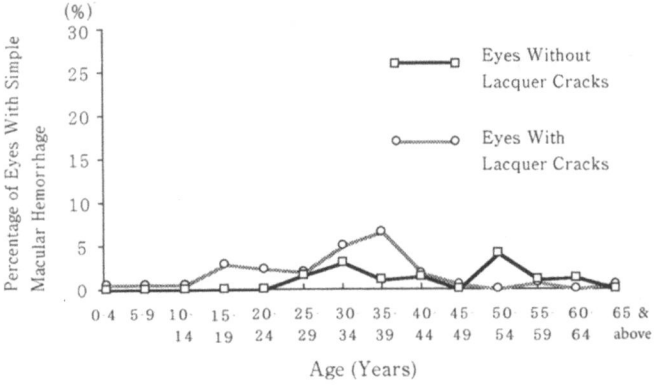

Fig. 4.11. Relationship between lacquer crack lesions and simple macular hemorrhage by age group, showing the frequency distribution of simple macular hemorrhage for each age group in eyes with (*circles*) or without (*squares*) lacquer crack lesions

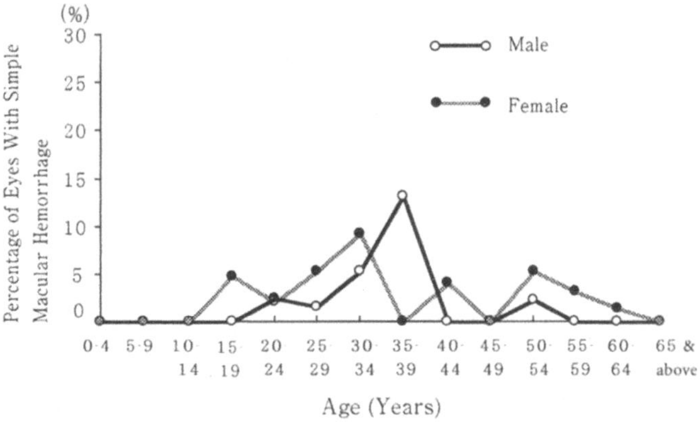

Fig. 4.12. Percentage of eyes with simple macular hemorrhage by gender and age. Age groups are divided into 5-year periods

From the percentages of simple macular hemorrhage recorded in each age group, it is known that most cases occur in the first half of the fourth decade (7.6%) and in the first half of the sixth decade (4.1%) (Fig. 4.10). This finding shows a similar distribution of two peaks observed with the lacquer crack (Lc) lesion (Fig. 4.5).

Simple macular hemorrhage can be divided into two types: one with and one without the Lc lesion. With this kind of classification, the distribution of the frequency of simple macular hemorrhage with Lc lesion by age group has only one peak in the second half of the fourth decade (Fig. 4.11). It has been suggested that this figure represents the first peak in the frequency distribution of all cases of simple macular hemorrhage. On the other hand, although the frequency distribution of simple macular hemorrhage without the Lc lesion shows two different peaks, the most frequent value occurs in the first half of

the sixth decade. This peak is believed to be the second peak of the distribution of all cases of simple macular hemorrhage. Therefore, simple macular hemorrhage is divided into two types: the juvenile type, which is related to the Lc lesion, and the senile type, which is unrelated to the Lc lesion.

In women, both the juvenile type and the senile type coexist. In men, however, we find that most of the simple macular hemorrhages appear at a young age (only the juvenile type exists) (Fig. 4.12).

4.1.4 Frequency of Peripapillary Atrophy by Age

Peripapillary atrophy is thought to originate from the enlargement of the annular crescent around the optic disc. This type of atrophy is closely related to age, axial length, posterior staphyloma, and chorioretinal atrophy in pathologic myopia. After observing peripapillary atrophy in different cases of high myopia for more than 10 years, we have confirmed that the area of peripapillary atrophy enlarges, although very slowly (see the atlas in the second half of this volume). To evaluate the area of peripapillary atrophy, we take the value (ratio) of the area of peripapillary atrophy to the area of optic disc. By measuring each area with a digitizer from color fundus photography, we show the relationship between this ratio (area of peripapillary atrophy/area of optic disc) and age (Fig. 4.13). Figure 4.13 confirms that this ratio increases significantly with aging. The mean value of the area of peripapillary atrophy increases about three times from age 20 to 60 years (219%, less than 20 years old; 578%, more than 60 years old). This ratio also differs between genders: it is 307% ± 188% (n = 212 eyes) in men and 422% ± 287% (n = 334 eyes) in women, which indicates that the ratio is larger in women than in men ($P < .0001$).

The crescent in the temporal, nasal, and inferior sides of the optic disc will develop an annular crescent that surrounds the peripapillary area. It is not clear, however, whether the annular crescent develops into peripapillary atrophy (although peripapillary atrophy is mainly formed from annular enlargement, it also may originate from enlargement of the inferior or nasal crescent). In Fig. 4.13, we show the peripapillary atrophy and not the optic nerve crescent. Excluding the 538 eyes with peripapillary atrophy, we demonstrated chorioretinal atrophy in 568 high myopic eyes with only a temporal, nasal, inferior, or annular crescent. In Fig. 4.14, the relationship between diffuse chorioretinal atrophy and nonannular crescent or annular crescent is shown. When diffuse chorioretinal atrophy changes from tessellated fundus → D_1 → D_2 → MA, the percentage of annular crescent also increases, from 3.4% to 23.7%, 56.2%, and 88.0%, respectively ($P < .001$).

The relationship between the Lc lesion and nonannular crescent or annular crescent was also investigated. Of the eyes without the Lc lesion, 20.2% had an annular crescent, while 28.6% of the eyes with Lc lesion had an annular crescent. Although the percentage of eyes

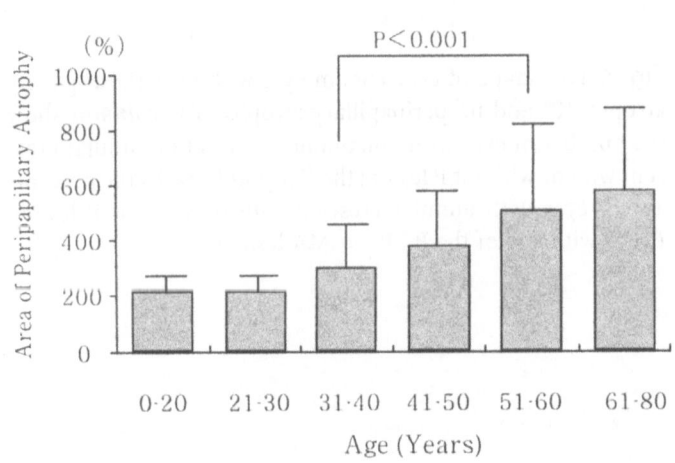

Fig. 4.13. Ratio of area of peripapillary atrophy to area of optic disc in all high myopic eyes by age. Each *column* shows the mean value of each ratio; the *vertical axis* shows the standard deviation

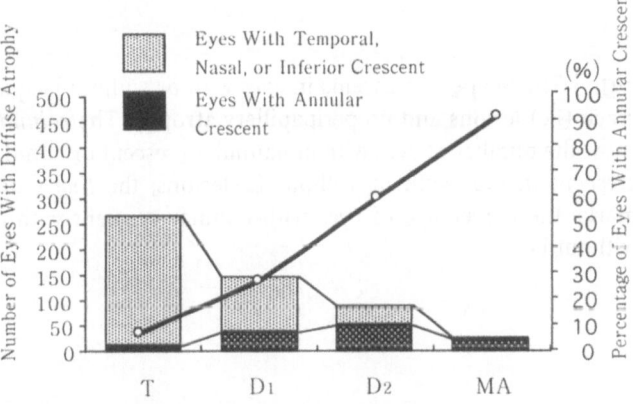

Fig. 4.14. Number of eyes with diffuse chorioretinal atrophy and crescents among eyes without peripapillary atrophy. Columns show the number of eyes with nonannular (temporal, nasal, inferior) crescent or annular crescent in each kind of diffuse chorioretinal atrophy; the line graph illustrates the percentage of eyes with annular crescent [the number of eyes with annular crescent/(the number of eyes with annular crescent + the number of eyes with nonannular crescent)] and diffuse chorioretinal atrophy

with annular crescent and Lc lesion is high, the difference between them is not significant (Fig. 4.15). In addition, the annular crescent is observed in 15.9% of eyes without patchy atrophy, although it occurs in 70.2% of eyes with patchy atrophy of the P_1, P_2, or MA lesion (Fig. 4.16) ($P < .01$).

The percentages of annular crescents in eyes with or without neovascular hemorrhage (choroidal neovascular membrane) are 42.7% and 18.4%, respectively ($P < .01$). The percentage of annular crescent in the eyes with or without simple macular hemorrhage is 33.3% and 20.4%, respectively (there is no significant difference) (Fig. 4.17). Therefore, it is understood that the peripapillary crescent will become annular if the chorioretinal atrophy is severe. On the other hand, the average age in eyes with annular and non-annular crescent is 52 years and 35 years, and the average axial length is 29.9 mm and 28.2 mm, respectively. Therefore, it is reasonable that the percentage of annular crescent will increase in eyes with aging and long axial length.

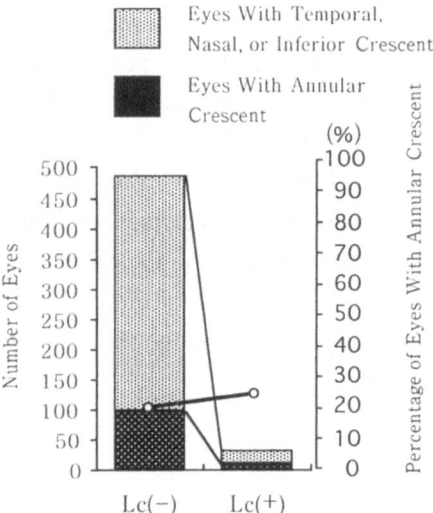

Fig. 4.15. Shape of crescents in eyes with or without lacquer crack (Lc) lesions and no peripapillary atrophy. The *columns* show the number of eyes with nonannular crescent or annular crescent in eyes with or without Lc lesions; the *line graph* marks the percentage of eyes with annular crescent with or without Lc

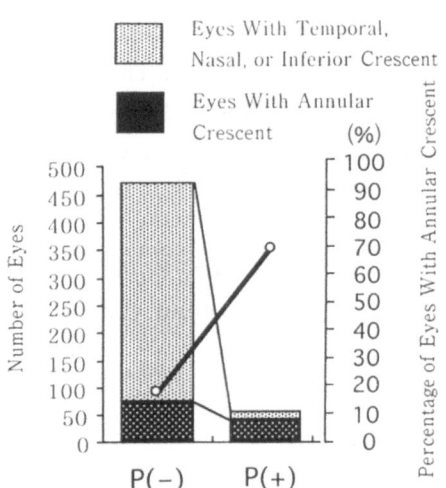

Fig. 4.16. Shape of crescents in eyes with or without patchy atrophy (P) and no peripapillary atrophy. The *columns* show the number of eyes with nonannular crescent or annular crescent with or without P lesion; the *line graph* marks the percentage of eyes with annular crescent with or without P lesion. P, eye with any of the P_1, P_2, or MA lesions

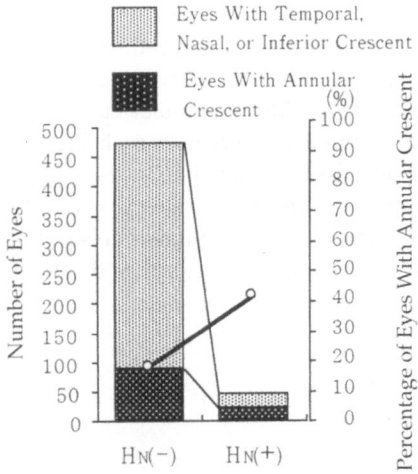

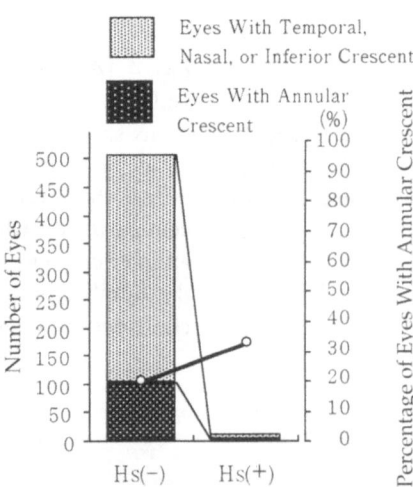

Fig. 4.17. Shape of crescents in eyes with or without neovascular macular hemorrhage (choroidal neovascular membrane)/simple macular hemorrhage and no peripapillary atrophy. The *columns* show the number of eyes with nonannular or annular crescent; the *line graph* illustrates the percentage of eyes with annular crescent

4.2 Percentage of Eyes with Chorioretinal Atrophy in Each Axial Length Group

4.2.1 Correlation Between Axial Length and Refraction

In myopia, there is a correlation between axial length and refraction, which indicates that the degree of myopia will be high if the axial length is long. It is known that an additional 1 mm in axial length will increase myopia an additional −3 D [3,37,38]. In our findings, the correlation between axial length and refraction has been investigated in 1106 myopic eyes that exceed −8.0 D. An excellent correlation was observed (correlation coefficient is 0.705) (Fig. 4.18).

The calculation that an additional 1 mm of axial length will produce an additional −3 D in refraction also holds true in high myopia. For the same −3.0 D increase in myopia above −15 D, however, the axial elongation is less than 1 mm, and the refraction tends to have a smaller influence on axial elongation when myopia increases [39]. The progression of high myopia is caused by axial elongation and the occurrence or progression of chorioretinal atrophy initiated by this elongation.

4.2.2 Percentage of Eyes with Diffuse Chorioretinal Atrophy by Axial Length

If the axial length is longer than 30 mm in high myopic eyes, chorioretinal atrophy and the functional impairment of the eye will become severe [1,3,22,23,28,40]. It is observed that about 90% of eyes with only tessellated fundus and no chorioretinal atrophy have an axial length less than 26 mm. This percentage decreases linearly in eyes with longer axial length and becomes 0 when the axial length is longer than 31 mm. Also, a 1-mm elongation in axial length will lead to about a 13% increase of chorioretinal atrophy from eyes with only tessellated fundus and no chorioretinal atrophy (Fig. 4.19).

The percentage of eyes with tessellated fundus and no chorioretinal atrophy in each axial length group differs by gender. The percentage of tessellated fundus is 10%–20% higher in men than in women if the axial length is the same. No eye with only tessellated fundus can be found when the axial length is more than 31.0 mm in men and more than 30.5 mm in women (Fig. 4.20). If all the eyes with high myopia that have only tessellated fundus are divided by age, the percentage of those with tessellated fundus in eyes under age 40 is greater than in those over age 40. It is a natural result of that finding that the

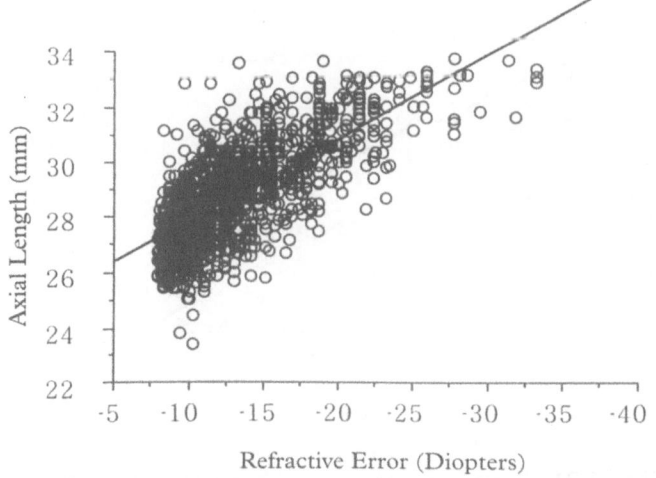

Fig. 4.18. Relationship between axial length (mm) and refraction (D), calculated by linear regression analysis

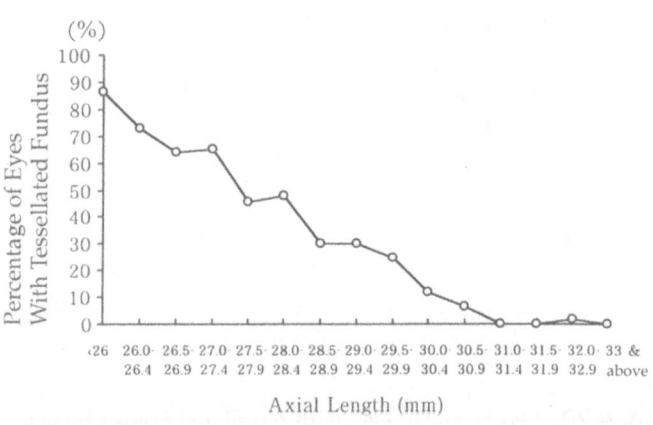

Fig. 4.19. Percentage of eyes with tessellated fundus in all high myopic eyes by axial length, divided into 0.5-mm lengths ranging from more than 26 to less than 32 mm

tessellated fundus changes to chorioretinal atrophy with aging (Fig. 4.21).

Taking the percentage of eyes with tessellated fundus and the scattergram of axial lengths less than 31 mm (because the percentage of tessellated fundus is 0% when the axial length is greater than 31 mm), a simple regression equation can be obtained by the method of least squares. With this gradient, the corresponding reduction rate of tessellated fundus in each axial length group can be calculated. The reduction rate of tessellated fundus is 13.3%/mm in all high myopic eyes, 14.8%/mm in men, 12.9%/mm in women, 14.8%/mm under age 40, and 10.4%/mm over age 40. In comparing the different percentages of eyes with tessellated fundus in these results, we found that the reduction rate in men under age 40 is greater than in women or in eyes over age 40. In other words, the reduction rate of tessellated fundus in men less than 40 years of age is higher than in women less than 40 years of age.

Regarding the relationship between axial length and D_1, it is known that the frequency of D_1 increases with axial elongation, if the axial length is less than 29 mm. The maximum percentage of D_1 (about 46%) occurs at about 29 mm in axial length. When the axial length exceeds 30 mm, the percentage of eyes with D_1 decreases with lengthening of the eye (Fig. 4.22). In other words, it is believed that D_1 has changed to D_2 when axial length exceeds 30 mm. When the percentage of eyes with D_1 is investigated by axial length in men and women, the maximum value appears at about 30 mm in men (61%) and about 29 mm in women (54%) (Fig. 4.23). There is no significant difference in the percentage of eyes with D_1 by gender.

If all eyes with high myopia are divided into groups under and over age 40, the percentage of eyes with D_1 deviates from a normal distribution. The maximum percentage of D_1 (about 78%) appears around 32 mm in those younger than age 40 years, while the maximum percentage of D_1 (about 65%) appears around 28 mm in those over the age of 40 years. A symmetric distribution of these two groups intersects at an axial length of about 29 mm. This finding indicates that the percentage of D_1 increases with lengthening of the eye under age 40, but D_1 decreases with lengthening of the eye over age 40 (Fig. 4.24). This information is consistent with the finding that the frequencies of D_2 and MA increase after 40 years of age.

There is some relationship between axial length and D_2. The percentage of eyes with D_2 is as low as 10% when the axial length is shorter than 28 mm. When the axial length increases beyond 28.5 mm, the percentage of eyes with D_2 will increase linearly in proportion to the lengthening of the eye, and it will stop increasing at about 32 mm. Beyond 32 mm, the percentage of eyes with D_2 decreases (Fig. 4.25). The percentage of eyes with D_2 differs by gender with axial length. The percentage of eyes with D_2 is 10% higher in women than in men (Fig. 4.26). Although the percentage of eyes with chorioretinal atrophy is high in women, the difference

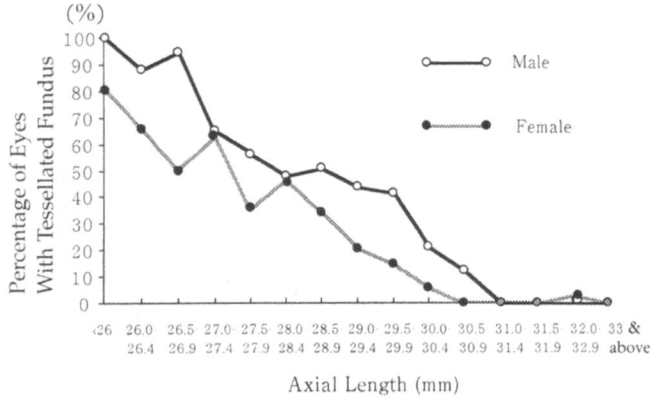

Fig. 4.20. Percentage of eyes with tessellated fundus by gender and axial length in millimeters

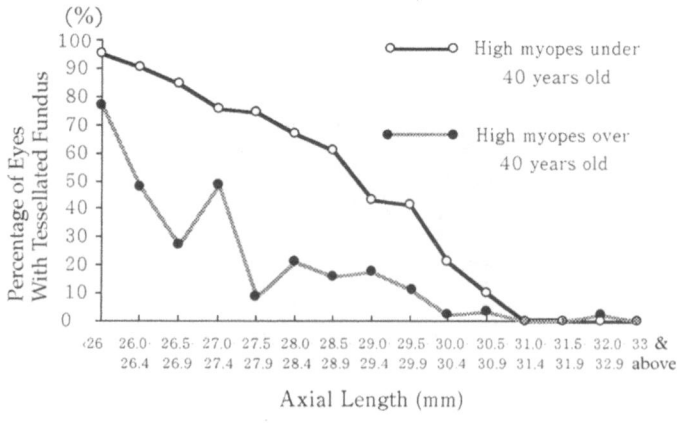

Fig. 4.21. Percentage of eyes with tessellated fundus in patients less than or more than 40 years of age by axial length

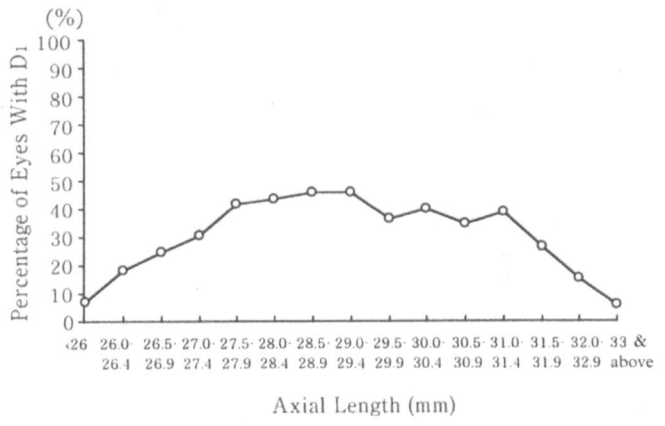

Fig. 4.22. Percentage of eyes with D₁ in all high myopic eyes by axial length

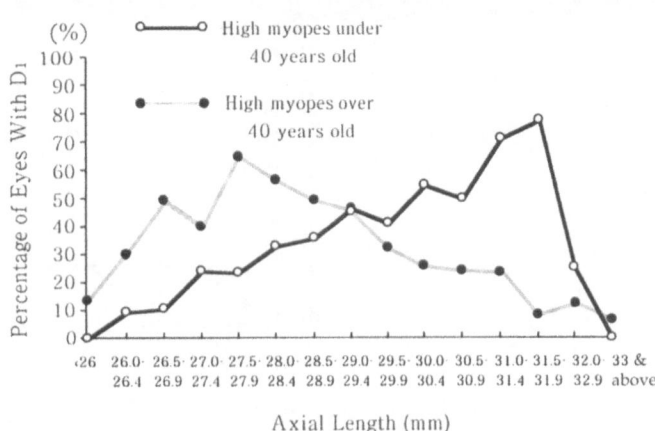

Fig. 4.24. Percentage of eyes with D₁ in patients less than or more than 40 years of age by axial length

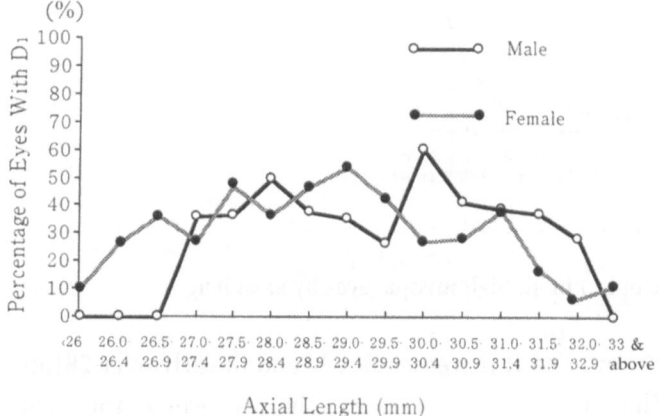

Fig. 4.23. Percentage of eyes with D₁ by gender and axial length

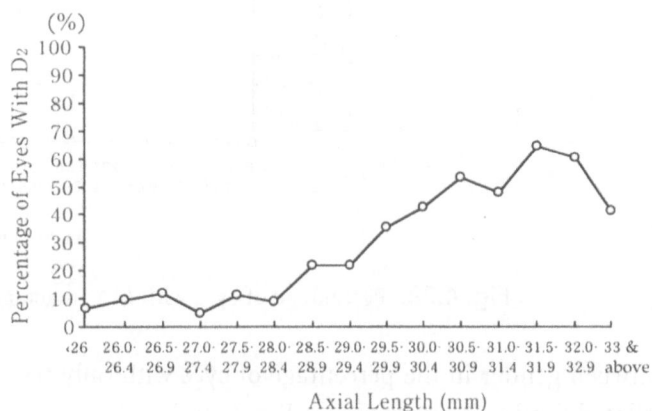

Fig. 4.25. Percentage of eyes with D₂ in all high myopic eyes by axial length from more than 26 to less than 33 mm

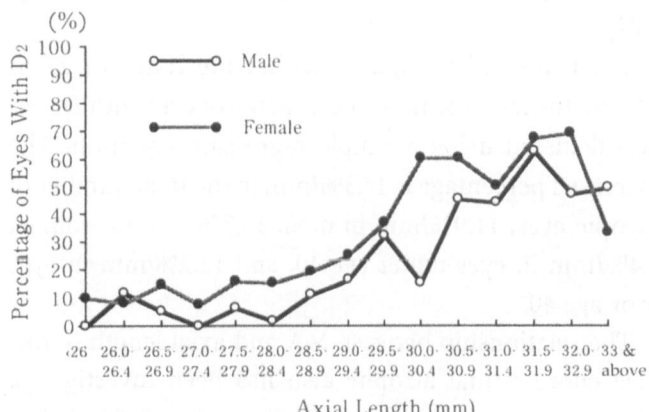

Fig. 4.26. Percentage of eyes with D₂ by gender and axial length

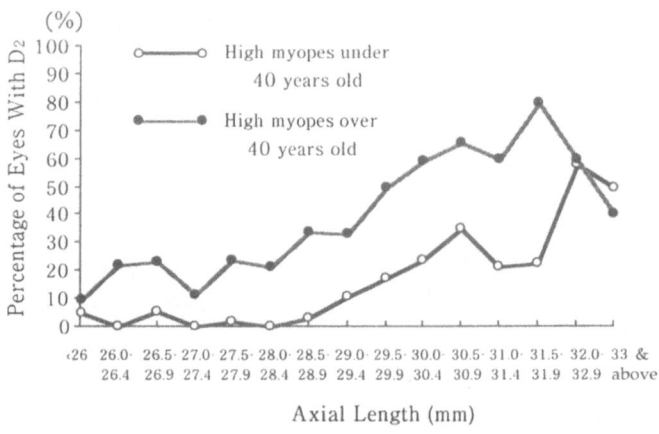

Fig. 4.27. Percentage of eyes with D_2 in patients less than or more than 40 years of age by axial length

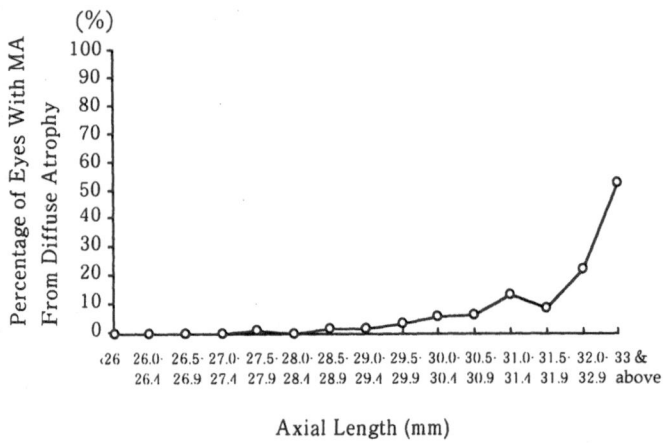

Fig. 4.28. Percentage of eyes with MA (macular atrophy) in all high myopic eyes by axial length

between gender in the percentage of eyes with only tessellated fundus is reversed (see Fig. 4.20).

When all the eyes with high myopia are divided into groups under and over age 40, the percentage of eyes with D_2 differs by axial length. Because diffuse chorioretinal atrophy progresses with aging, the percentage of eyes with D_2 after age 40 is much higher than that before age 40 when the axial length is the same. In other words, chorioretinal atrophy is more common with aging, no matter how long the axial length (Fig. 4.27).

When the axial length is within the range of 27 to 33 mm, the increase in the percentage of eyes with D_2 can be calculated using a simple regression equation. The increased percentage is 13.3%/mm in the total number of myopic eyes, 11.9%/mm in men, 13.3%/mm in women, 9.4%/mm in eyes under age 40, and 12.2%/mm in eyes over age 40.

The relationship between MA and axial length in diffuse chorioretinal atrophy also has been investigated. The percentage of eyes with MA is almost 0% below

28 mm, and it increases slowly and linearly over 28 mm. The percentage increases sharply when the axial length exceeds 32 mm (Fig. 4.28). There is no difference in gender or in age (i.e., less than or more than 40 years of age).

4.2.2.1 Percentage of Eyes with Lacquer Crack Lesions by Axial Length

The frequency distribution of Lc has been evaluated by axial length. The largest number of eyes with Lc appears between 29 and 29.4 mm (Fig. 4.29). If all high myopic eyes are divided into three groups of similar size according to axial length, the percentages of those with Lc are 2.2% in eyes shorter than 28 mm (364 eyes), 8.3% in those between 28 and 29.5 mm (356 eyes), and 11.9% in those longer than 29.5 mm (383 eyes). Lc reaches maximum value when the axial length is longer than 29.5 mm. The frequency of Lc differs by gender according to axial length. No Lc is seen in men whose axial length is shorter than 28.5 mm, although it occurs in women with short axial lengths (Fig. 4.30). The incidence of Lc by each axial length group (shorter than 28 mm, between 28 and 29.5 mm and longer than 29.5 mm) is 0%, 7.4%, and 11.4% in men, and 3.6%, 9.0%, and 12.3% in women.

If the percentage of eyes with Lc in each axial length group is divided by age, that is, under and over age 40, the frequency distribution of eyes with Lc by axial length under age 40 is similar to that in men, with a maximum value of about 27% in eyes between 32 and 33 mm in axial length. No Lc is observed when the axial length is shorter than 28.5 mm. On the other hand, the frequency distribution of eyes with Lc by axial length in those over age 40 is similar to that in women, with a maximum value of about 17% in eyes between 29.5 and 30 mm in axial length (Fig. 4.31).

The incidence of Lc in three groups of axial length is 0%, 7.5%, and 18.0% in patients less than 40 years of age. The corresponding rates are 5.3%, 9.3%, and 7.9% in patients more than 40 years of age. Lc appears only in those with a longer axial length in their eyes under age 40, but it can appear in eyes with a shorter axial length in patients over age 40.

Furthermore, of the 30 male eyes with Lc, 17 occurred in eyes of patients younger than 40 years and 13 in eyes older than 40 years. Of the 51 female eyes with Lc, 24 were in those younger than 40 years and 27 in eyes older than 40 years. There is no significant difference between groups less than and more than age 40 by gender. Therefore, the frequency distribution of Lc by axial length in men is similar to that in eyes under age 40, and the frequency distribution of Lc in each axial length group in women is similar to that in eyes over age 40. Why this is true is unclear, but it is not because there are more men who are younger than age 40 or more women who are older than age 40.

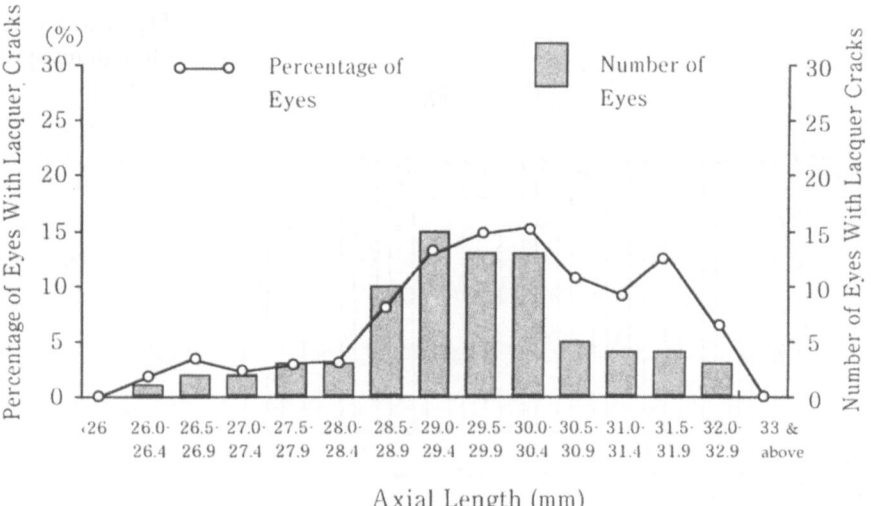

Fig. 4.29. Percentage of eyes with lacquer crack (Lc) lesions in all high myopic eyes by axial length

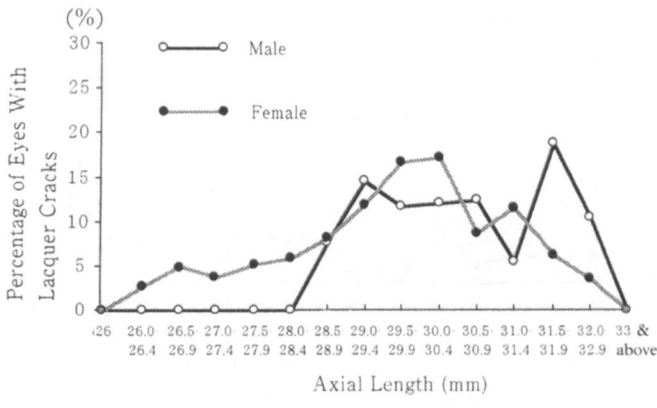

Fig. 4.30. Percentage of eyes with lacquer crack lesions by gender and axial length

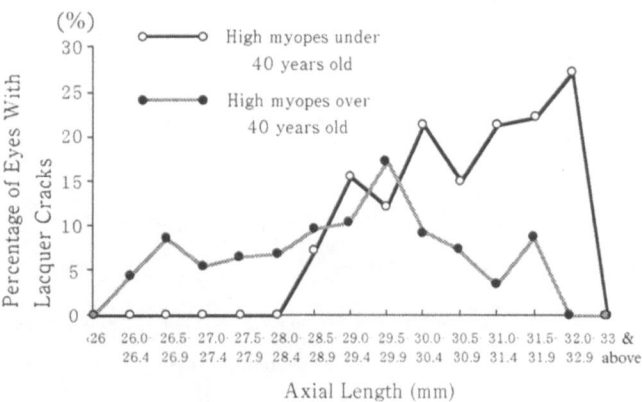

Fig. 4.31. Percentage of eyes with lacquer crack lesions in patients less than or more than 40 years of age by axial length

4.2.3 Percentage of Eyes with Patchy Atrophy by Axial Length

An investigation into the relationship between axial length and patchy atrophy showed that the percentage of patchy atrophy is low when the axial length is shorter than 27 mm; it is 3.3% from 27 to 27.9 mm. The percentage of patchy atrophy then increases linearly with lengthening of the eye. The percentage of patchy atrophy exceeds 25% if the axial length is longer than 31 mm, and it exceeds 50% if the axial length is longer than 32 mm (Fig. 4.32).

The relationship between axial length and P_1 was also investigated. Almost no eyes with P_1 can be observed when the axial length is shorter than 27 mm, but beyond 28.5 mm it increases linearly with lengthening of the eye, reaching 15.4% in 32 mm (Fig. 4.33). There is a tendency for the percentage of P_1 to be higher in women than in men.

The incidence of P_1 under age 40 is almost 0% when the axial length is shorter than 28 mm. The incidence of P_1 increases under age 40 when the axial length is longer than 32 mm. In other words, patchy atrophy will not occur in young people with short axial lengths. Eyes with P_1 appear in a variety of axial lengths, however, after age 40. The incidence of P_1 after age 40 is 4.5% even when the axial length is shorter than 27 mm, and it is 15.4% when the axial length is longer than 33 mm (Fig. 4.34).

The relationship between axial length and P_2 reveals that the incidence of P_2 is low when the axial length is shorter than 29 mm. It then begins to increase from 29 mm. When the axial length exceeds 30 mm, the incidence of P_2 increases sharply and reaches 33.3% when the axial length is longer than 33 mm. This frequency curve

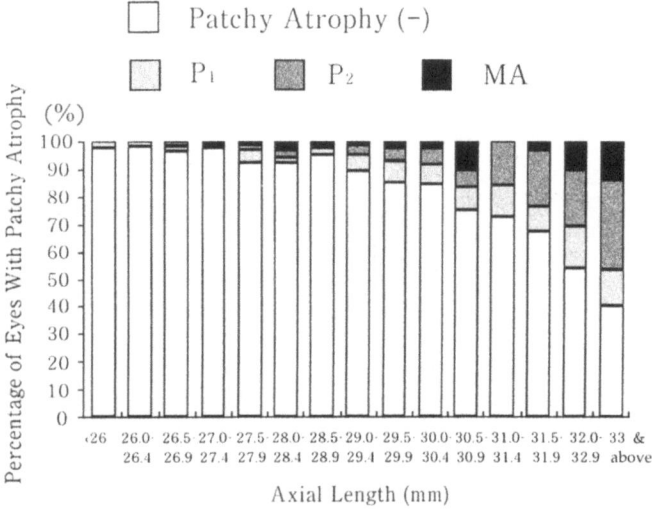

Fig. 4.32. Percentage of eyes with patchy atrophy (P_1 or P_2) in all high myopic eyes by axial length

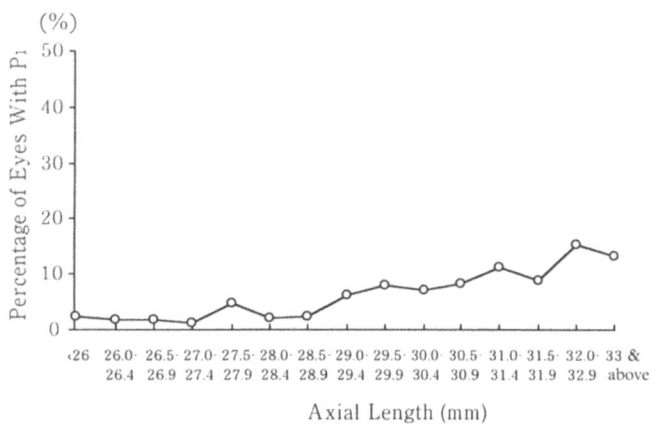

Fig. 4.33. Percentage of eyes with P_1 in all high myopic eyes by axial length

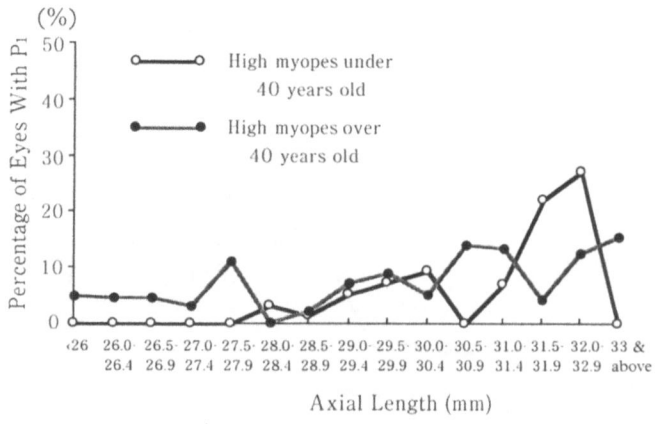

Fig. 4.34. Percentage of eyes with P_1 in patients less than or more than 40 years of age by axial length

Fig. 4.35. Percentage of eyes with P_2 in all high myopic eyes by axial length

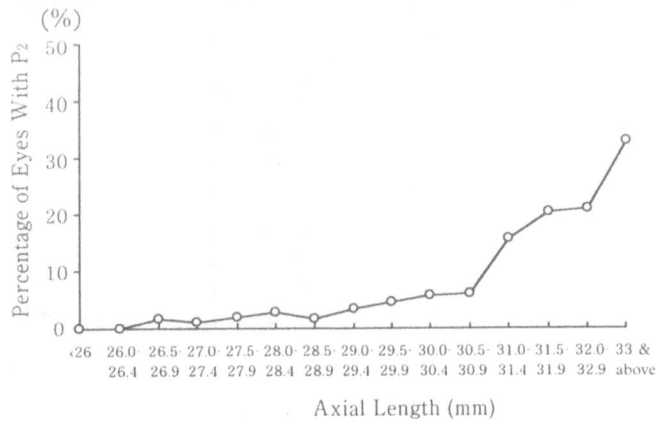

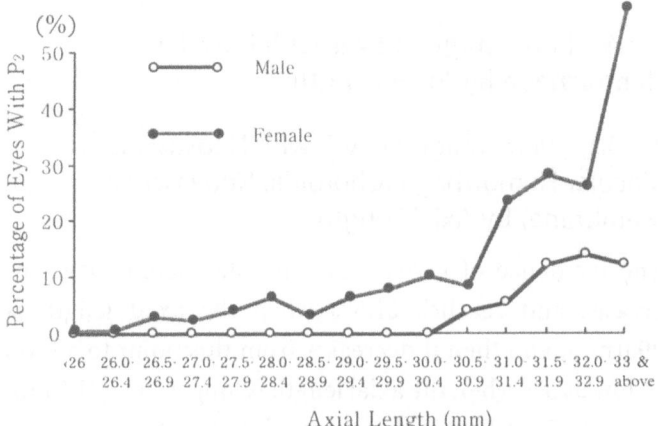

Fig. 4.36. Percentage of eyes with P_2 by gender and axial length

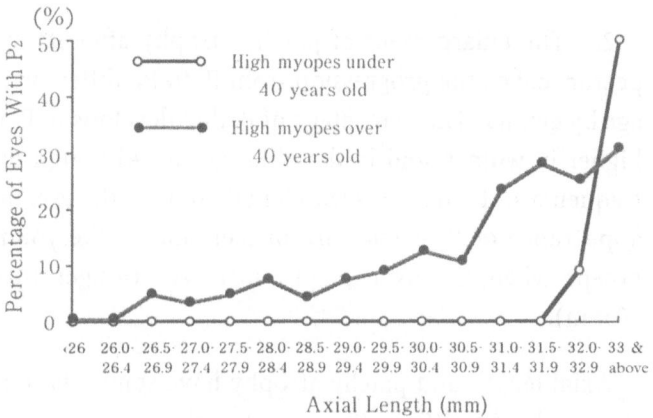

Fig. 4.37. Percentage of eyes with P_2 in patients less than or more than 40 years of age by axial length

is closer to a quadratic curve than a straight line (Fig. 4.35).

Looking at the relationship between axial length and P_2 by gender, we find that the incidence of P_2 in women is much higher than in men, reaching a maximum value of 57.1% when the axial length is longer than 33 mm. Conversely, the incidence of P_2 in men is 0% when the axial length is shorter than 30 mm. It begins to increase when the axial length is longer than 30 mm. Therefore, the incidence of P_2 by axial length is quite different between men and women (Fig. 4.36).

The incidence of P_2 in eyes under and over age 40 demonstrates that when the axial length is longer than 26 mm, the incidence of P_2 in eyes over age 40 increases together with lengthening of the eye. On the other hand, the incidence of P_2 under age 40 is 0% when the axial length is shorter than 32 mm. It is not unusual to find that P_2 before the age of 40 years begins to appear when the axial length is longer than 32 mm (Fig. 4.37).

Curtin and co-workers divided all patients with patchy atrophy into three groups: age 19 years and less, between ages 20 and 39 years, and age 40 years and older. The authors found that age affected patchy atrophy in that the incidence of patchy atrophy increases with aging [28]. Figures 4.36 and 4.37 show that the incidence of P_2 in women and in the older group increases with lengthening of the eye. Also, P_2 is difficult to observe in men and in young people when the axial length is short.

The incidence of P_1 in women and in eyes over age 40 years is also somewhat higher than in men and in young people under age 40. The incidence is consistent with corresponding percentages of P_2. Therefore:

1. The appearance of P_1 depends on axial length. The incidence of P_1 increases with lengthening of the eye. Also, the incidence of P_1 in women and in those more than 40 years old is also slightly higher than the incidence of P_1 in men and in those less than 40 years of age.

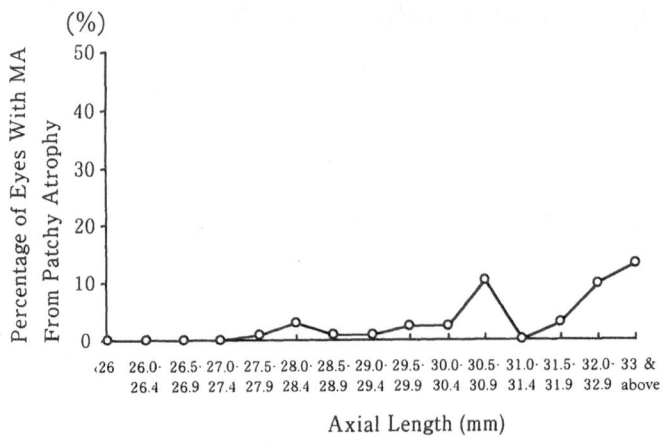

Fig. 4.38. Percentage of eyes with MA from patchy atrophy in all high myopic eyes by axial length

2. The enlargement of patchy atrophy after its appearance, i.e., the progression from P_1 to P_2, differs with age by gender. The percentage of P_1 that develops to P_2 is higher in women and in the older group. Although the frequency of P_2 increases with lengthening of the eye, the appearance of P_2 is still rare in men and in the young except when the axial length increases (longer than 30 mm).

Axial length and patchy atrophy have some relationship with MA. When the axial length is shorter than 27 mm, the percentage of MA is 0%, but it increases linearly with the lengthening of the eye when the axial length is longer than 27 mm (Fig. 4.38). The frequency of MA in eyes under and over age 40 years was also investigated by gender. The frequency of MA in men and in eyes under age 40 is lower than that in women and in eyes over age 40. Also, almost no MA is seen in eyes under age 40. This finding is consistent with the relationship between axial length and P_2. It is possible that P_2 and MA do not readily occur in men and in the young.

4.2.4 Percentage of Eyes with Macular Hemorrhage by Axial Length

4.2.4.1 Percentage of Eyes with Neovascular Macular Hemorrhage (Choroidal Neovascular Membrane) by Axial Length

The incidence of neovascular macular hemorrhage increases and reaches 21.5% when the axial length is 29.0 mm, and then it decreases from this point to a level as low as 5% when the axial length is longer than 31.5 mm (Fig. 4.39). Choroidal neovascular membrane in the fovea is very important because it can severely impair visual function.

Excluding eyes with choroidal neovascular membrane that have an axial length longer than 31.5 mm, a linear regression can be determined from the scattergram of choroidal neovascular membrane and eyes with an axial length shorter than 31 mm. The gradient of the linear regression obtained is then 2.5%/mm. The percentage of choroidal neovascular membrane in the total number of eyes with high myopia is 5%–6% when the axial length is

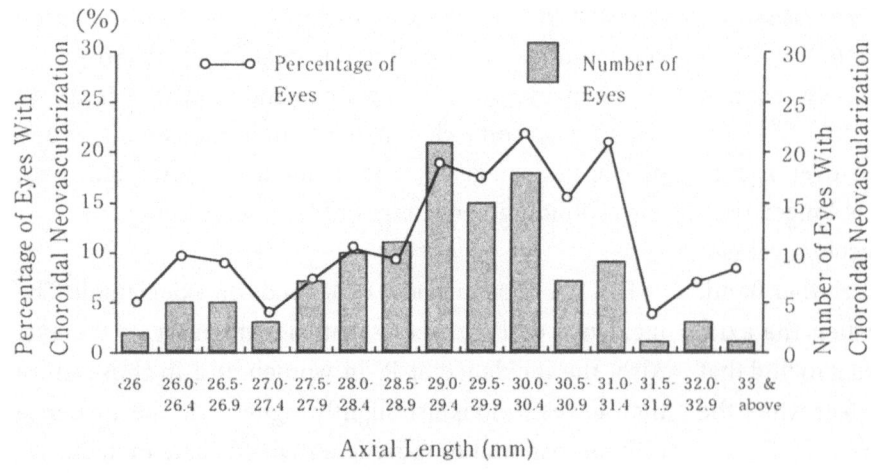

Fig. 4.39. Percentage of eyes with neovascular macular hemorrhage (choroidal neovascular membrane) in all high myopic eyes by axial length

Fig. 4.40. Scattergram of neovascular macular hemorrhage (choroidal neovascularization) by axial length and gender was calculated by axial length and frequency of neovascular macular hemorrhage by gender; the linear regression is obtained in axial lengths under 31 mm

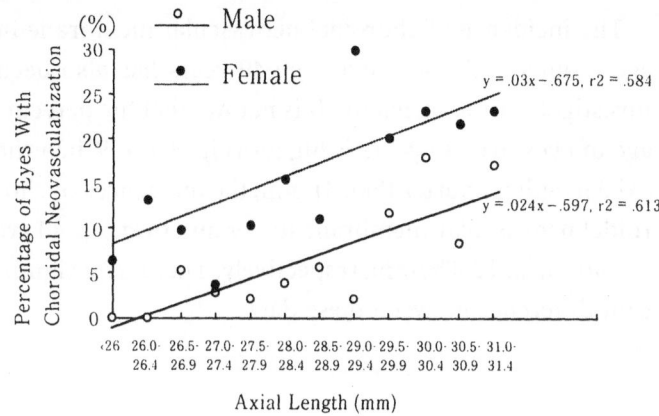

Fig. 4.41. Ratio of frequency of eyes with neovascular macular hemorrhage (neovascularization) by gender and axial length, shows by line graph. No eyes with an axial length greater than 31.5 mm is represented

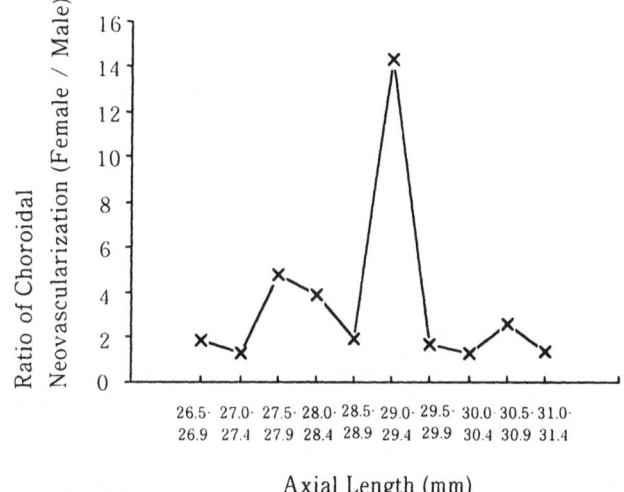

shorter than 26 mm. Because the percentage of macular hemorrhage increases 2.5% with 1 mm of axial elongation, this percentage reaches about 20% when the axial length is 31 mm (Fig. 4.40).

The percentage of choroidal neovascular membrane has been investigated by age, and it was found that choroidal neovascular membrane increases linearly with aging (see Figs. 4.8, 4.9). When the percentage of eyes with choroidal neovascular membrane is examined by axial length, the incidence is noted to decrease sharply with axial lengths longer than 31.5 mm, as mentioned earlier (see Fig. 4.39). The reason for this finding may reflect the difficulty in identifying choroidal neovascular membrane with ophthalmoscopy and with fluorescein fundus angiography when diffuse and patchy chorioretinal atrophy becomes highly developed. It also becomes difficult to distinguish chorioretinal atrophy of the macula, which progresses from choroidal neovascular membrane or from large patchy lesions of patchy atrophy that appear with lengthening of the eye. It is also possible that chor-

oidal neovascular membrane occurs less frequently because of the high degree of chorioretinal atrophy.

The incidence of choroidal neovascular membrane differs by gender. It reaches a maximum value of 17% in men when the axial length is longer than 30 mm and shorter than 30.4 mm. On the other hand, when the axial length is longer than 29 mm and shorter than 29.4 mm, the maximum value in women is 30%, which is higher than in men. In eyes with axial lengths less than 31 mm, a linear regression can be obtained from the scattergram of choroidal neovascular membrane and axial length. The incidence determined from the gradient of the linear regression is 2.4%/mm in men and 3.0%/mm in women (Fig. 4.40).

The ratio of women to men is shown in Fig. 4.41. Choroidal neovascular membrane occurs more often in women than in men in eyes with a variety of axial lengths. The incidence of choroidal neovascular membrane in women is two to six times that in men in eyes of all axial lengths except at 29.0–29.5 mm.

Percentage of Eyes with Chorioretinal Atrophy in Each Axial Length Group   **41**

The incidence of choroidal neovascular membrane in age groups under and over age 40 years has also been investigated by axial length. It is natural that the percentage of eyes over 40 years is higher (Fig. 4.42). When the axial length is shorter than 31 mm, the incidences of choroidal neovascular membrane under and over age 40 are 2.2%/mm and 2.4%/mm, respectively. There is no significant difference between these data.

4.2.4.2 Percentage of Eyes with Simple Macular Hemorrhage by Axial Length

Simple macular hemorrhage is uncommon and occurs in fewer than 10 eyes per axial length group. No simple macular hemorrhage has been observed in eyes with axial lengths less than 27 mm (Fig. 4.43). The difference is not significant by gender. The incidence of simple macular hemorrhage under age 40 is higher than that over 40;

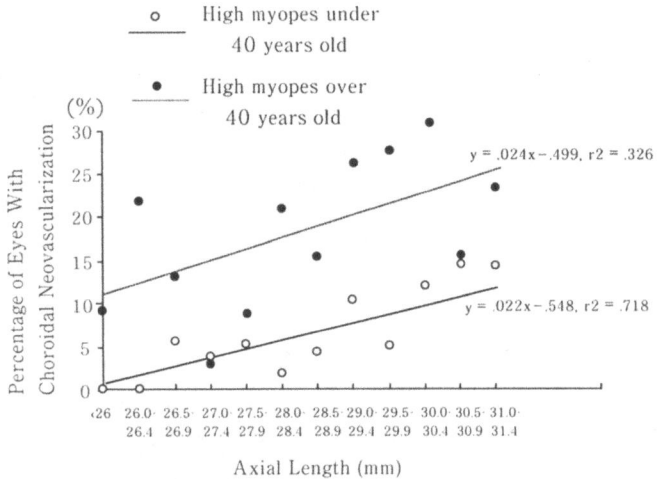

Fig. 4.42. Scattergram of neovascular macular hemorrhage (choroidal neovascularization) in patients less than or more than 40 years of age by axial length, calculated by axial length and frequency of neovascular macular hemorrhage; the linear regression was obtained for axial lengths less than 31 mm

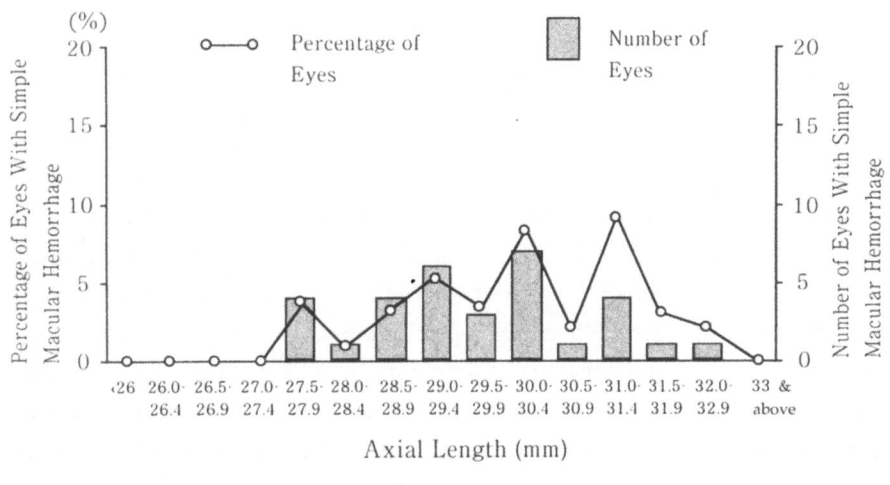

Fig. 4.43. Percentage of eyes with simple macular hemorrhage in all high myopic eyes by axial length

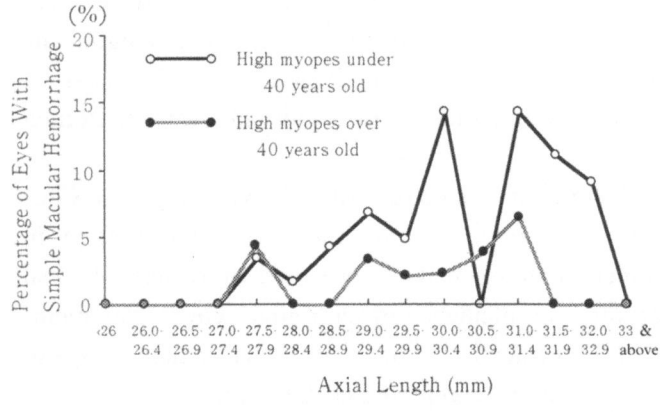

Fig. 4.44. Percentage of eyes with simple macular hemorrhage in patients less than or more than 40 years of age by axial length

i.e., more young patients have simple macular hemorrhage (Fig. 4.44). This finding is different from that of diffuse and patchy atrophy.

4.2.5 Relationship Between Axial Length and Area of Peripapillary Atrophy

No relationship could be found between axial length and area of papillary atrophy. In other words, there is no tendency for peripapillary atrophy to progress with lengthening of the eye (Fig. 4.45).

4.3 Percentage of Chorioretinal Atrophy With or Without Posterior Staphyloma

4.3.1 Distribution of Axial Length and Percentage of Posterior Staphyloma by Axial Length

It is conceivable that posterior staphyloma is closely related to chorioretinal atrophy [41,42]. In general, the axial length is long if posterior staphyloma exists. The percentage of posterior staphyloma is about 10% in eyes with axial lengths less than 26 mm, and it reaches about 90% in eyes with axial lengths more than 33 mm (Fig. 4.46). In a report by Curtin et al., the minimum percentage of staphyloma was 1.4% when the axial length was 26.5–27.4 mm, and the maximum value was 76.4% when the axial length was 33.5–36.6 mm. The percentage of staphyloma increases linearly with lengthening of the eye in the range of 27.4 to 33.5 mm [28]. These results are similar to ours.

Fig. 4.45. Ratio of area of peripapillary atrophy to area of optic disc in all high myopic eyes by axial length, divided into 1-mm lengths. *Columns* show the mean value for each ratio; the *vertical axis* shows the standard deviation

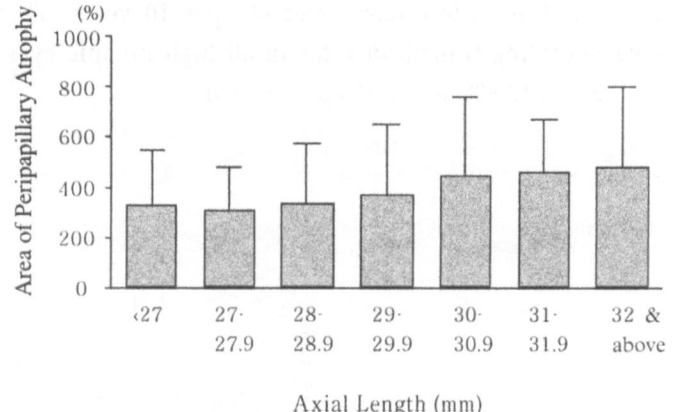

Fig. 4.46. Axial length for all high myopic eyes with or without posterior staphyloma. Axial lengths are divided into 0.5-mm intervals ranging from more than 26 to less than 32 mm. Distribution by number of eyes is nearly normal. *Shaded areas*, eyes with posterior staphyloma; *white areas*, eyes without posterior staphyloma. The percentage of eyes with posterior staphyloma is shown by the *line graph*

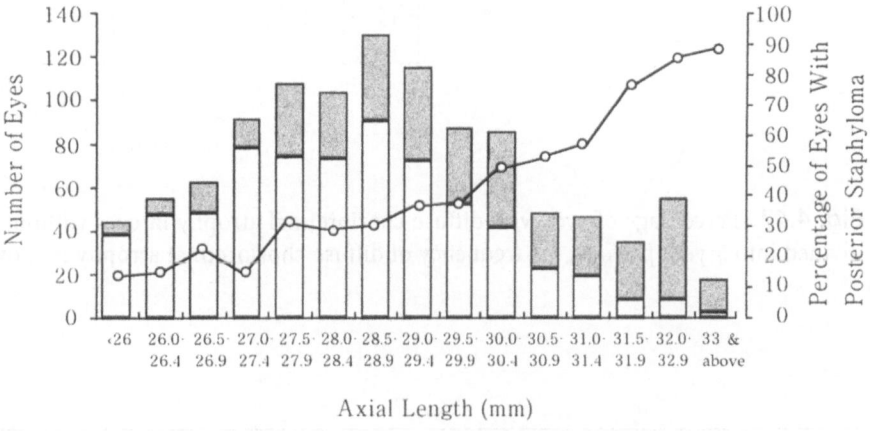

4.3.2 Diffuse Chorioretinal Atrophy With or Without Posterior Staphyloma

4.3.2.1 Diffuse Chorioretinal Atrophy Without Posterior Staphyloma (662 Eyes)

The percentage of diffuse chorioretinal atrophy without staphyloma has been evaluated in 668 eyes. The percentage of eyes with only tessellated fundus was 56.5%, D_1 was 33.8%, D_2 was 9.5%, and MA was 0.2%. Therefore, the percentage of eyes with only tessellated fundus and D_1 is higher and the percentage of eyes with D_2 and MA without posterior staphyloma is lower than in the total number of eyes. Almost no MA occurs in eyes without staphyloma (Fig. 4.47). It is believed that these findings may be influenced by the fact that the distribution of eyes without staphyloma is greater in young people.

The reduction rate of tessellated fundus is 11.5% per 10 years. The rate of increase of D_1 and D_2 is 5.0% and 6.6% per 10 years, respectively, and the rate of increase of MA is 0% per 10 years (Fig. 4.48). On the other hand, the transition rate of tessellated fundus $\rightarrow D_1$, $D_1 \rightarrow D_2$, and $D_2 \rightarrow$ MA is 11.5%, 6.5%, and 0% per 10 years. The corresponding transition rates in all high myopic eyes are 13.8%, 13.8%, and 3.1% per 10 years.

In comparison of the transition rate without staphyloma with that in all high myopic eyes:

1. The percentage of eyes with progression of diffuse chorioretinal atrophy and no staphyloma is lower than that in all myopic eyes (the transition rate is small).

2. The transition rate of tessellated fundus $\rightarrow D_1$ in eyes without staphyloma is somewhat lower than in all eyes, but the transition rate of $D_1 \rightarrow D_2$ and $D_2 \rightarrow$ MA in eyes without staphyloma is much lower than in all eyes. Meanwhile, the progression of D_1 and D_2 continues to increase, which is a characterstic feature of this lesion (see Fig. 4.4).

4.3.2.2 Diffuse Chorioretinal Atrophy with Posterior Staphyloma (423 Eyes)

The percentage of eyes with diffuse chorioretinal atrophy and staphyloma has been investigated. The percentage of eyes with only tessellated fundus was 6.9%, D_1 was 33.3%, D_2 was 48.7%, and MA was 11.1%. The incidence of tessellated fundus in eyes under age 30 years is quite rare, and it stabilizes to a low percentage in those over age 40. A dramatic reduction in the frequency of D_1 occurs linearly over age 30. The frequency of D_2 is low under age 20 years, but increases sharply in those above age 25, and continues to increase, albeit at a slow pace (Fig. 4.49).

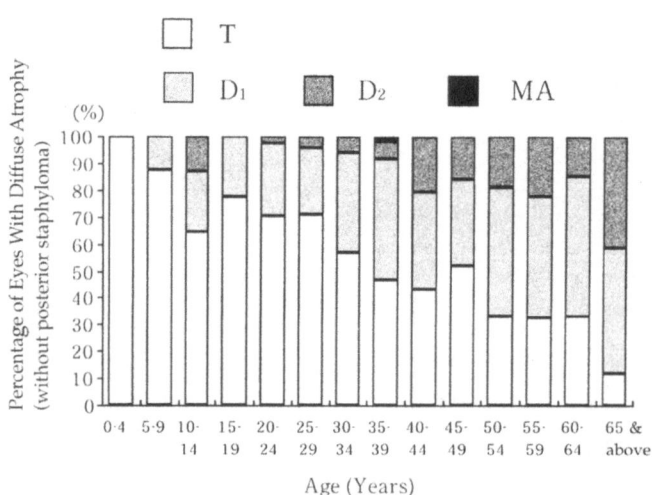

Fig. 4.47. Percentage of eyes with diffuse chorioretinal atrophy in eyes without posterior staphyloma by age group. Ages are divided into 5-year periods; the frequency of diffuse chorioretinal atrophy is shown for each group

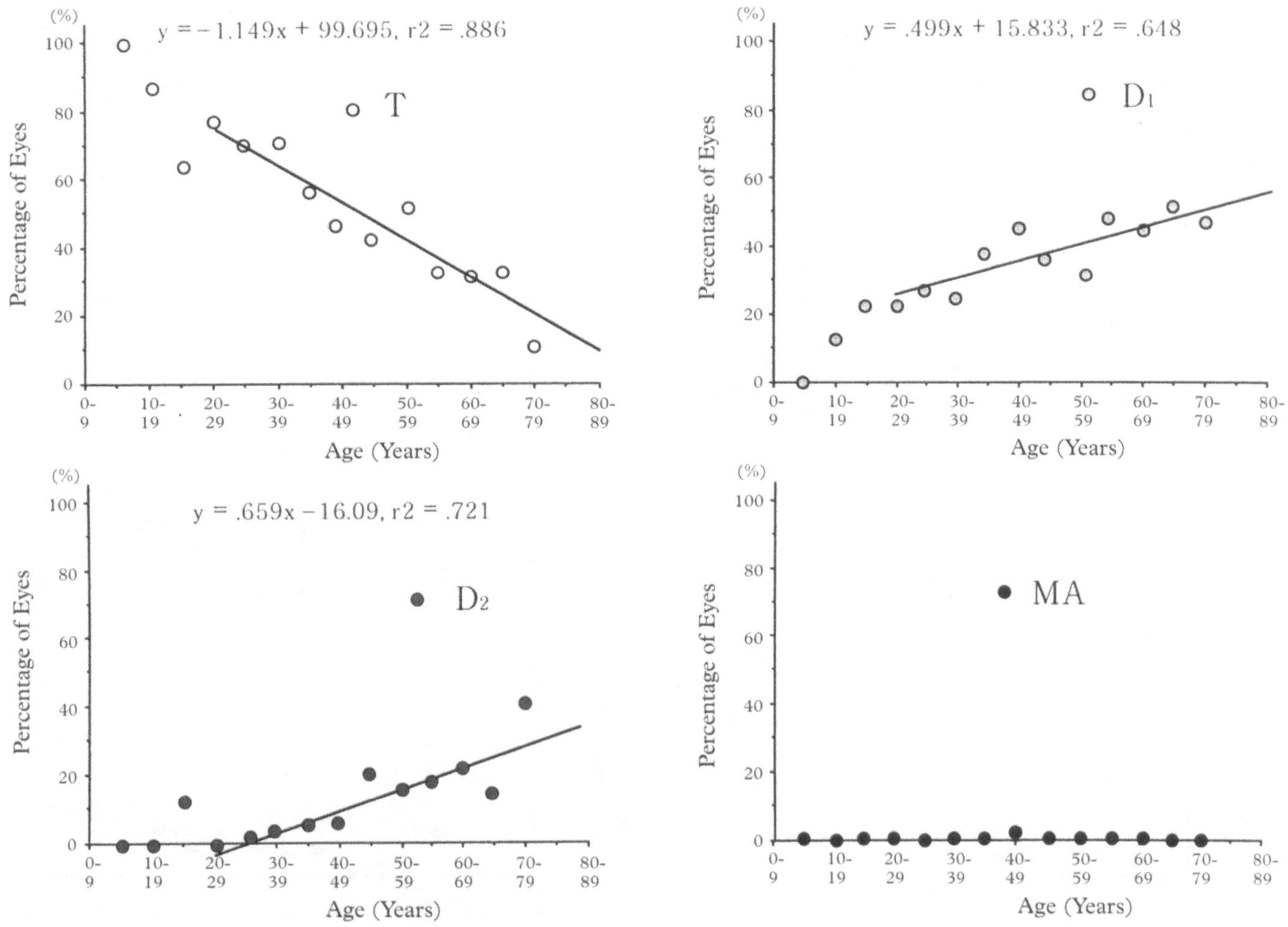

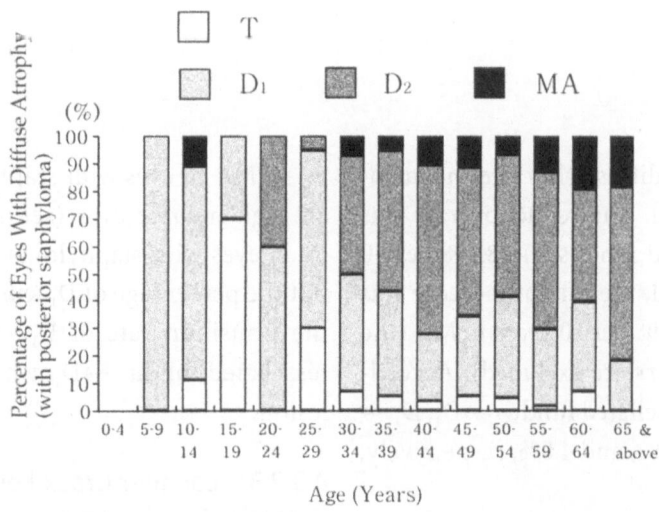

Fig. 4.48. Scattergrams show each kind of diffuse chorioretinal atrophy by age in eyes without posterior staphyloma, with linear regression analyses calculated for each type

Fig. 4.49. Percentage of eyes with diffuse chorioretinal atrophy in eyes with posterior staphyloma by age group. Ages are divided into 5-year periods; frequency of diffuse chorioretinal atrophy is shown for each group

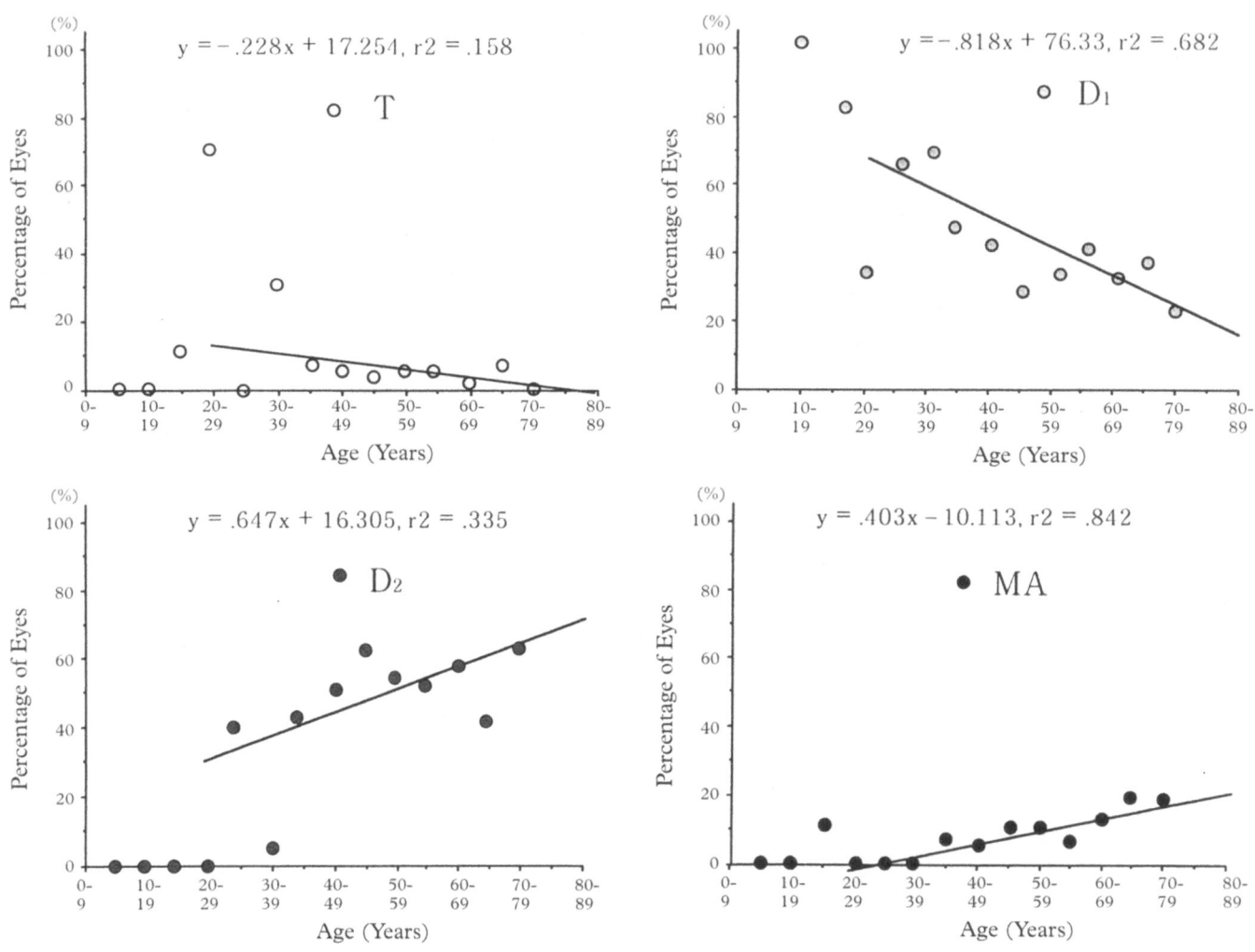

Fig. 4.50. Scattergrams show each kind of diffuse chorioretinal atrophy by age in eyes with posterior staphyloma, with linear regression analyses calculated for each type

The change in each type of diffuse chorioretinal atrophy also has been investigated. The reduction rate was 2.3% per 10 years in tessellated fundus and 8.2% per 10 years in D_1. On the other hand, the rate of increase was 6.5% per 10 years in D_2 and 4.0% per 10 years in MA (the data for eyes under age 20 years are excluded). Accordingly, the transition rate of tessellated fundus $\rightarrow D_1$, $D_1 \rightarrow D_2$, and $D_2 \rightarrow$ MA is 2.3%, 10.5%, and 4.0%, respectively, per 10 years (Fig. 4.50).

The transition rate of tessellated fundus $\rightarrow D_1$ in eyes with staphyloma is much lower than that in all high myopic eyes, but the transition rates of $D_1 \rightarrow D_2$ and

$D_2 \rightarrow$ MA in eyes with staphyloma are similar to that in all high myopic eyes (see Fig. 4.4). The percentage of D_1 in eyes with staphyloma is high even at a young age, but the percentage of D_1 will decrease with aging because the transition rate of $D_1 \rightarrow D_2$ is higher than that of tessellated fundus $\rightarrow D_1$, which is a characteristic of this lesion.

4.3.2.3 Lacquer Crack Lesion With or Without Posterior Staphyloma

It has been reported that Lc is easily formed in eyes with staphyloma [14,30]. The percentage of eyes with Lc le-

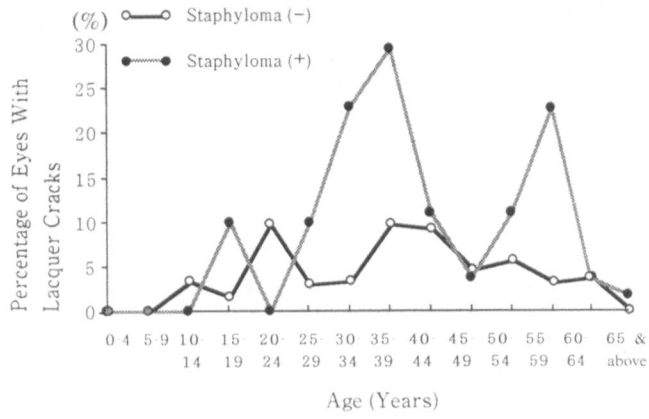

Fig. 4.51. Percentage of eyes with lacquer crack (Lc) lesions, with or without posterior staphyloma, by age in 5-year intervals

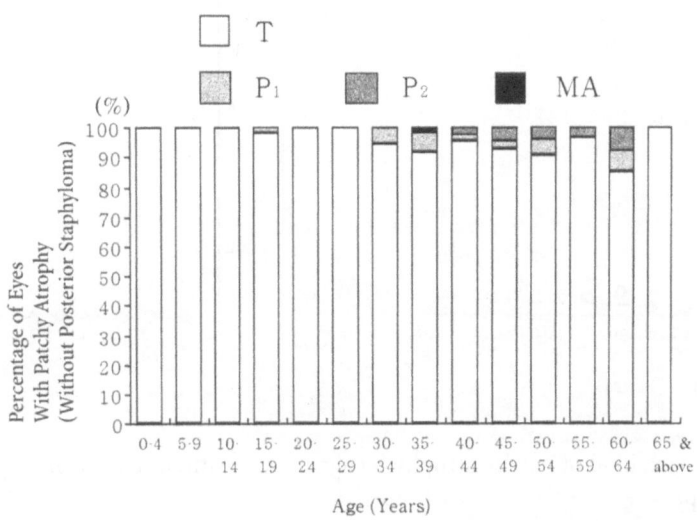

Fig. 4.52. Percentage of eyes with patchy atrophy and no posterior staphyloma by age in 5-year intervals

sions with or without staphyloma has also been investigated (Fig. 4.51). The percentage of Lc in eyes without staphyloma is as low as 5%–10% and does not show a distribution of two peaks. Conversely, the frequency distribution of Lc in eyes with staphyloma shows two peaks at around the age of 40 years and at about age 60 years. In other words, this finding reflects the characteristics of frequency distribution of Lc with age in eyes with posterior staphyloma.

4.3.3 Patchy Atrophy With or Without Posterior Staphyloma

Of all high myopic eyes without posterior staphyloma (668 eyes), 96.1% had no patchy atrophy (643 eyes), 1.2% (8 eyes) had P_2, and 0.1% (1 eye) had MA (Fig. 4.52).

The reduction rate of eyes without patchy atrophy was 1.2% per 10 years, the rate of increase of eyes with P_1 was 0% per 10 years, the rate of increase of eyes with P_2 was 1.0% per 10 years, and the rate of increase of eyes with MA was 0% per 10 years (Fig. 4.53). Accordingly, the transition rate of no patchy atrophy $\rightarrow P_1$, $P_1 \rightarrow P_2$, and P_2

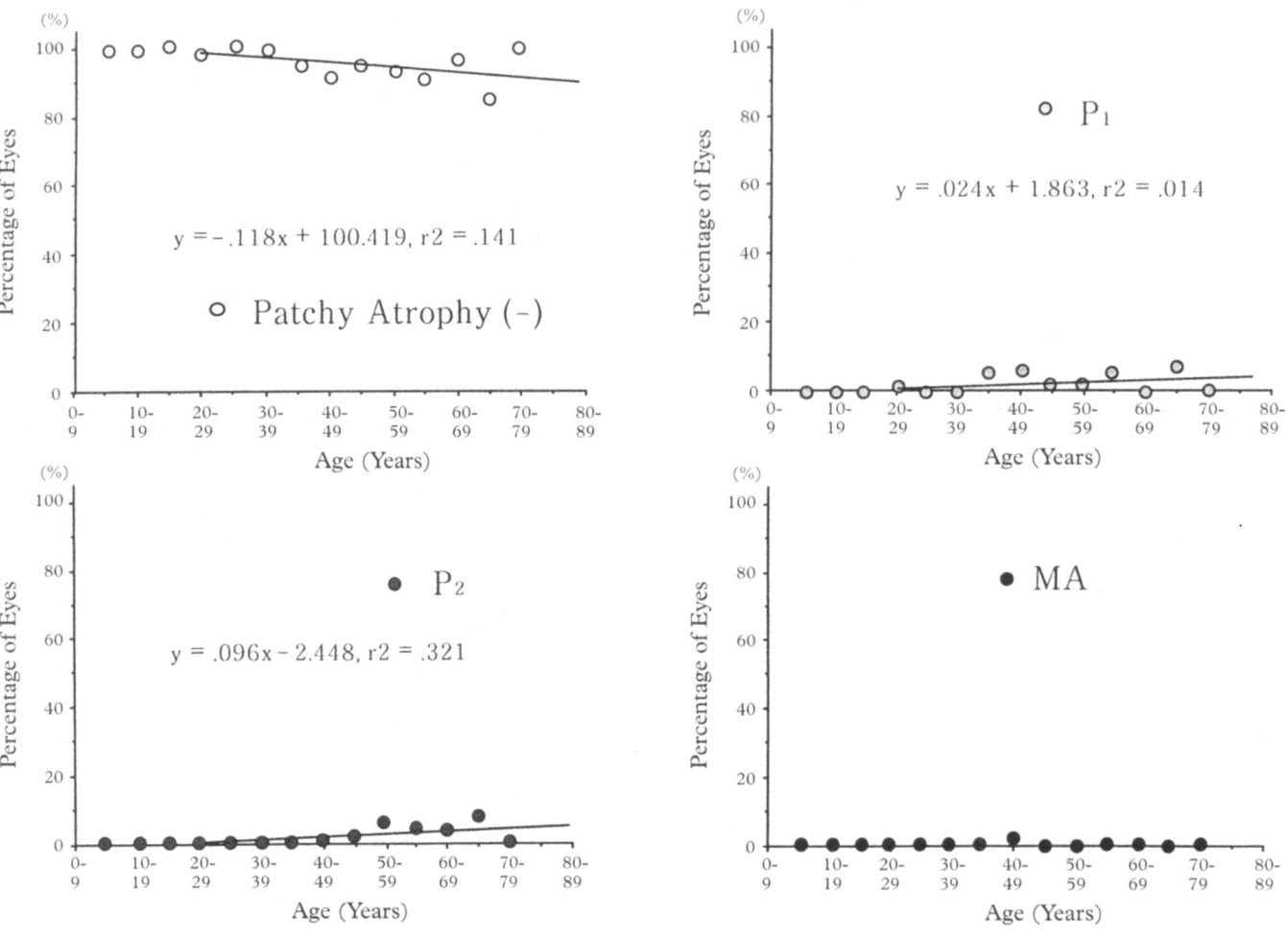

Fig. 4.53. Scattergrams show each kind of patchy atrophy by age in eyes without posterior staphyloma, with linear regression analyses calculated for each type

→ MA was 1.2%, 1.2%, and 0% per 10 years, respectively. It is believed that the formation of patchy atrophy without posterior staphyloma is much lower than that of all high myopic eyes (see Fig. 4.7).

As many as 74.5% (307 of 412 eyes) of high myopic eyes with posterior staphyloma do not have patchy atrophy. We found P_1 in 9.5% (39 of 412 eyes), P_2 in 11.6% (48 of 412 eyes), and MA in 6.5% (27 of 412 eyes) (Fig. 4.54). More cases of patchy atrophy were observed in eyes with than in eyes without posterior staphyloma.

The reduction rate of eyes withotu patchy atrophy was 8.5% per 10 years, the increasing percentage of P_1 was 0%

per 10 years, of P_2, 4.6% per 10 years, and of MA, 3.4% per 10 years (Fig. 4.55). Accordingly, the transition rate of no patchy atrophy $\rightarrow P_1$, $P_1 \rightarrow P_2$, and $P_2 \rightarrow$ MA in eyes with staphyloma was 8.5%, 8.5%, and 3.4% per 10 years, respectively. The transition rate of patchy atrophy in the total number of high myopic eyes was 7.4%, 5.9%, and 2.3% per 10 years, respectively (Fig. 4.55). The progression of patchy atrophy with posterior staphyloma tends to be faster than in all high myopic eyes.

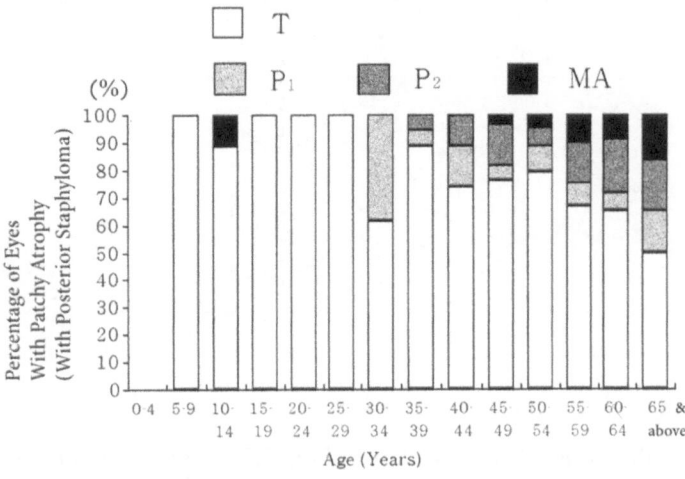

Fig. 4.54. Percentage of eyes with patchy atrophy and posterior staphyloma by age in 5-year intervals

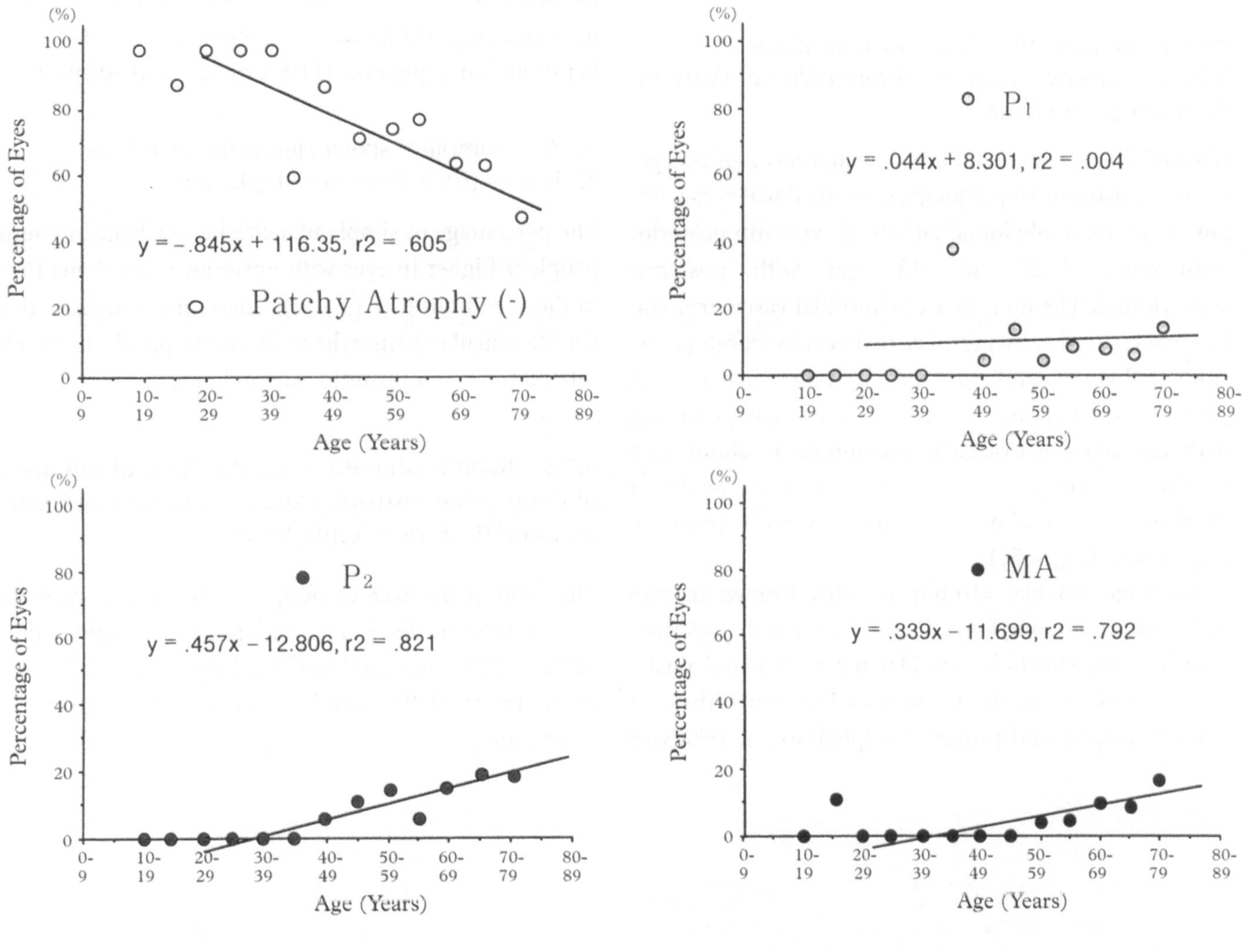

y = −.845x + 116.35, r2 = .605

Patchy Atrophy (-)

y = .044x + 8.301, r2 = .004

P₁

y = .457x − 12.806, r2 = .821

P₂

y = .339x − 11.699, r2 = .792

MA

Fig. 4.55. Scattergrams show each kind of patchy atrophy by age in eyes with posterior staphyloma, linear regression analyses calculated for each type

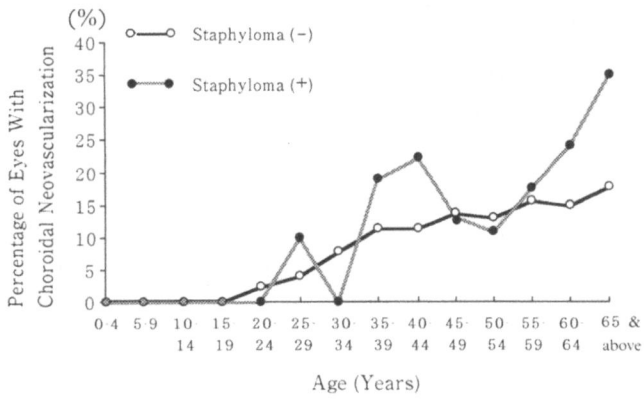

Fig. 4.56. Percentage of eyes with choroidal neovascularization, with or without posterior staphyloma, by age in 5-year intervals

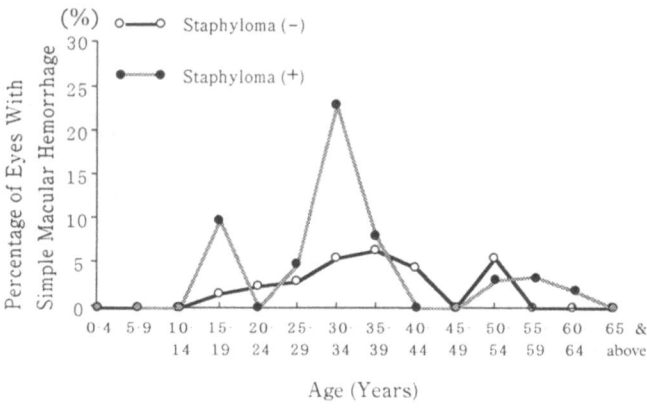

Fig. 4.57. Percentage of eyes with simple macular hemorrhage, with or without posterior staphyloma, by age in 5-year intervals

4.3.4 Macular Hemorrhage in Eyes With or Without Posterior Staphyloma

4.3.4.1 Neovascular Macular Hemorrhage (Choroidal Neovascular Membrane) With or Without Posterior Staphyloma

Choroidal vascular membrane was observed in 50 eyes without posterior staphyloma (7.5% of all 668 eyes without posterior staphyloma) and in 72 eyes with posterior staphyloma (17.5% of 412 eyes with posterior staphyloma). The incidence of choroidal vascular membrane increased 3.1% per 10 years in eyes without posterior staphyloma and 5.7% per 10 years in eyes with posterior staphyloma. Therefore, the percentage of eyes with choroidal neovascular membrane is about 20% in the seventh decade of those without posterior staphyloma and about 35% in eyes with posterior staphyloma (Fig. 4.56).

Although macular atrophy is easily formed in eyes with posterior staphyloma, it is not clear if the relationship between choroidal vascular membrane and posterior staphyloma is similar to that between diffuse or patchy atrophy and posterior staphyloma. A relatively high percentage of choroidal neovascular membranes forms even in eyes without posterior staphyloma. The incidence of choroidal vascular membrane in eyes with posterior staphyloma was 50% higher in the total number of high myopic eyes (11.3% or 122 of 1080 eyes).

4.3.4.2 Simple Macular Hemorrhage in Eyes With or Without Posterior Staphyloma

The percentage of simple macular hemorrhage in young people is higher in eyes with posterior staphyloma than in those without it (Fig. 4.57). Therefore, it appears that simple macular hemorrhage in young people is closely related to Lc and posterior staphyloma.

4.3.5 Relationship Between the Ratio of the Area of Peripapillary Atrophy and the Area of the Optic Disc and Posterior Staphyloma

The ratio of the area of peripapillary atrophy over the area of the optic disc in eyes with posterior staphyloma is 457% ± 297% (n = 262), which is larger than the 303% ± 193% (n = 279) found in eyes without posterior staphyloma.

5 Visual Acuity and Chorioretinal Atrophy

5.1 Distribution of Visual Acuity and Axial Length

The distribution of the best corrected visual acuity is illustrated in Fig. 5.1. The mean visual acuity in a logMAR is 0.31 (visual acuity in decimals is 0.49). Of the total number of high myopic eyes, 27.9% had a visual acuity of 1.0 or better, 61% better than 0.5, and 13.7% worse than 0.1. The mean visual acuity in a logMAR is 0.38 (visual acuity in decimals, 0.42) in women and 0.21 (visual acuity in decimals, 0.61) in men. The relationship between corrected visual acuity and axial length is shown in Fig. 5.2. Visual acuity can also be influenced by factors in addition to axial length [3,6,12,40,43] such as age, gender, and chorioretinal atrophy. If we concentrate only on the relationship between visual acuity and axial length, we find that corrected visual acuity becomes less with lengthening of the eyes (Fig. 5.2). The best visual acuity in eyes with choroidal neovascular membrane was 0.5 (2 eyes); all others were less than 0.4.

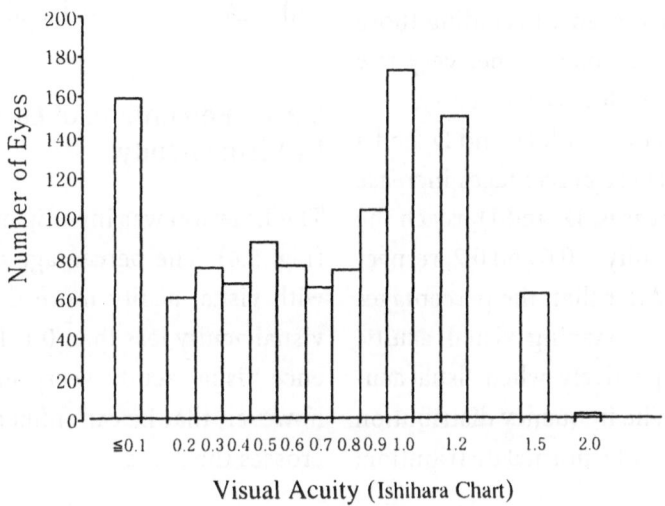

Fig. 5.1. Distribution of corrected visual acuity for all high myopic eyes. Corrected visual acuity below 0.1 includes counting fingers

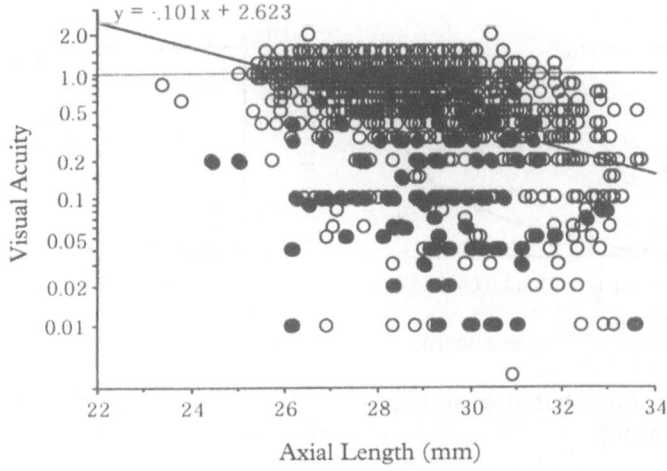

Fig. 5.2. Relationship between corrected visual acuity and axial length in all high myopic eyes. Visual acuity is presented in a logarithm; the *line graph* shows the linear regression chanalysis. *White circles*, eyes without choroidal neovascular membrane; *black circles*, eyes with choroidal neovascular membrane

5.2 Percentage of Diffuse Chorioretinal Atrophy by Visual Acuity

The total number of myopic eyes has been divided into several groups according to visual acuity, and the percentage of diffuse chorioretinal atrophy has been evaluated in each visual acuity group (Fig. 5.3). The visual acuity in 77% of eyes with tessellated fundus was better than 1.5. This percentage, however, decreases with worsening of visual acuity. It was observed that almost no eyes with tessellated fundus have visual acuity less than 0.1. Of the 408 eyes with tessellated fundus in the total number of high myopic eyes, 63% had visual acuity greater than 1.0, and 95% had visual acuity greater than 0.5. Fewer than 1.1% of eyes with tessellated fundus had visual acuity less than 0.1. When eyes with tessellated fundus have low visual acuity, they usually are associated with choroidal neovascular membrane. Excluding those cases with choroidal neovascular membrane, very few eyes with tessellated fundus have low visual acuity.

As few as 21.9% and 1.6% of eyes with D_1 and D_2 had a visual acuity of 1.5 or better. These percentages increase gradually as visual acuity decreases. D_1 and D_2 reach the maximum value when visual acuity is 0.6 and 0.2, respectively (D_1, 56.9%; D_2, 62.8%). After that, the percentages of D_1 and D_2 decrease with worsening visual acuity, reaching 16.7% and 33.3%, respectively, when visual acuity is less than 0.01 (Fig. 5.3). The frequency distribution of D_1 and D_2 by visual acuity is not a normal distribution;

instead, the frequency distribution of D_1 is symmetric and that of D_2 indicates some skewness to the right. This kind of distribution is similar to that of D_1 and D_2 with axial length (see Figs. 4.22, 4.25). On the other hand, the distribution of the percentage of D_1 and D_2 to age was also investigated, and D_1 and D_2 actually decrease with age. The percentage of D_1 and D_2 with age is quite consistent, as shown in a simple regression equation (see Figs. 4.4, 4.48, 4.50). The distribution of the percentage of D_1 and D_2 by axial length or visual acuity is different from the distribution by age.

No MA of diffuse choroidal atrophy was observed in eyes with visual acuity greater than 0.6. The percentage of MA was 2.4% in eyes with visual acuity of 0.5. This percentage increases with worsening of visual acuity and reaches a maximum of 50% in eyes with visual acuity less than 0.01 (Fig. 5.3). Also, 50% of the total number of eyes with MA have a visual acuity less than 0.1.

5.2.1 Percentage of Lacquer Crack Lesions by Visual Acuity

The Lc lesion was investigated in relation to visual acuity (Fig. 5.4). The percentage of Lc was about 10% in eyes with visual acuity more than 0.2 and 5% in eyes with visual acuity less than 0.1. In general, Lc does not influence visual acuity veery much. It has been suggested, however, that Lc can influence visual acuity so long as it crosses the fovea.

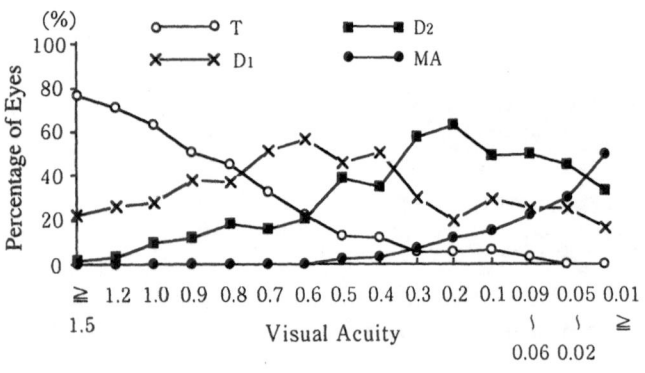

Fig. 5.3. Percentage of eyes with diffuse chorioretinal atrophy in all high myopic eyes by visual acuity

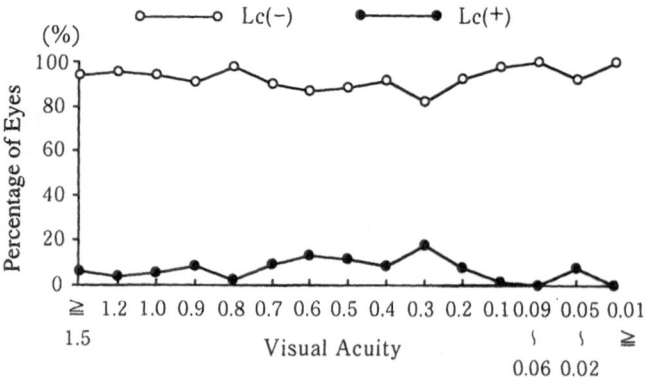

Fig. 5.4. Percentage of eyes with lacquer crack lesions (*Lc*) by visual acuity

5.3 Percentage of Patchy Atrophy by Visual Acuity

Patchy atrophy ($P_1 + P_2 + MA$) in each visual acuity group was investigated (Fig. 5.5). The percentage of eyes with patchy atrophy was lowest (1.6%) in eyes with visual acuity greater than 1.5. This percentage increased almost linearly with worsening visual acuity until it reached a level of about 0.2–0.3. From that point, the rate increased, reaching a maximum of 66.5% in eyes with visual acuity less than 0.01. We had 145 eyes with patchy atrophy, 60% of which have visual acuity greater than 0.2; the other 40% had visual acuity less than 0.1. The percentage of eyes with patchy atrophy increased with aging (see Figs. 4.6, 4.7) and also with lengthening of the eyes (Figs. 4.32, 4.33, 4.35, 4.38).

5.4 Percentage of Eyes with Macular Hemorrhage

5.4.1 Percentage of Eyes with Neovascular Macular Hemorrhage (Choroidal Vascular Membrane) by Visual Acuity

The percentage of choroidal vascular membrane by visual acuity is shown in Fig. 5.6. The percentage of choroidal vascular membrane is less than 5% in eyes with visual acuity above 0.6. This percentage, however, increased gradually with worsening of visual acuity and reached a maximum of 58% in eyes with visual acuity between 0.01 and 0.05. Among the 128 eyes with choroidal vascular membrane, 50% had visual acuity less than 0.1, and about 75% had visual acuity less than 0.3. The frequency distribution of choroidal vascular membrane by visual acuity is similar to that by axial length (Fig. 4.39), but differs from the linear distribution of choroidal vascular membrane by age (See Fig. 4.8). The percentage of choroidal vascular membrane is low in eyes with visual acuity less than 0.01.

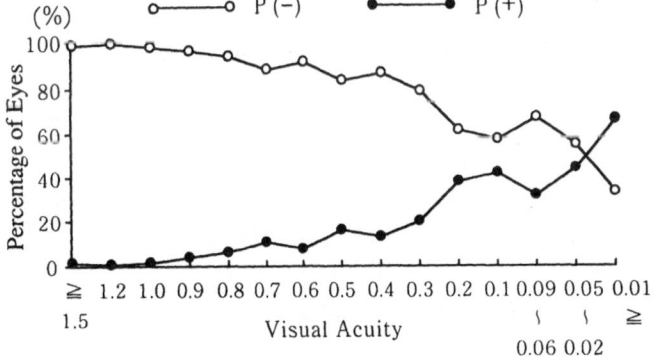

Fig. 5.5. Percentage of eyes with patchy atrophy (*P*) by visual acuity

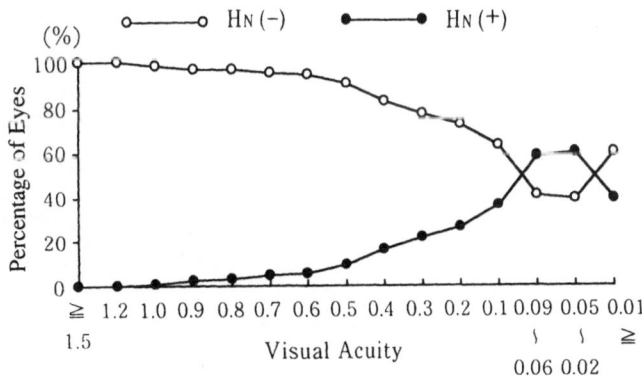

Fig. 5.6. Percentage of eyes with neovascular macular hemorrhage (choroidal neovascular membrane) by visual acuity

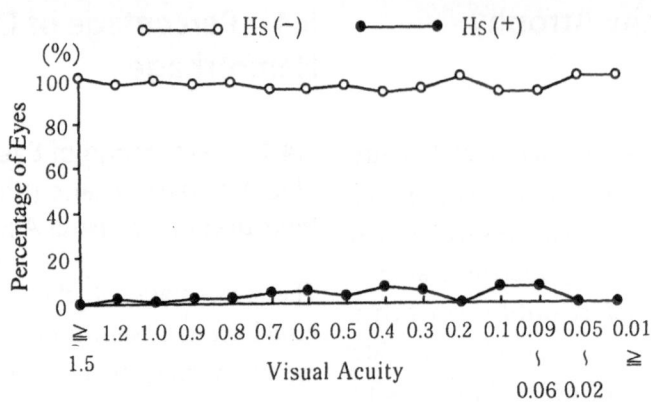

Fig. 5.7. Percentage of eyes with simple macular hemorrhage (*Hs*) by visual acuity

5.4.2 Percentage of Simple Macular Hemorrhage in Each Vision Group

The percentage of simple macular hemorrhage by visual acuity is shown in Fig. 5.7. The percentage is as low as about 5% in eyes regardless of visual acuity. This distribution of simple macular hemorrhage is similar to that of Lc (see Fig. 5.4), and suggests that, like Lc, simple macular hemorrhage does not influence visual acuity very much.

5.5 Visual Acuity and Area of Peripapillary Atrophy

Although visual acuity (log MAR) has a tendency to decrease with the enlargement of an area of peripapillary atrophy, the correlation is low (correlation coefficient, .422).

6 Progression of Chorioretinal Atrophy in Cases of Long-Term Observation

The progression of chorioretinal atrophy was investigated in 389 eyes of 221 patients who have been observed for more than 3 years (cases of monocular high myopia are also included, unlike those discussed in Chapters 3–5). The distribution of age, refraction, and axial length at the initial examination has been determined (Fig. 6.1).

6.1 Diffuse Chorioretinal Atrophy

The progression of diffuse chorioretinal atrophy in 81 eyes (17.7%) was observed. We found $T \to D_1$ (Lc) in 14 eyes, $D_1 \to D_2$ in 10 eyes, and an enlargement of D_2 in 57 eyes. Among the eyes with D_1, lacquer crack (Lc) is a special lesion that can progress to other kinds of lesions. Among 51 patients with Lc, 64 eyes have been followed up for a long time. Some changes were observed in 36 eyes (56.2%); these included an increase to Lc in 23.4%, $Lc \to P$ in 20.3%, $Lc \to D_2$ in 14.1%, and $Lc \to HN$ in 3.1%. Also, simple macular hemorrhage that does not accompany neovascular membrane is often observed with the progression of chorioretinal atrophy. Among 23 eyes of 21 patients that formed Lc during the period of observation, 11 eyes (47.8%) of 10 patients originally had simple macular hemorrhage. Lc formed in half the eyes in which simple macular hemorrhage occurred. It is not clear, however, whether Lc or simple macular hemorrhage is the original lesion.

6.2 Patchy Atrophy

The progression of patchy atrophy was observed in 79 eyes (17.2%), including D_1 (Lc) $\to P$ in 9 eyes, $P_1 \to P_2$ in 10 eyes, and enlargement of P_2 in 60 eyes.

6.3 Choroidal Neovascular Membrane

We observed 24 eyes of 21 patients for more than 5 years. In 18 (75%) of these eyes, atrophic lesions expanded beyond the choroidal neovascular membrane and developed into macular atrophy after an average of 7.5 years. The visual acuity in 22 (91.7%) of the 24 eyes decreased below 0.1 during the period of observation, suggesting a poor prognosis.

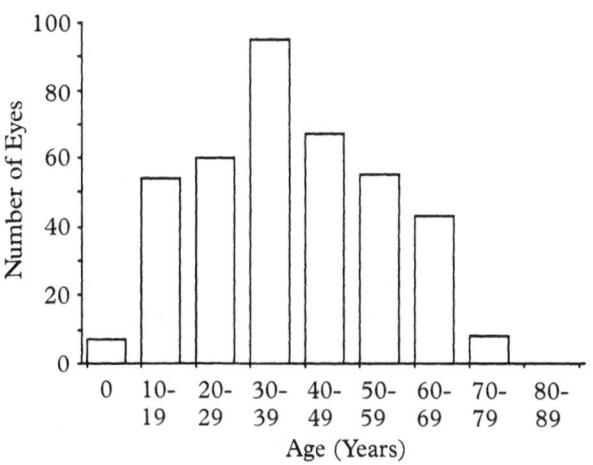

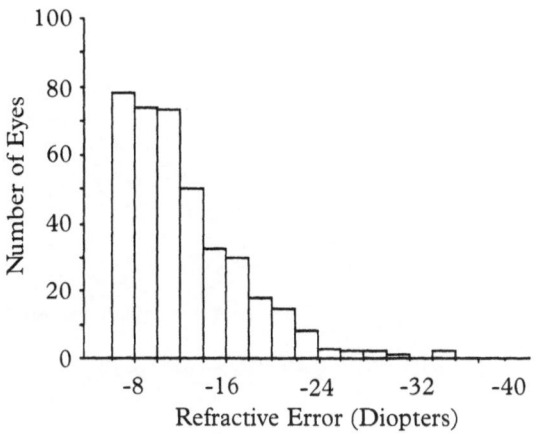

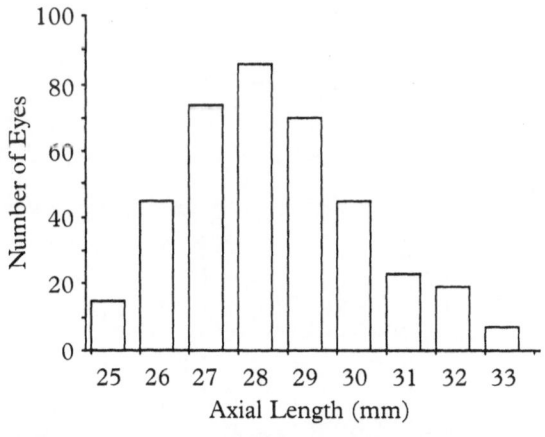

Fig. 6.1. Distribution of age (*top*), refraction (*middle*), and axial length (*bottom*) in high myopic eyes after observation for more than 3 years. Ages are divided into 10-year groups; refractions are divided into 2-D groups; axial lengths are divided into 1-mm groups

7 Progression of Fundus Changes in the Posterior Pole

Lesions that cause visual loss are choroidal neovascular membrane, patchy atrophy, and diffuse chorioretinal atrophy. These lesions are also among those seen as chorioretinal atrophy in the posterior pole. The main cause of visual loss is axial elongation. Also, aging has an influence on fundus changes in the posterior pole.

Aging plays an important part in the development of posterior staphyloma in axial elongation of high myopia. Posterior staphyloma is clearly caused by thinning of the sclera, but also it accompanies other choroidal changes, disappearance of retinal pigment epithelial (RPE) cells, and decrease in visual cells, among others [11,44–52]. Therefore, chorioretinal atrophy in the posterior pole must be severe in eyes with posterior staphyloma.

It takes a long time for chorioretinal atrophy to progress in high myopia. We have determined the mode of progression by observing the same case over a long period of time. The primary forms of the progression are as follows:

1. Tessellated fundus (T) → spotty or linear lesion of diffuse atrophy (D_1) [including lacquer crack lesion (Lc)] → enlarged lesion of diffuse atrophy (D_2) → chorioretinal atrophy of the macula (MA)

2. Tessellated fundus (T) → spotty lesion of patchy atrophy (P_1) → patchy lesion of patchy atrophy (P_2) → chorioretinal atrophy of the macula (MA)

3. Tessellated fundus (T) → active stage of neovascular macular hemorrhage (HN_1) → scar stage of neovascular macular hemorrhage (HN_2) → atrophic stage of neovascular macular hemorrhage (MA)

4. Tessellated fundus (T) → active stage of simple macular hemorrhage (HS_1) → scar stage of simple macular hemorrhage (HS_2) [10]

Some other forms of progression exist, such as from simple macular hemorrhage (HS_1) to spotty or linear lesion of diffuse atrophy (D_1), especially to Lc, and from spotty or linear lesion of diffuse atrophy (D_1 or Lc) to active stage of simple macular hemorrhage (HS_1) or spotty lesion of patchy atrophy (P_1). The model of chorioretinal atrophy progression is shown in Fig. 7.1 [40]. Among these lesions, macular hemorrhage, that is, neovascular macular hemorrhage or choroidal neovascular membrane, can greatly influence the prog-

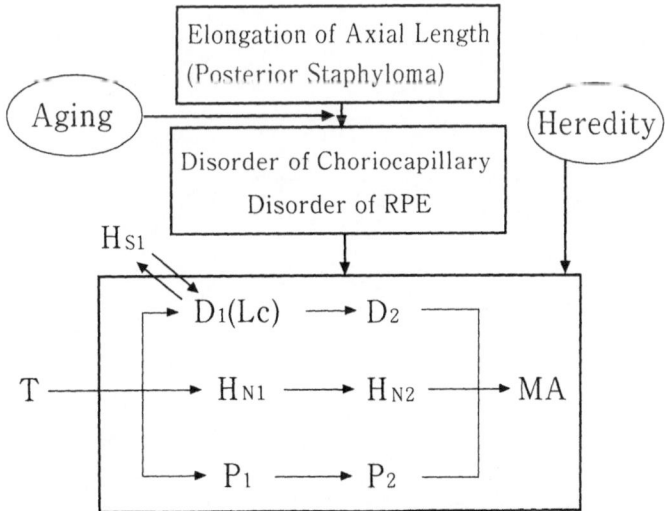

Fig. 7.1. Model illustrating the progression of chorioretinal atrophy in high myopic eyes. *T*, tessellated fundus; *D$_1$*, spotty or linear lesion of diffuse chorioretinal atrophy; *Lc*, lacquer crack lesion; *D$_2$*, enlarged lesion of diffuse chorioretinal atrophy; *MA*, chorioretinal atrophy of the macula; *HS$_1$*, simple macular hemorrhage; *HN$_1$*, active stage of neovascular macular hemorrhage; *HN$_2$*, scar stage of neovascular macular hemorrhage; *P$_1$*, spotty lesion of patchy atrophy; *P$_2$*, patchy lesion of patchy atrophy; *RPE*, retinal pigment epithelial cell

nosis for visual acuity. Therefore, it is important to determine the best course of treatment to prevent the occurrence or spreading of choroidal neovascular membrane.

During the progression of chorioretinal atrophy, whether the primary damage originates from the RPE or choriocapillaris is an interesting question [40]. According to electrophysiological examination (electrooculogram, EOG), the reduction of the EOG ratio and the prolongation of the peak time in EOG can be observed when refraction is high or axial length is long, suggesting the functional impairment of RPE [53–57]. An experiment with pigmented rabbit, injected intravenously with sodium iodate or injected with ornithine into the vitreous cavity, showed that damage to the choriocapillaris was secondary to that of the RPE [58–60]. From fluorescein angiographic (FAG) and indocyanine green angiographic (IA) findings, however, it is believed that RPE and choriocapillaris both can undergo primary damage [61,62]. For example, if primary damage originates in the RPE, it is still unknown whether this damage is caused by mechanical action by axial elongation or choroidal circulatory failure.

Also, it is possible that the hyperpermeability of the inner side of the blood–retinal barrier in high myopia is

one of the factors that induce this damage [63,64]. In any event, it is believed that the interaction of mechanical extension, circulatory failure, and aging can influence the occurrence and progression of chorioretinal atrophy.

7.1 Classification of Stage of Fundus Change in the Posterior Pole

Stage 1: Tessellated fundus (T)
Stage 2: Spotty or linear lesion of diffuse atrophy (D_1)
Spotty lesion of patchy atrophy (P_1)
Simple macular hemorrhage (HS_1, HS_2)
Stage 3: Enlarged lesion of diffuse atrophy (D_2)
Paramacular patchy lesion of patchy atrophy (P_2)
Neovascular macular hemorrhage (HN_1, HN_2)
Stage 4: Chorioretinal atrophy of the macula (MA)

Note:
Even if only one lesion exists in a certain stage, this fundus change is classified in this stage. If there are multiple lesions that belong to different stages, the fundus changes are classified in the most severe stage. For example, the change should be classified as stage 3 if P_1 and D_2 coexist.

Appendix: Relationship Between Fundus Changes in the Posterior Pole and Visual Acuity

A.1 Factors That Can Explain the Present Visual Acuity

From the multiple regression analysis to the factors that can influence the present visual acuity, a model equation is determined as $\log V = 1.528 - 0.002Y - 0.115D - 0.161P - 0.314F - 0.028A$. Here, V is age (years), A is axial length (mm), D_1 is diffuse chorioretinal atrophy (none = 1, T = 2, D_1 = 3, D_2 = 4, MA = 5), and F is choroidal neovascular membrane (Fuchs' spot) (none = 1, HN_1 = 2, HN_2 = 3, MA = 4).

When the factors with large contribution rates to visual acuity undergo multivariant analysis by quantification I, the reasons for visual loss are choroidal neovascular membrane (partial correlation coefficient, 0.463), diffuse chorioretinal atrophy (0.298), patchy atrophy (0.191), axial length (0.178), and age (0.107), in descending order. These factors strongly influence chorioretinal atrophy in the posterior pole [65].

Using the same equation, the presumed visual acuity can be obtained from explanatory variables. The visual acuity presumed and the visual acuity measured are compared in Fig. A.1. The tendency is for the presumed visual acuity to be better than the visual acuity measured in eyes with low visual acuity, but the coefficient of determination is 0.608 with the multiple correlation coefficient of 0.780. About 60% of fluctuation in visual acuity can be explained with this equation.

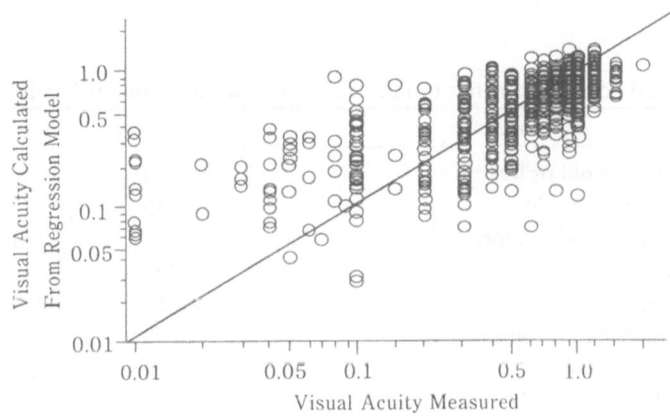

Fig. A.1. Relationship between visual acuity calculated from the model equation and measured visual acuity. *Vertical axis*, visual acuity in a logarithm presumed from multiple regression equations; *horizontal axis*, measured visual acuity in a logarithm

A.2 Prognosis of Visual Acuity According to Multivariant Analysis by Quantification II

We observed 162 patients with high myopia for longer than 3 years (excluding monocular cases). All received periodic examinations, and their refraction and visual function were recorded. There were 265 eyes, 115 eyes in 68 men and 150 eyes in 94 women. The contributing factors of future visual loss were age, sex, axial length, corneal curvature, visual field, diffuse chorioretinal atrophy, chorioretinal patchy atrophy, and choroidal neovascular membrane (Fuchs' spot). Each factor was investigated with multivariant analysis by quantification II; logistic regression analysis was then used for those variants of the eye that cause visual loss. Finally, the value of the corresponding partial correlation coefficient was obtained.

The category score for each contributing factor was done for the following factors; age (23 years and under, 24–55 years, 56 years and over), gender (male, female), axial length (26.9 mm and less, 27.0–29.9 mm, 30 mm and more), corneal curvature (7.39 mm and less, 7.40–7.89 mm, 7.90 mm and more), visual field (normal, enlargement of blind spot of Mariotte, paracentral scotoma, central scotoma), diffuse chorioretinal atrophy (tessellated fundus, D_1, D_2, MA), patchy atrophy (no patchy atrophy, P_1, P_2), and choroidal neovascular membrane (present, absent).

The value and range of the category score for each contributing factor and the partial correlation coefficient are shown in Table A.1. From these partial correlation coefficient of contributing factors (Table A.1), it is known that Fuchs' spot has excellent correlation with visual acuity, followed by diffuse chorioretinal atrophy, patchy atrophy, axial length, and age. The difference in gender has the least influence on visual loss. Visual loss, however, is easily induced when each category score is high.

From these category scores calculated at the beginning of the observation, the score distribution can be obtained (Fig. A.2). Of 265 eyes, 81 had a score higher than 0.3,

Table A.1. Presumption of visual acuity according to multivariant analysis by quantification II

Item	Category	Category score	Range	Partial correlation coefficient
Age	23 years old or less	−0.2970		
	24–25 years old	0.0045		
	26 years old or more	0.5296	0.8266	.1480
Gender	Male	0.1123		
	Female	−0.1414	0.2537	.0813
Axial length	Less than 27.0 mm	−0.3508		
	27.0–29.9 mm	0.2137		
	30.0 mm or more	−0.3470	0.5646	.1712
Radius of corneal curvature	Less than 7.40 mm	0.2176		
	7.40–7.89 mm	0.0968		
	7.90 mm or more	−0.3246	0.5422	.1339
Visual field	Normal	−0.0908		
	Enlargement of Mariotte's blind spot	0.3640		
	Paracentral scotoma	0.5096		
	Central scotoma	1.2453	1.3361	.1428
Diffuse atrophy	(−)	−0.2821		
	D_1	−0.0121		
	D_2	0.5558		
	MA	0.2612	0.8379	.1764
Patchy atrophy	(−)	0.0395		
	P_1	0.5085		
	P_2	−1.0321	1.5406	.1773
Fuchs' spot	(−)	−0.1493		
	(+)	1.7775	1.9268	.2792

(−), absent; (+), present.

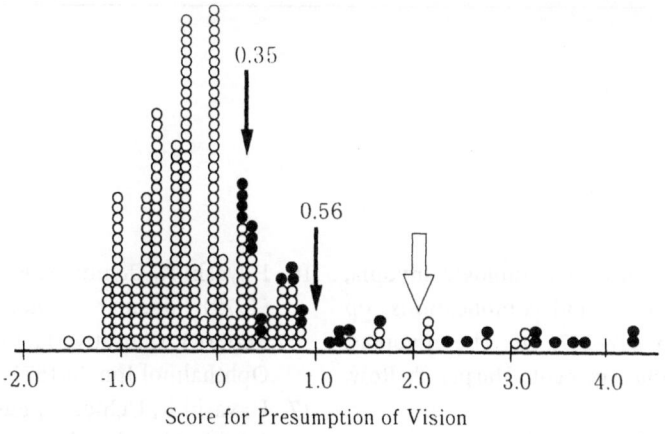

Fig. A.2. Relationship between visual loss after 3 years and score for presumption of vision (multivariant analysis by quantification II) at the initial observation of high myopic eyes. Score for presumption of vision was calculated from the category score with multivariant analysis by quantification II. *Circles* represent eyes that have been observed for more than 3 years: *white circles*, those without visual loss; *black circles*, those with visual loss. The *black arrows* show the positions with the score for presumption of vision of 0.3 and 1.0, and the *numerals* show the percentage of eyes with visual loss. The *white arrow* shows the position with the score value of 1.9986 for presumption of visual acuity, which is calculated in the text

which has a possibility of visual loss during the observation of more than 3 years. We found that visual loss occurred in 29 (35%) of 81 eyes during our period of observation. Also, among the 27 eyes that had a score higher than 1.0, 15 eyes (56%) developed visual loss. It is possible that the score for presumption of visual acuity can be used to forecast future visual loss.

An example is given to show how to calculate the score for presumption of visual acuity (Table A.1). This case shows a woman (-0.1414) who is 73 years old ($+0.5296$). Her axial length is 30.3 mm (-0.3470), corneal curvature is 8.01 mm (-0.3246), and visual field is normal (-0.0908). The fundus finding is diffuse chorioretinal atrophy D_2 ($+0.5558$), with no patchy atrophy ($+0.0395$). There is a Fuchs' spot ($+1.7775$). The summation of all categorized quantitative data within the parentheses is $-0.1414 + 0.5296 - 0.3470 - 0.3246 - 0.0908 + 0.5558 + 0.0395 + 1.7775 = 1.9986$

The corresponding score for presumption of visual loss is shown in Fig. A.2. According to the score for presumption of visual loss derived at the beginning of the period of observation, it is expected that after 3 years visual loss will occur in 59% (10 of 17 eyes).

References

1. Curtin BJ (1985) (a) The nature of pathologic myopia, pp 237–245. (b) Ocular findings and complications, pp 277–332. (c) Pathology, pp 247–267. In: The myopias. Basic science and clinical management. Harper & Row, Philadelphia

2. Duke-Elder S (1970) Pathological refractive errors. System of ophthalmology, vol V. Ophthalmic optics and refraction. In: Mosby, St. Louis, pp 297–373

3. Tokoro T, Hayashi K, Sato K, Uchida A, Sato Y (1977) Studies on anomalies of visual function of high myopia. J Jpn Ophthalmol Soc 81:330–339

4. Tokoro T, Hayashi K, Uchida A, Sato K, Ito Y (1978) Standardization for diagnosis of pathological myopia by axial length. Report of research committee on chorioretinal degenerations, The Ministry of Health and Welfare of Japan, Tokyo, pp 7–12

5. Tokoro T (1988), On the definition of pathologic myopia in group studies. Acta Ophthalmol 66 (suppl 185):107–108

6. Tokoro T, Hayashi K, Sato Y (1979) Visual disturbance of pathological myopia. Report of research committee on chorioretinal degenerations, The Ministry of Health and Welfare of Japan, Tokyo, pp 14–18

7. Maruo T, Ogura Y, Kubota N (1984) Frequency of pathological myopia in elementary, junior and senior high school. Report of research committee on chorioretinal degenerations, The Ministry of Health and Welfare of Japan, Tokyo, pp 22–25

8. Sato A, Hayashi K, Uchida A, Tokoro T (1982) Nationwide survey of pathologic myopia. Report of research committee on chorioretinal degenerations, The Ministry of Health and Welfare of Japan, pp 32–35

9. Maruo T (1982) Pathological myopia. Jpn Rev Clin Ophthalmol 76:1–13

10. Tokoro T, Maruo T, Kanai A, Hayashi K (1987) Manual for diagnosis of pathological myopia. Report of research committee on chorioretinal degenerations, The Ministry of Health and Welfare of Japan, Tokyo, pp 1–14

11. Black RK, Jay B (1965) The glaucomatous disc in degenerative myopia. Trans Ophthalmol Soc UK 85:161–168

12. Hayashi K (1978) Macular lesions in pathological myopia. Jpn J Clin Ophthalmol 32:271–284

13. Klein RM, Curtin BJ (1975) Lacquer crack lesion in pathologic myopia. Am J Ophthalmol 79:386–392

14. Ohno-Matsui K, Tokoro T (1966) The progression of lacquer cracks in pathologic myopia. Retina 16:29–37

15. Ohno-Matsui K, Morishima N, Ito M, Tokoro T (1995) Indocyanine green angiographic features of lacquer crack lesion in high myopia. Jpn J Clin Ophthalmol 49:593–597

16. Hayashi K, Uchida A, Fukushita K, Takizawa E, Tokoro T (1979) Macular hemorrhage in pathological myopia. Report I: Causative factors of macular hemorrhage. Folia Ophthalmol Jpn 30:1571–1576

17. Hayashi K, Uchida A, Fukushita K, Takizawa E, Tokoro T (1980) Macular hemorrhage in pathological myopia. Report II: The clinical features of macular hemorrhage without neovascular tissue. Folia Ophthalmol Jpn 31:459–467

18. Fuchs E (1901) Der centrale Fleck bei Myopie. Z Augenheilk 5:171–178

19. Ohtake Y, Ito M, Tokoro T, Iwabuchi M, Toki T (1993) Prognostic factors of choroidal neovascularization in degenerative myopia. Jpn J Clin Ophthalmol 47:345–348

20. Ohno-Matsui K, Ito M, Tokoro T (1996) Subretinal bleeding without choroidal neovascularization in pathologic myopia—a sign of new lacquer crack formation. Retina 16:196–202

21. Karlin DB, Curtin BJ (1976) Peripheral chorioretinal lesions and axial length of the myopic eye. Am J Ophthalmol 81:625–635

22. Curtin BJ (1982) Posterior staphyloma development in pathologic myopia. Ann Ophthalmol 14:655–658

23. Hayashi K, Tokoro T, Muto M, Sato K, Takizawa E (1976) Relationship between axial length and posterior fundus changes of high myopia. Folia Ophthalmol Jpn 27:962–967

24. Avila MP, Weiter JJ, Jalkh AE, Trempe CL, Pruett RC, Schepens CL (1984) Natural history of choroidal neovascularization in degenerative myopia. Ophthalmology 91:1573–1581

25. Morita H, Funata M, Tokoro T (1995) A clinical study of the development of posterior vitreous detachment in high myopia. Retina 15:117–124

26. Nakase Y, Hayashi K, Tokoro T (1982) Follow-up studies on high myopia. Report of research committee on chorioretinal degenerations, The Ministry of Health and Welfare of Japan, Tokyo, pp 19–21

27. Ito M, Sato A, Tokoro T (1987) Long term follow-up study of chorioretinal atrophy and axial length in high myopia. Report of research committee on chorioretinal degenerations, The Ministry of Health and Welfare of Japan, Tokyo, pp 41–43

28. Curtin BJ, Karlin DB (1971) Axial length measurements and fundus changes of the myopic eye. Am J Ophthalmol 71:42–53

29. Tokoro T, Hayashi K (1985) Chorioretinal atrophy accompanied with high myopia. Ganka Mook 26:174–183

30. Tokoro T, Yoshino Y (1984) Clinical classification of myopic chorioretinal atrophy. Report of research commit-

tee on chorioretinal degenerations, The Ministry of Health and Welfare of Japan, Tokyo, pp 31–33

31. Tokoro T, Hayashi K, Yoshino Y, Sato A (1985) Classification of myopic chorioretinal atrophy. Report of research committee on chorioretinal degenerations, The Ministry of Health and Welfare of Japan, Tokyo, pp 23–26

32. Klein RM, Green S (1988) The development of lacquer cracks in pathologic myopia. Am J Ophthalmol 106:282–285

33. Shapiro M, Chandra SR (1985) Evolution of lacquer cracks in high myopia. Ann Ophthalmol 17:231–235

34. Watanabe C, Yamaji S, Yoshihara M (1976) Fluorographic findings in high myopia. Folia Ophthal Jpn 27:645–650

35. Levy JH, Pollock HM, Curtin BJ (1977) The Fuchs' spot: an ophthalmic and fluorescein angiographic study. Ann Ophthalmol 9:1433–1443

36. Brancato R, Pece A, Avanza P, Radrizzani E (1990) Photocoagulation scar expansion after laser therapy for choroidal neovascularization in degenerative myopia. Retina 10:239–243

37. Tokoro T, Muto M, Hayashi K (1975) Refractive components in high myopia. Folia Ophthalmol Jpn 26:554–559

38. Tokoro T, Uesugi E (1976) Relationship between refraction and axial length. Jpn Rev Clin Ophthalmol 70:739–742

39. Tokoro T, Uesugi E (1976) Relationship between refraction (3D) and axial length (1 mm). Jpn Rev Clin Ophthalmol 70:739–742

40. Tokoro T (1994) Mechanism of axial elongation and chorioretinal atrophy in high myopia. Jpn J Ophthalmol Soc 98:1213–1237

41. Curtin BJ, Teng CC (1957) Scleral changes in pathological myopia. Trans Am Acad Ophthalmol Oto-Laryngol 62:777–788

42. Steidl SM, Pruett RC (1977) Macular complications associated with posterior staphyloma. Am J Ophthalmol 123:181–187

43. Tokoro T (1977) Etiology of myopia and its treatment. Asian Med J 40:416–422

44. Curtin BJ (1977) The posterior staphyloma of pathologic myopia. Trans Am Ophthalmol Soc 75:67–86

45. Curtin BJ (1979) Normal and staphylomatous sclera of high myopia. An electron microscopic study. Arch Ophthalmol 97:912–915

46. Apple DJ, Rabb MF (1985) Clinical applications and self-assessment. In: Ocular pathology. Mosby, St. Louis, pp 38–44

47. Spencer WHÅ (1985) Ophthalmic pathology, 3rd edn, vol 2. Saunders, Philadelphia, pp 912–924

48. Grossniklaus HE, Green WR (1992) Pathologic findings in pathologic myopia, Retina 12:127–133

49. Chonan T (1959) A histopathologic study of myopic eye. J Jpn Ophthalmol Soc 63:2144–2163

50. Ohno H (1983) Electron microscopic studies of myopic retinochoroidal atrophies. I. Choroidal changes. Folia Ophthalmol Jpn 34:1244–1253

51. Ohno H (1984) Election microscopic studies of myopic retinochoroidal atrophies. II. Retinal pigment epithelial changes. Folia Ophthalmol Jpn 35:1152–1160

52. Okisaka S (1981) Pathohistological studies on myopic chorioretinal atrophy. Ophthalmology (Ganka) 23:143–155

53. Uchida A (1977) Studies on electrical activities of the eye in high myopia. J Jpn Ophthalmol Soc 81:1328–1350

54. Blach RK, Jay B, Kolb H (1966) Electrical activity of the eye in high myopia. Br J Ophthalmol 50:629–641

55. Mikawa T (1974) EOG ratio in myopia. J Jpn Ophthalmol Soc 78:265–276

56. Arden GB, Barrada A, Kelsey JH (1962) New clinical test of retinal function based upon the standing potential of the eye, Br J Ophthalmol 46:449–467

57. Uchida A, Tokoro T, Hayashi K, Fukushita K (1979) EOG in high myopia under osmotic stress. Folia Ophthalmol Jpn 30:1794–1798

58. Henkind P, Gartner S (1983) The elationship between retinal pigment epithelium and choriocapillaris. Trans Ophthalmol Soc UK 103:444–447

59. Korte GE, Reppucci U, Henkind P (1984) RPE destruction causes choriocapillary atrophy. Invest Ophthalmol Visual Sci 25:1135–1145

60. Mori S (1993) Effect of retinal pigment epithelial damage on choroidal circulation I. Change in choroidal blood flow for 4 weeks after ornithine administration to rabbits. Folia Ophthalmol Jpn 44:1130–1139

61. Behrendt T, Duane TD (1966) Investigation of fundus oculi with spectral reflectance photography. I. Depth and integrity of fundal structures. Arch Ophthalmol 75:375–379

62. Hayashi K (1985) Infared fundus photography. Ophthalmology (Ganka) 27:1541–1550

63. Yoshida A: Blood-ocular barrier permeability in myopia. Folia Ophthalmol Jpn 40:109–117

64. Ishiko S, Yoshida A, Hosaka A (1991) Changes in ocular structures and in blood-ocular barrier permeability of experimental myopia induced in monkeys. J Jpn Ophthalmol Soc 95:522–529

65. Krumpaszky HG, Klauß V (1996) High-grade myopia as a cause of blindness. Epidemiology of blindness and eye disease. Ophthalmologica 210:45–50

Cases of Chorioretinal Atrophy

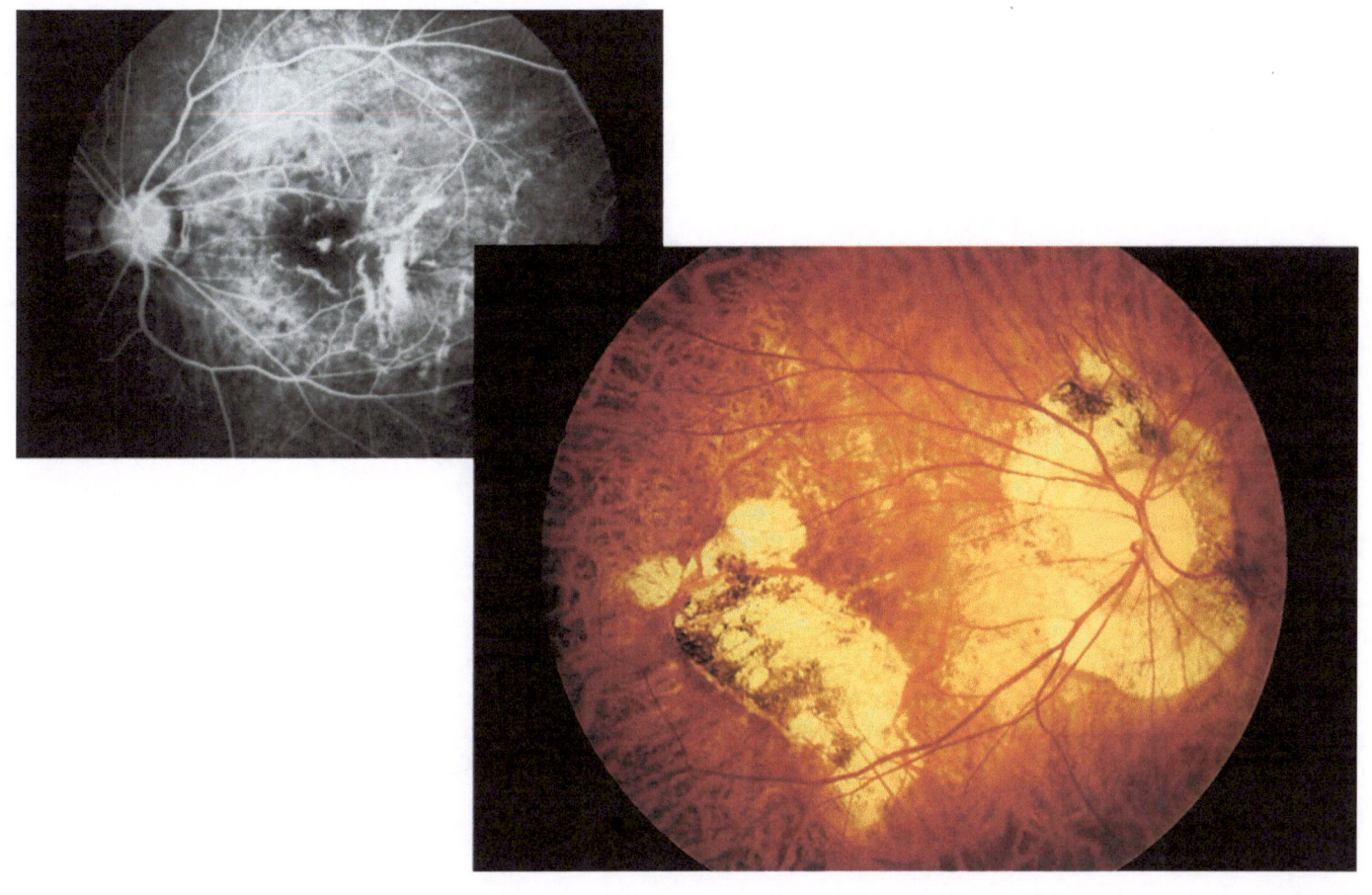

Diffuse Chorioretinal Atrophy

Spotty and linear lesions of diffuse atrophy appear in the early developmental stage of highly myopic eyes. They appear first around the optic disc or in the region between the macula and the optic disc. With time, they coalesce and progress into an enlarged lesion of diffuse atrophy. Their progression is very slow. It may be difficult to detect the progression without periodic observation and a continuous series of fundus photographs. Although diffuse atrophy tends to progress in elderly patients who have longer axial lengths, diffuse atrophy sometimes appears and progresses in extremely myopic eyes of young patients as well.

Diffuse atrophy tends to progress with the development of the posterior staphyloma. The progression of diffuse atrophy may be the result of continuous mechanical expansion within the posterior staphyloma found in highly myopic eyes.

It is well known that progressive diffuse chorioretinal atrophy usually does little to impair vision and has a relatively good visual prognosis among the various forms of myopic chorioretinal degeneration. However, the lesions are significant as possible precursors of more advanced myopic chorioretinal atrophies. Highly myopic eyes with diffuse atrophy sometimes exhibit other types of myopic macular changes (including patchy atrophy or choroidal neovascularization). Regular follow-up examinations are recommended in highly myopic patients with rapidly progressing diffuse atrophy.

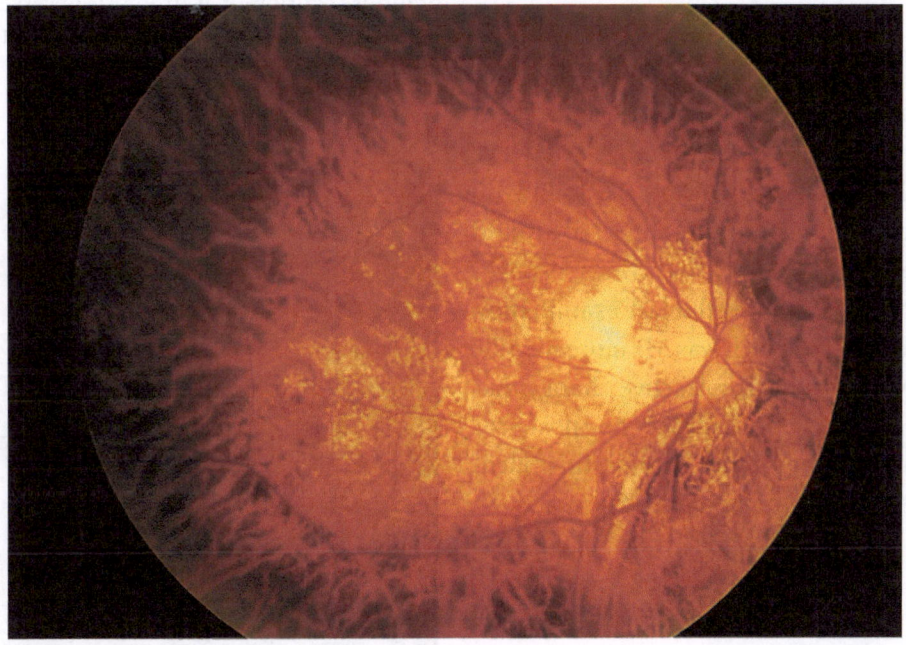

Fig. 13C. *(see page 95)*

Cases 1–15 ▶

Abbreviations *T*: Tessellated fundus; *D*: Diffuse chorioretinal atrophy; *Lc*: Lacquer crack lesion; *P*: Patchy atrophy; *NS*: Simple macular hemorrhage; *HN*: Neovascular macular hemorrhage; *MA*: Chorioretinal atrophy of the macula. For details, refer to Table 3.1 and Fig. 7.1.

Case 1

A 32-year-old woman presented on February 4, 1983, with a 2- to 3-month history of floaters in her left eye. She began wearing glasses for distance vision when she was 12 years old. Her prescription was changed several times because of progressive myopia. Her medical history was noncontributory. No family members had severe myopia.

In the initial examination, the patient's best corrected visual acuity was 0.7 in both eyes. The refractive error was −12.00 D sphere[1] in the right eye and −11.25 D sphere in the left. The axial length measurements were 28.6 mm in the right eye and 28.3 mm in the left. Intraocular pressures and anterior segments were normal in both eyes. We describe here the long-term fundus changes in her left eye.

Summary

This patient was followed up for 10 years, beginning at age 32 years. In the initial examination, her left eye showed only tessellated fundus. During the follow-up period, linear lesions of diffuse atrophy appeared around the optic disc in her left fundus.

The patient's refractive error at the last examination was −14.25 D in the left eye, which was 3 D more myopic than it was initially. Despite this refractive change, her visual acuity remained stable because no posterior staphyloma developed and no other chorioretinal atrophy appeared in her left eye to impair vision.

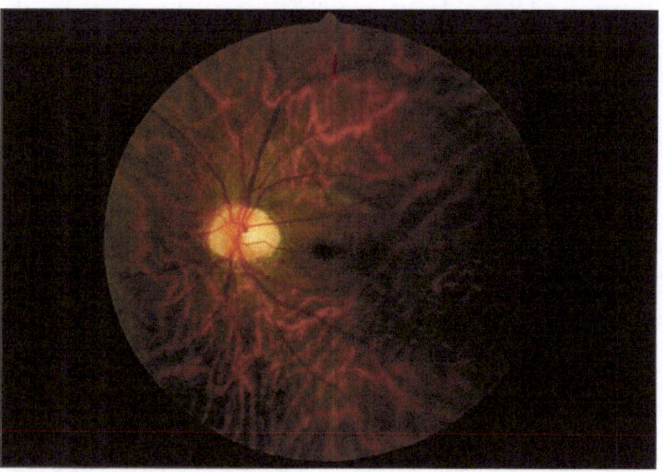

Fig. 1A. Left fundus at the initial examination (February 1983) shows tessellated fundus only. No posterior staphyloma or diffuse chorioretinal atrophy is observed. The optic disc tilts inferiorly. A crescent is seen inferior to the optic disc. Visual acuity is 0.7, and the refractive error is −11.25 D

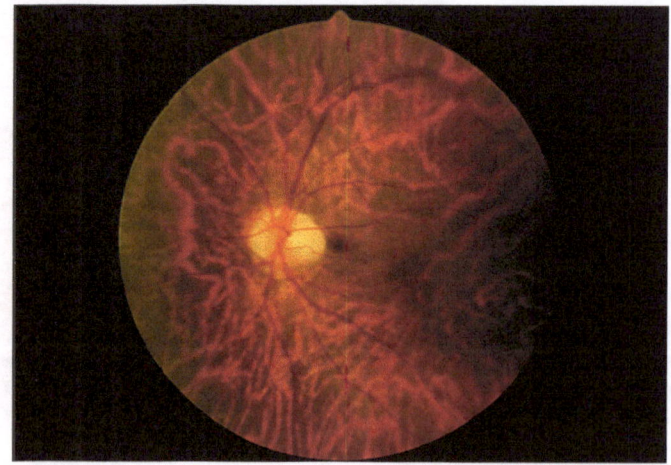

Fig. 1B. Three years later (January 1986), the left eye shows only tessellated fundus. No other chorioretinal atrophy is seen

---

[1] Refractive errors in all subjects are shown as the value in the spherical equivalent.

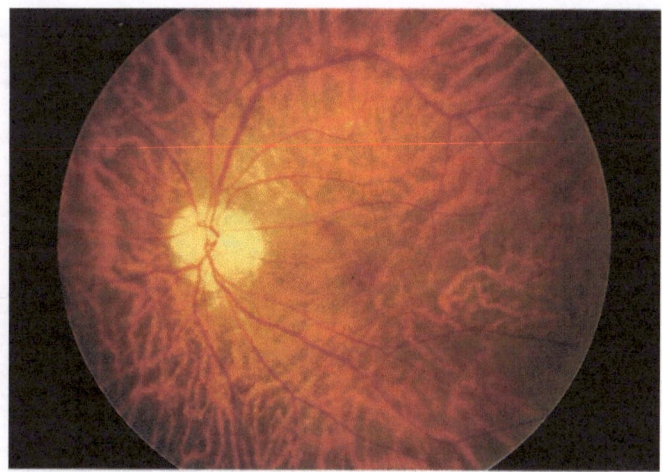

Fig. 1C. Eight years after the initial examination (January 1991), linear lesions of diffuse chorioretinal atrophy appear around the left optic disc

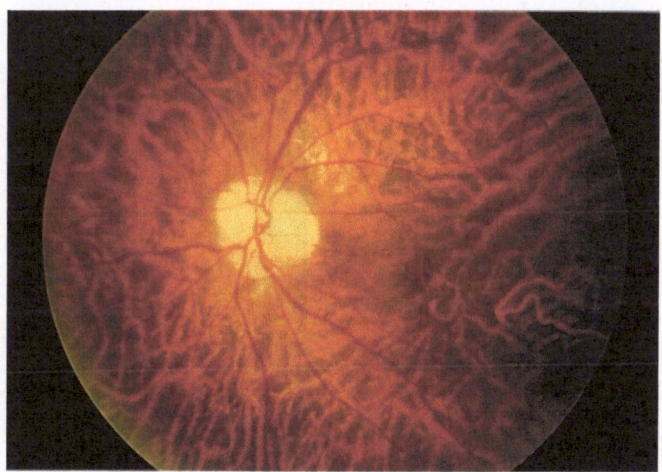

Fig. 1D. Ten years after the initial examination (March 1993), linear lesions of diffuse atrophy are clearly visible, especially superior to the optic disc. Visual acuity is 1.0, and the refractive error is −14.25 D

Case 2

A 57-year-old man was examined for high myopia on May 30, 1986. His myopia began when he was in elementary school. He started wearing glasses at age 12 years. His myopia progressed until age 40. His medical history was noncontributory. No family members had severe myopia.

In the initial examination, the patient's best corrected visual acuity was 0.7 in the right eye and 0.8 in the left. The refractive error was −20.50 D sphere in the right eye and −22.00 D sphere in the left, and the axial length measurements were 30.6 mm in the right eye and 30.7 mm in the left. Intraocular pressures and anterior segments were normal in both eyes. We describe the long-term fundus changes in his right eye.

Summary

This patient has been followed up for 10 years, since 1986. In the fundus photographs taken 1, 6, and 7 years after the initial examination, the linear lesions of diffuse atrophy temporal to the optic disc have gradually enlarged and coalesced. In the fundus photographs taken 7 years after the initial examination, new linear lesions of diffuse atrophy appeared temporal to the macula. As seen in this patient, the progression of diffuse atrophy is usually slow and takes about 10 years to detect.

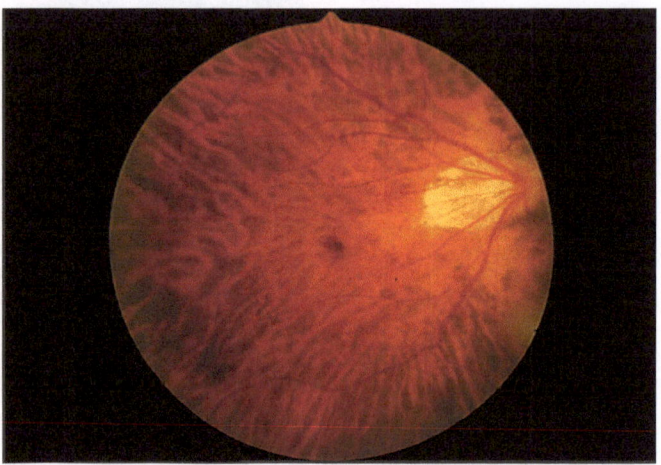

Fig. 2A. Right fundus at the initial examination (May 1986) shows spotty or linear lesions of diffuse atrophy temporal to the optic disc. The optic disc tilts temporally. A temporal peripapillary crescent is seen. A type I posterior staphyloma (according to Curtin's classification; see Fig. 2G) is present

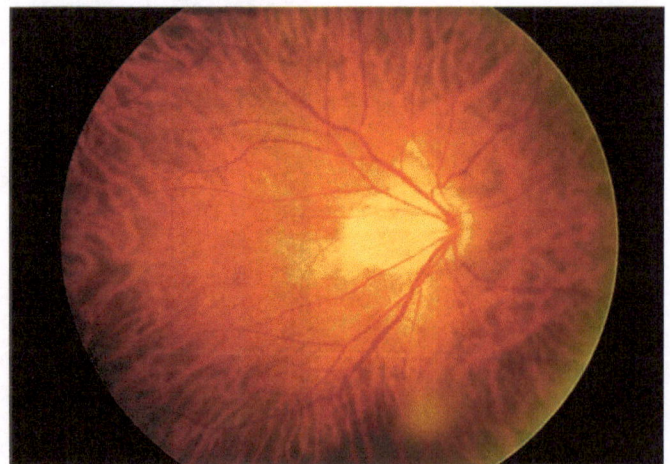

Fig. 2B. One year later (June 1987), spotty or linear lesions of diffuse atrophy have increased around the peripapillary crescent

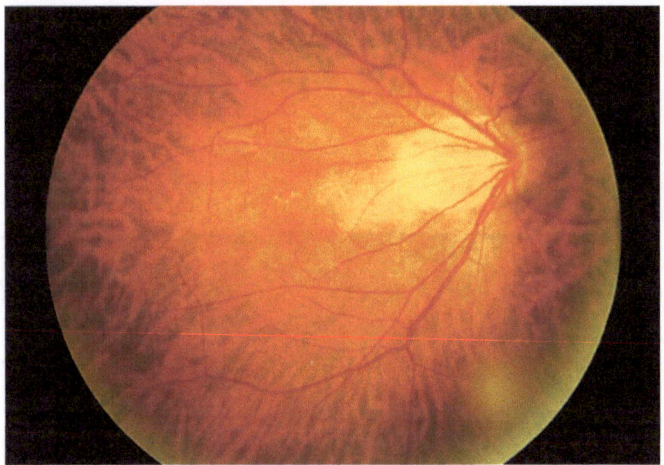

Fig. 2C. Six years after the initial examination (June 1992), spotty or linear lesions of diffuse atrophy have increased further. Visual acuity is 0.7, and the refractive error is −20.00 D

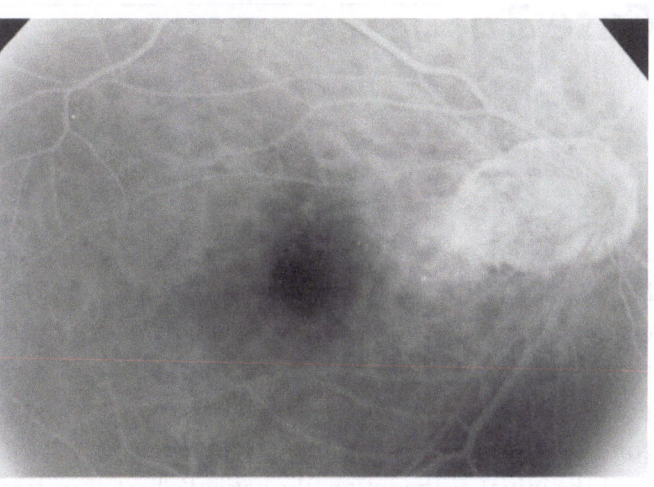

Fig. 2E. Fluorescein fundus angiogram 6 years after the initial examination (July 1992). At 6 min after dye injection, hyperfluorescence caused by diffuse atrophy temporal to the peripapillary crescent is seen

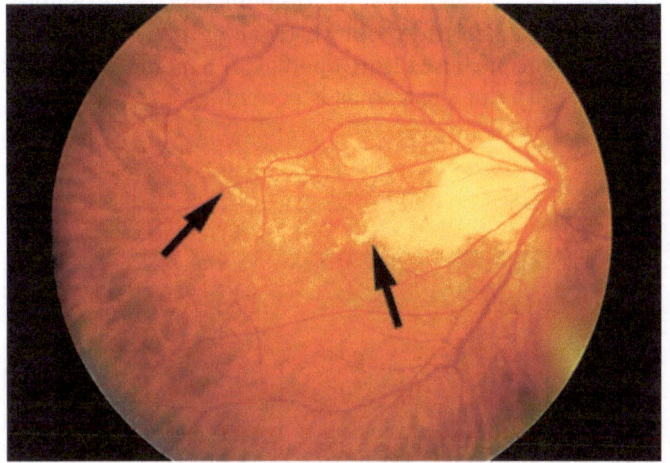

Fig. 2D. Seven years after the initial examination (August 1993), new linear lesions of diffuse atrophy (lacquer crack lesions) appear temporal to and in the macula (*arrows*). Spotty or linear lesions of diffuse atrophy around the peripapillary crescent have increased and have gradually coalesced. Visual acuity is 0.6, and the refractive error is −20.00 D

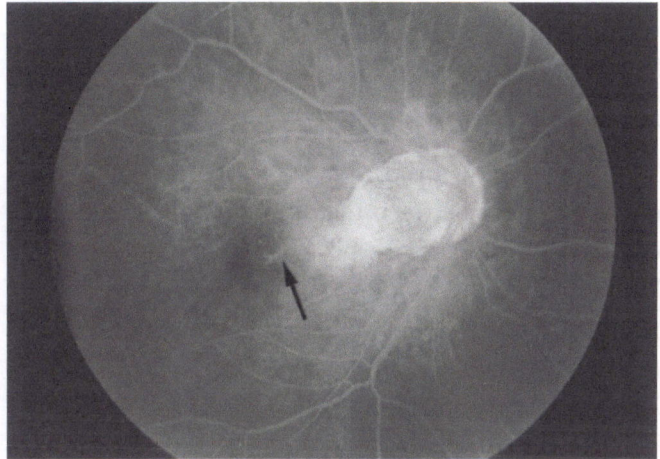

Fig. 2F. Fluorescein fundus angiogram 7 years after the initial examination (August 1993). At 6 min after dye injection, linear hyperfluorescence is visible corresponding to the lacquer crack lesion in the macula (*arrow*). Diffuse atrophy temporal to the optic disc is also hyperfluorescent

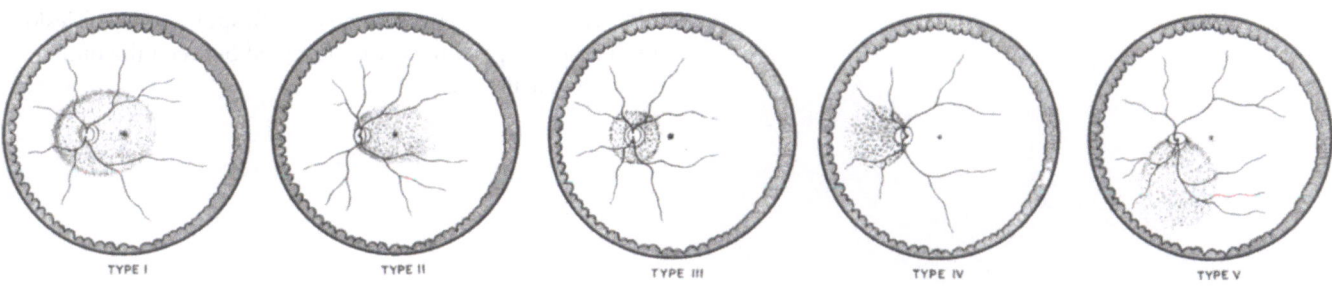

Fig. 2G. Shematic drawings of Curtin's classification of posterior staphyloma. (From [44], with permission)

Case 3

A 31-year-old man was examined for high myopia on May 22, 1987. He reported visual disturbances in distance vision at age 9 years. Since then, his glasses prescription has been changed several times because of progressive myopia. His medical history was noncontributory. No family members had severe myopia.

In the initial examination, the patient's best corrected visual acuity was 1.0 in both eyes. The refractive error was −12.00 D sphere in the right eye and −14.00 D sphere in the left eye, and the axial length measurements were 27.7 mm in the right eye and 28.2 mm in the left eye. Intraocular pressures and anterior segments were normal. We describe the long-term fundus changes in both his eyes.

Summary

This patient was followed up for 9 years, since 1987. During the follow-up period, spotty or linear lesions of diffuse atrophy between the optic disc and the macula enlarged and gradually progressed into an enlarged lesion of diffuse atrophy. The progressive pattern of myopic fundus changes in this patient was from D_1 to D_2 bilaterally. It is expected that the entire macula will be covered with typical D_2 lesions in several years. No other myopic fundus changes were noted in either eye. No decreased visual acuity was found during the follow-up period.

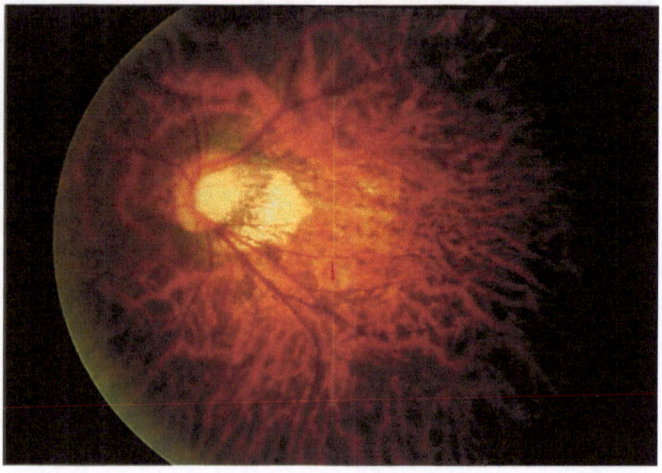

Fig. 3A. Left fundus at the initial examination shows spotty or linear lesions of diffuse atrophy between the optic disc and the macula. The optic disc tilts temporally. A temporal crescent is seen. No posterior staphyloma is present

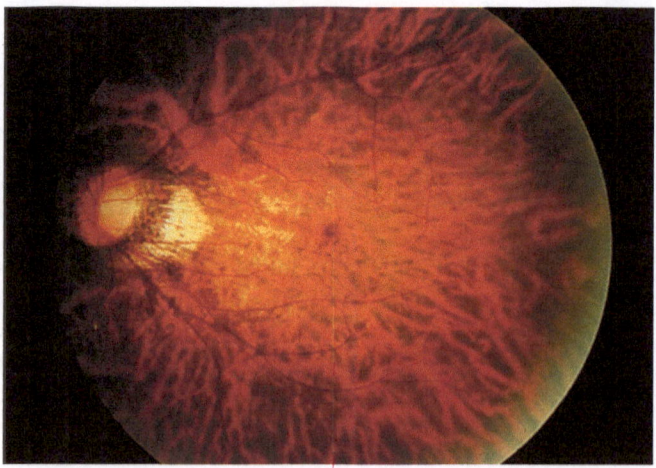

Fig. 3B. One year later (August 1988), spotty or linear lesions of diffuse atrophy are clearly observed between the optic disc and the macula

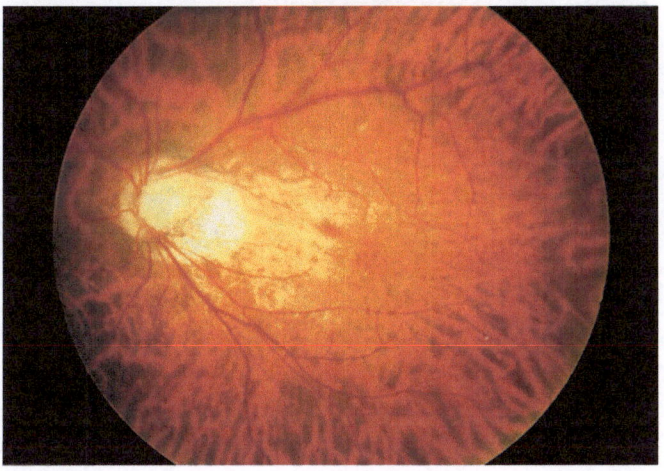

Fig. 3C. Three years after the initial examination (February 1990), spotty or linear lesions have enlarged

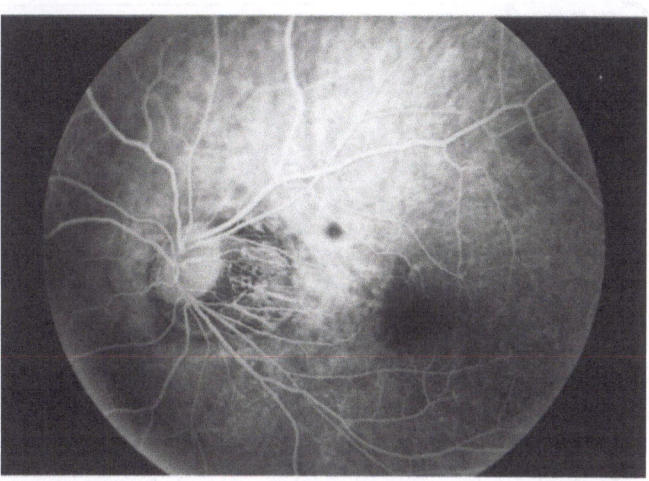

Fig. 3F. Fluorescein fundus angiogram 7 years after the initial examination (July 1994). At 1 min after dye injection, the surrounding tissue of choroidal vessels shows tissue staining

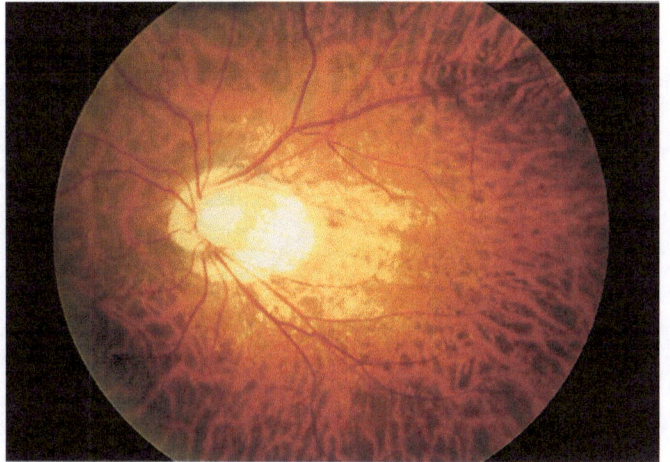

Fig. 3D. Seven years after the initial examination (July 1994), spotty or linear lesions have coalesced and progressed into an enlarged lesion of diffuse atrophy (D_2). Visual acuity is 1.2, and the refractive error is −13.25 D

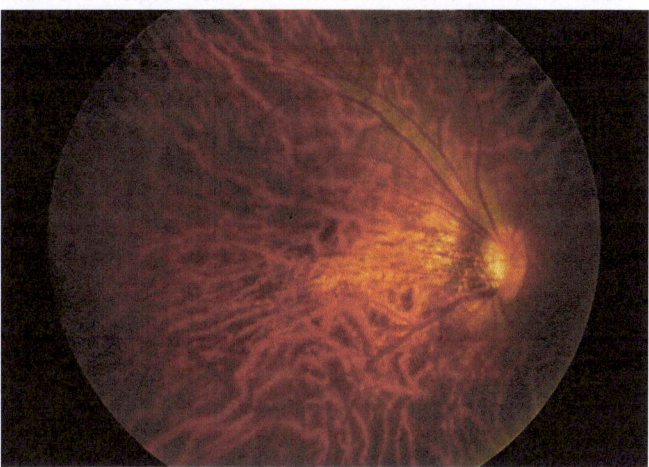

Fig. 3G. Right fundus at the initial examination shows spotty or linear lesions between the optic disc and the macula. The optic disc tilts temporally. No posterior staphyloma is present. Visual acuity is 1.0, and the refractive error is −12.0 D

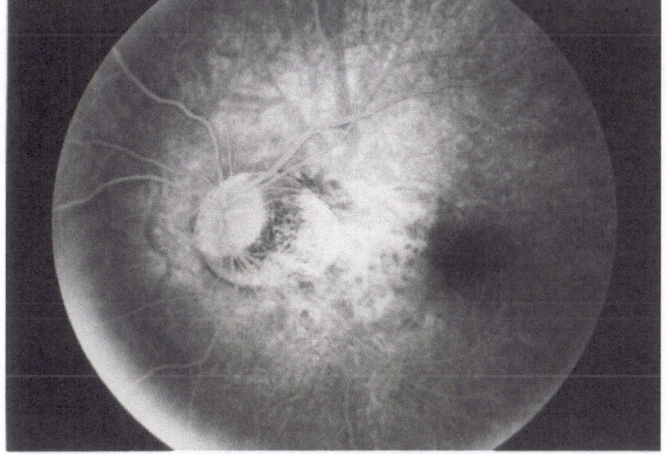

Fig. 3E. Fluorescein fundus angiogram 5 years after the initial examination (November 1992). At 11 min after dye injection, spotty or linear lesions between the optic disc and macula show tissue staining

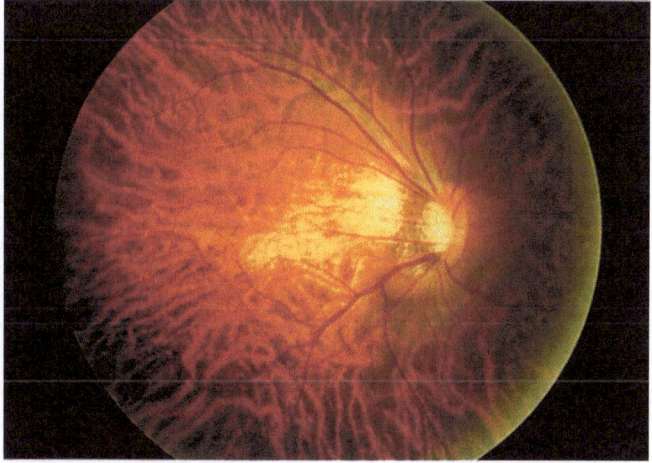

Fig. 3H. Right fundus 7 years after the initial examination (July 1994) shows the enlarged spotty or linear lesions of diffuse atrophy between the optic disc and the macula. Visual acuity is 1.2, and the refractive error is −13.25 D

Case 4

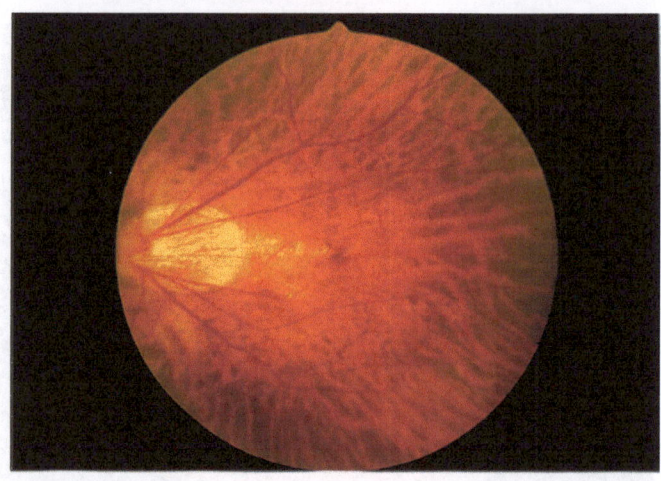

Fig. 4A. Left fundus at the initial examination shows linear lesions of diffuse atrophy between the optic disc and the macula. The optic disc tilts temporally. Temporal peripapillary crescent is seen. Type II posterior staphyloma is present

A 57-year-old man was examined for high myopia on May 30, 1986. He noticed decreased visual acuity in elementary school. He began wearing glasses for distance vision at age 12 years. His myopia progressed until age 40. His medical history was noncontributory. No family members had severe myopia.

In the initial examination, the patient's best corrected visual acuity was 0.5 in the right eye and 0.8 in the left. The refractive error was −21.5 D sphere in the right eye and −22.00 D sphere in the left, and the axial length measurements were 30.6 mm in the right eye and 30.7 mm in the left. Intraocular pressures and anterior segments were normal. We describe the long-term fundus changes in his left eye.

Summary

This patient was followed up for 10 years, since 1986. Spotty and linear lesions of diffuse atrophy increased between the optic disc and the macula. With time, they coalesced and progressed into an enlarged lesion of diffuse atrophy. Lacquer crack lesions appeared temporal to the macula and increased in number. Finally, they lost definition with the enlargement of surrounding diffuse atrophy.

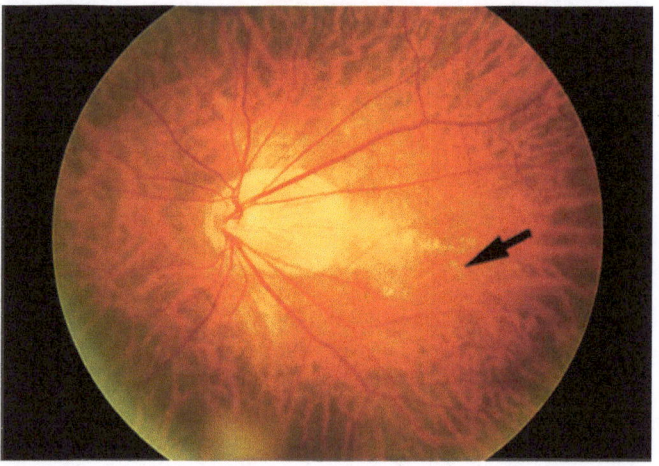

Fig. 4B. One year later (June 1987), linear lesions of diffuse atrophy have elongated temporally. A new lacquer crack lesion has appeared temporal to the macula (*arrow*)

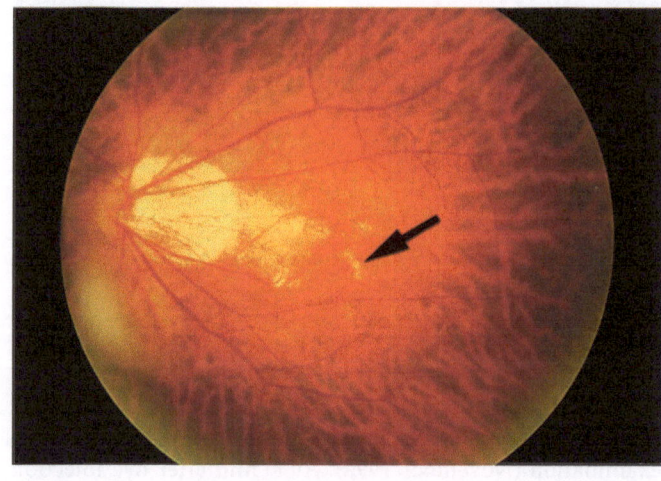

Fig. 4C. Three years after the initial examination (June 1989), spotty or linear lesions of diffuse atrophy around the peripapillary crescent have coalesced. A lacquer crack lesion temporal to the macula has elongated (*arrow*). Visual acuity is 0.7, and the refractive error is −22.0 D

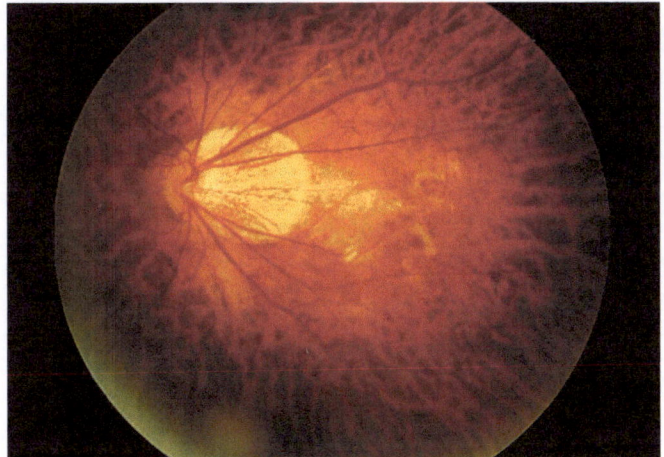

Fig. 4D. Five years after the initial examination (July 1991), lacquer crack lesions have increased temporal to the macula. Spotty lesions of diffuse atrophy have also enlarged in the macula

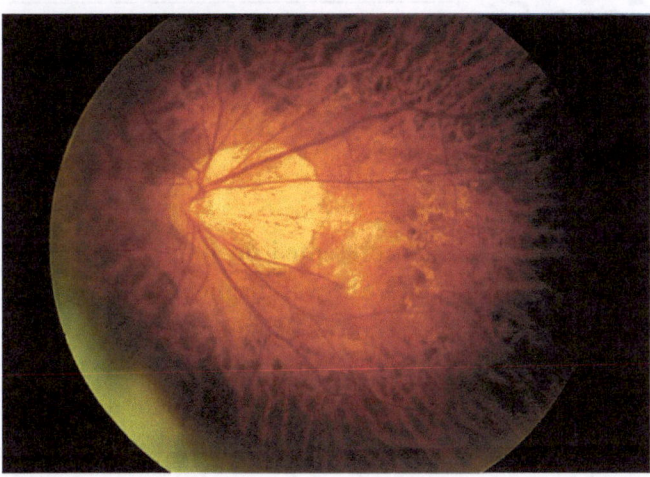

Fig. 4F. Eight years after the initial examination (August 1994), lacquer crack lesions are becoming less obvious as the surrounding spotty lesions of diffuse atrophy enlarge. Spotty or linear lesions of diffuse atrophy between the optic disc and macula have coalesced and progressed into an enlarged lesion of diffuse atrophy. Visual acuity is 0.8, and the refractive error is $-22.0\,D$

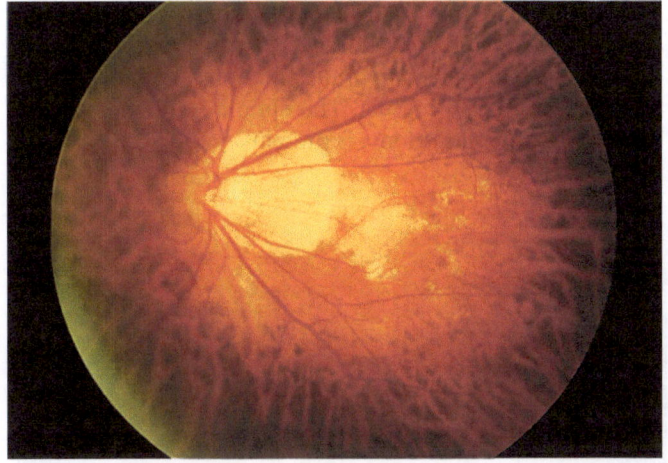

Fig. 4E. Seven years after the initial examination (June 1993), spotty lesions of diffuse atrophy have enlarged between the optic disc and the macula

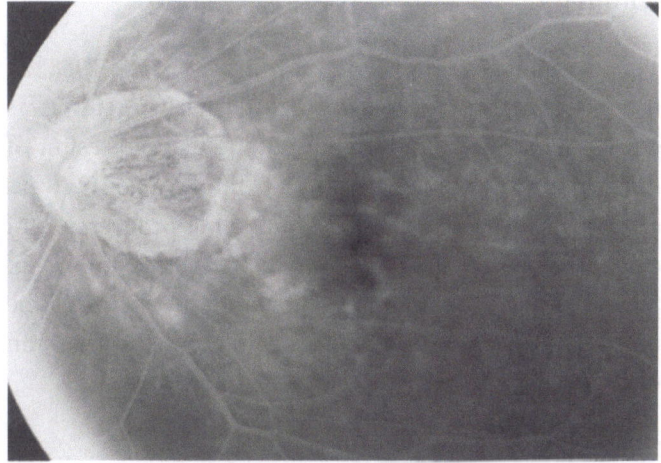

Fig. 4G. Fluorescein fundus angiogram 6 years after the initial examination (July 1992). At 4 min after dye injection, lacquer crack lesions show linear hyperfluorescence in the macula. Spotty or linear lesions of diffuse atrophy between the optic disc and the macula also appear hyperfluorescent because of tissue staining

Fig. 4H. Fluorescein fundus angiogram 7 years after the initial examination (August 1993). At 8 min after dye injection, spotty or linear lesions of diffuse atrophy between the optic disc and the macula show intense hyperfluorescence because of tissue staining. Linear hyperfluorescence corresponding to the lacquer crack lesions is less noticeable

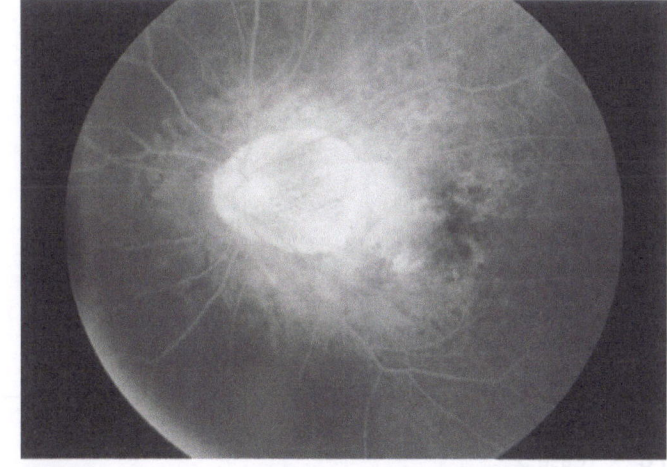

Case 5

A 45-year-old woman presented on June 7, 1988, with decreased visual acuity. She was diagnosed with myopia at age 7 years. She began wearing glasses for distance vision at age 10 years. Her medical history was non-contributory. No family members had severe myopia.

In the initial examination, the patient's best corrected visual acuity was 0.5 in the right eye and 1.0 in the left. The refractive error was −11.00 D sphere in both eyes, and the axial length measurements were 26.7 mm in the right eye and 26.2 mm in the left. Intraocular pressures and anterior segments were normal in both eyes. We describe the long-term fundus changes in her left eye.

Summary

This woman was followed up for 8 years, since 1988. At the initial examination, her corrected visual acuity was good and her left fundus showed an enlarged lesion of diffuse atrophy. Linear lesions of diffuse atrophy were also seen in the macula. No remarkable progression of diffuse atrophy was observed during the follow-up period. Visual acuity was well maintained during the period of 8 years. As seen in this patient, the progression of diffuse atrophy is very slow.

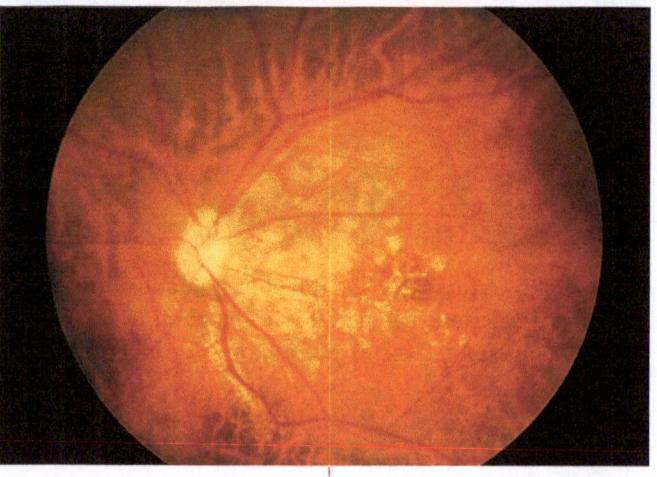

Fig. 5A. Left fundus at the initial examination (June 1988) shows an enlarged lesion of diffuse atrophy between the optic disc and the macula. Spotty or linear lesions of diffuse atrophy are also seen in the macula. The optic disc tilts temporally. Type I posterior staphyloma is present

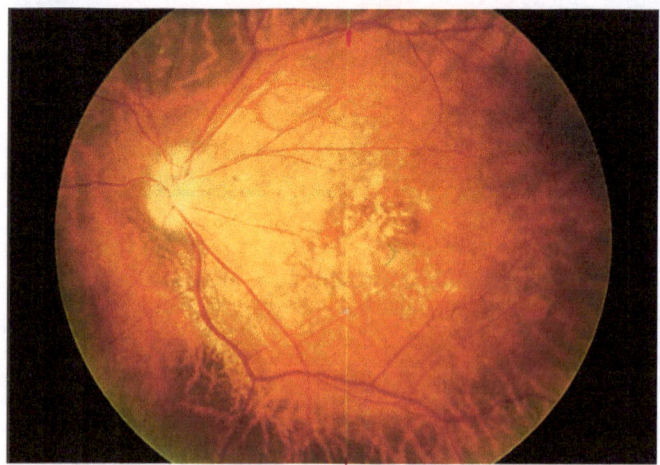

Fig. 5B. Six years after the initial examination (June 1994), no progression of diffuse atrophy is seen. Visual acuity is 1.0, and the refractive error is −12.00 D

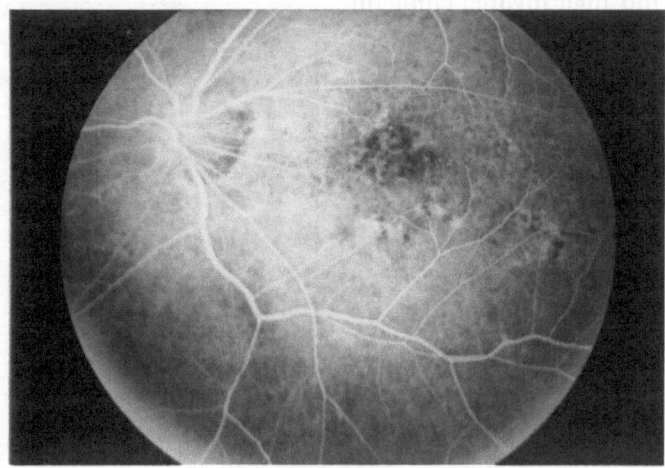

Fig. 5C. Fluorescein fundus angiogram 6 years after the initial examination (April 1994). At 25 sec after dye injection, irregular hyperfluorescence corresponding to the diffuse atrophy is seen in the macula. No patchy atrophy or choroidal neovascularization is detected angiographically

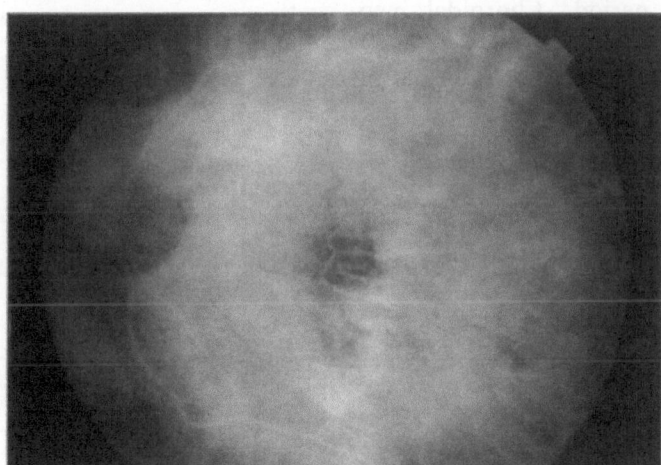

Fig. 5D. Indocyanine green fundus angiogram 8 years after the initial examination (April 1996). Macular area shows hypofluorescence in the late phase of the angiogram. Large choroidal vessels are seen within the hypofluorescence

Case 6

A 58-year-old woman visited our high myopia clinic on February 17, 1984, for further examination of her myopia. She noticed decreased visual acuity after entering junior high school. She began wearing glasses for distance vision at age 15 years. Her medical history was noncontributory. No family members had severe myopia.

In the initial examination, the patient's best corrected visual acuity was 0.9 in the right eye and 0.9 in the left. The refractive error was $-9.75\,D$ sphere in the right eye and $-8.00\,D$ in the left, and the axial length measurements were 27.3 mm in the right eye and 26.5 mm in the left. Intraocular pressures and anterior segments were normal in both eyes. We describe the long-term fundus changes in her right eye.

Summary

This woman has been followed up for 11 years, since 1984. Her right fundus showed diffuse atrophy only throughout the follow-up period. Choroidal neovascularization did not occur, and her right vision was well maintained for 11 years. The progressive pattern of myopic fundus changes in this patient was from D_1 to Lc to D_2. It was difficult to determine the exact date of the progression from D_1 to D_2 because both were continuous lesions.

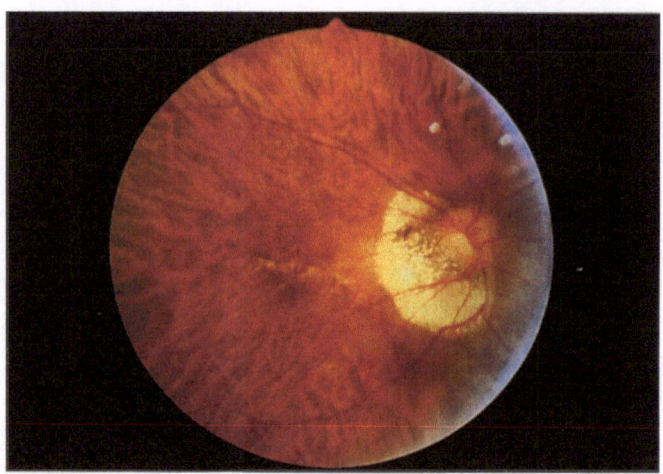

Fig. 6A. Right fundus at the initial examination (February 1984) shows a wide lacquer crack (Lc) lesion in the macula. Spotty or linear lesions of diffuse atrophy are also seen temporal to the optic disc. The optic disc tilts temporally. A temporal peripapillary crescent is seen. Type II posterior staphyloma is present

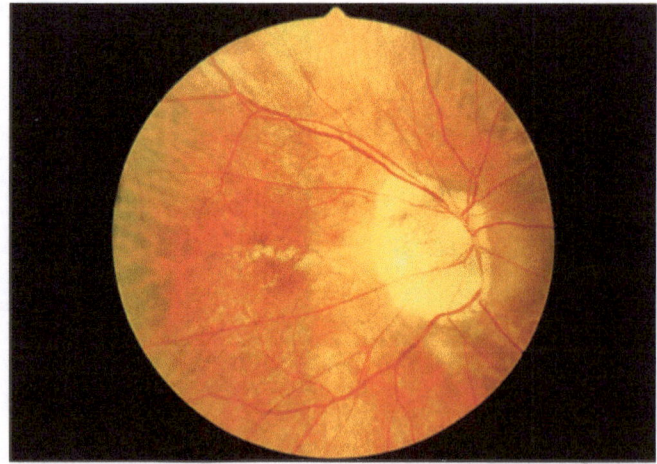

Fig. 6B. Two years later (April 1986), the lacquer crack lesion has slightly increased in width. Visual acuity is 0.9, and the refractive error is $-9.50\,D$

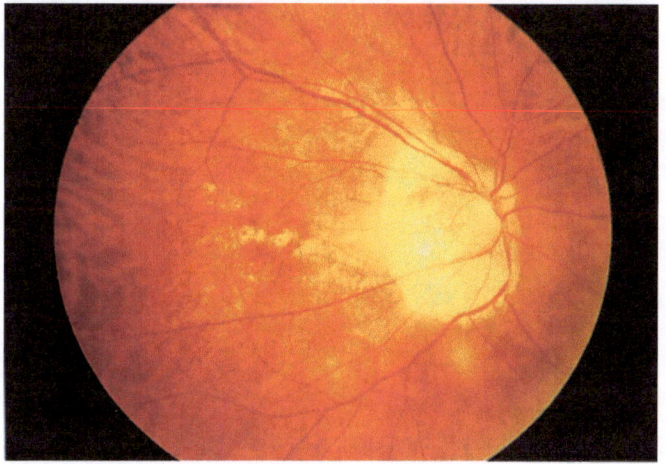

Fig. 6C. Five years after the initial examination (April 1989), the lacquer crack lesion has widened further. Spotty and linear lesions of diffuse atrophy have enlarged in the posterior fundus. Visual acuity is 0.8, and the refractive error is −9.75 D

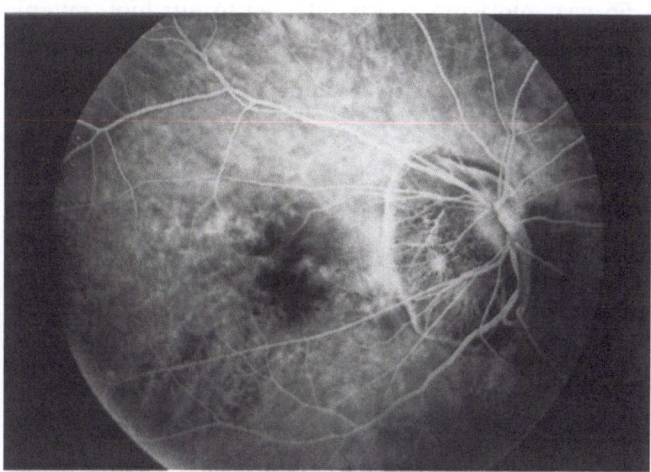

Fig. 6E. Fluorescein fundus angiogram 8 years after the initial examination (July 1992). At 2 min after dye injection, irregular hyperfluorescence is seen corresponding to the diffuse atrophy. The lacquer crack lesion does not show typical linear hyperfluorescence

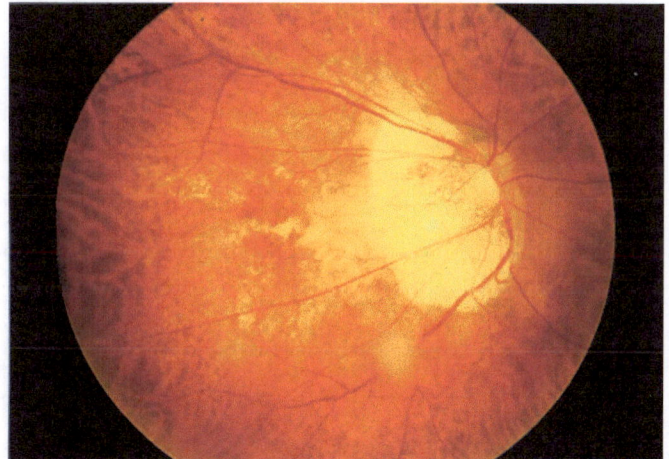

Fig. 6D. Ten years after the initial examination (April 1994), diffuse atrophy has enlarged and progressed into an enlarged lesion. An enlarged lesion of diffuse atrophy covers the entire posterior fundus. The peripapillary crescent has also enlarged. The lacquer crack lesion is less obvious, surrounded by an enlarged lesion of diffuse atrophy. Visual acuity is 0.8, and the refractive error is −10.50

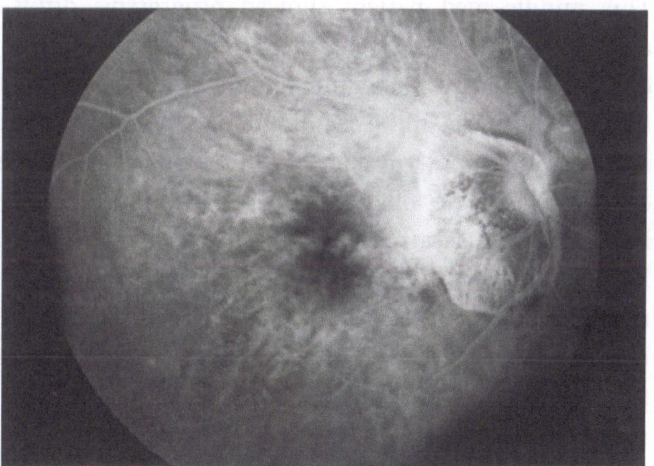

Fig. 6F. Fluorescein fundus angiogram 8 years after the initial examination (July 1992). At 8 min after dye injection, diffuse atrophy still shows irregular hyperfluorescence in the late phase

Case 7

A 56-year-old woman was referred to our high myopia clinic on December 7, 1984, for myopic fundus change in both her eyes. The patient reported no decreased visual acuity as a child. She began wearing glasses at age 17 years for distance vision. Recently, she visited a general practitioner for a feeling of heaviness in her left eye. She was diagnosed with bilateral high myopia. Her medical history was noncontributory. No family members had severe myopia.

In the initial examination, the patient's best corrected visual acuity was 0.9 in the right eye and 0.4 in the left. The refractive error was $-9.75\,D$ sphere in the right eye and $-13.00\,D$ sphere in the left, and the axial length measurements were 27.1 mm in the right eye and 28.9 mm in the left. Intraocular pressures and anterior segments were normal in both eyes. We describe the long-term fundus changes in both her eyes.

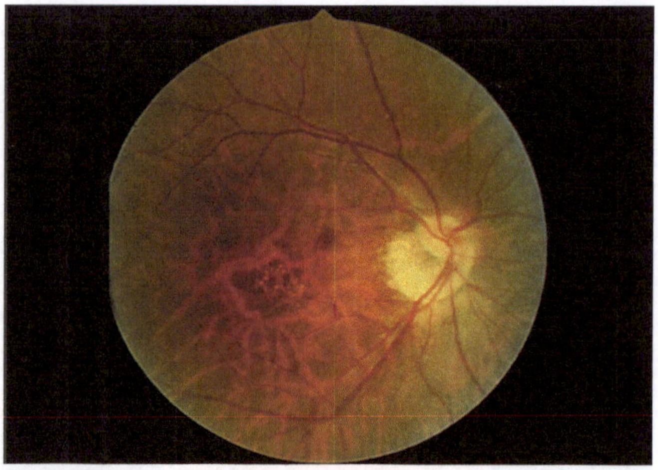

Summary

This middle-aged patient showed progressive diffuse atrophy in the right eye and the development of choroidal neovascularization within a lesion of diffuse atrophy in the left eye. The initial examination of the right fundus revealed small spotty lesions of diffuse atrophy near the central fovea. The left fundus showed spotty or linear lesions of diffuse atrophy covering the entire macula. During the 8-year follow-up period, spotty lesions in the right fundus increased until they covered the entire macula. The progression of diffuse atrophy in the right fundus suggests the possible future development of choroidal neovascularization, as seen in the left fundus.

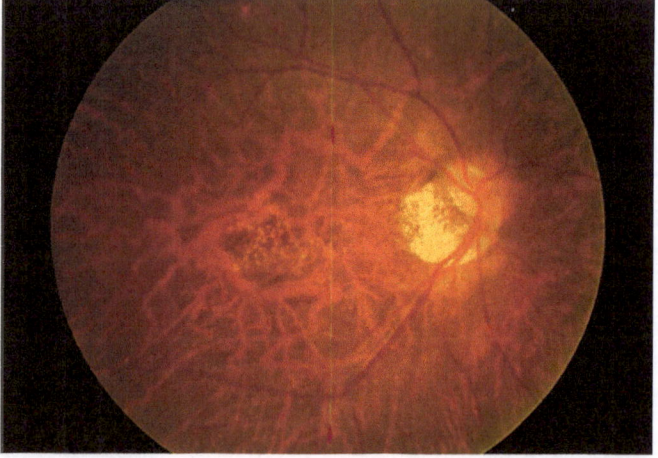

Fig. 7A. Right fundus at the initial examination (December 1984) shows spotty lesions of diffuse atrophy in the macula. The optic disc tilts toward the lower temporal region. A temporal peripapillary crescent is seen. Type II posterior staphyloma is present

Fig. 7B. Five years after the initial examination (January 1989), spotty lesions of diffuse atrophy have increased in the macula. Visual acuity is 0.8, and the refractive error is $-10.50\,D$

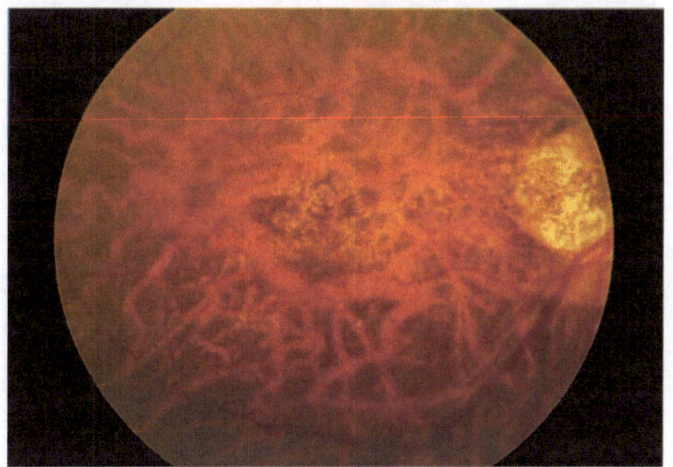

Fig. 7C. Seven years after the initial examination (February 1991), spotty lesions of diffuse atrophy have increased further. Visual acuity is 0.6, and the refractive error is −11.50 D

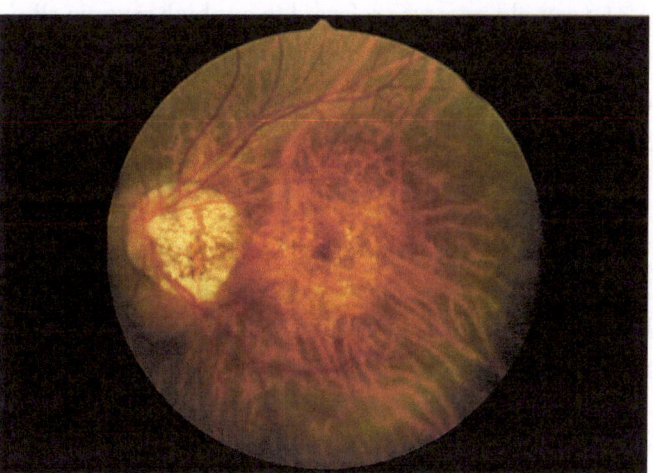

Fig. 7E. Left fundus at the first examination (December 1984). Visual acuity is 0.4 in the left eye and the refractive error is −13.00 D in the left. Diffuse atrophy already covers the entire macula. Left fundus shows advanced diffuse atrophy in the macula at this point

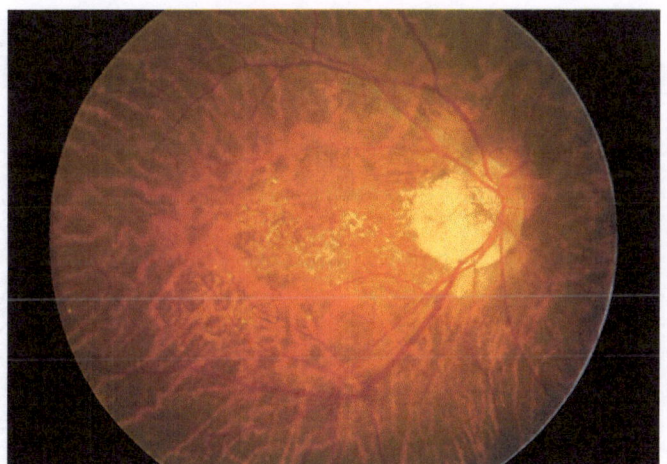

Fig. 7D. Eight years after the initial examination (June 1992), spotty lesions of diffuse atrophy have covered the entire macula. Visual acuity is 0.6, and the refractive error is −11.50 D

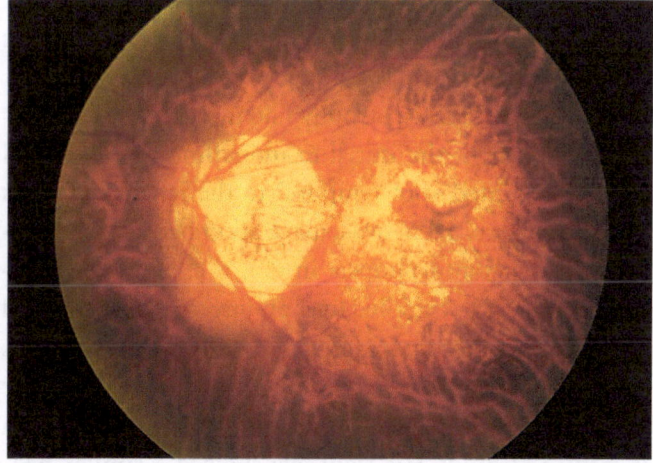

Fig. 7F. Left fundus 8 years after the initial examination (June 1992). Choroidal neovascularization has suddenly appeared within diffuse atrophy in the macula. In the left eye, visual acuity has dropped to 0.02, and the refractive error is −15.00 D

Case 8

A 31-year-old man was referred to our high myopia clinic on May 12, 1986, for metamorphopsia in the left eye. The patient's noncorrected visual acuity was 0.9 in both eyes at the age of 7. One year later, it dropped to 0.3 bilaterally. His refractive error in the left eye was −6.50 D at age 13 years, and his refractive error was −15.50 D at age 29 years. In April 1986, he noticed metamorphopsia in his left eye and visited a general practitioner. His medical history was noncontributory. His father is highly myopic.

In the initial examination, the patient's best corrected visual acuity was 1.0 in the right eye and 0.9 in the left. The refractive error was −15.50 D sphere in the right eye and −17.00 D sphere in the left, and the axial length measurements were 29.4 mm in the right eye and 29.9 mm in the left. Intraocular pressures and anterior segments were normal in both eyes. We describe the long-term fundus changes in both his eyes.

Summary

This patient has been followed up for 10 years, since 1986. At 6 years after the initial examination, spotty or linear lesion of diffuse atrophy had increased in the posterior fundus. At the initial examination, we suspected that a pigmented spot temporal to the left macula was regressed choroidal neovascularization because he complained of metamorphopsia in that eye. However, fluorescein angiography failed to show any signs of choroidal neovascularization. A series of fluorescein fundus angiograms clearly showed the progression of irregular hyperfluorescence corresponding to an enlarged lesion of diffuse atrophy. His right eye showed a similar progressive pattern of diffuse atrophy. Visual function was maintained in both his eyes for a long period.

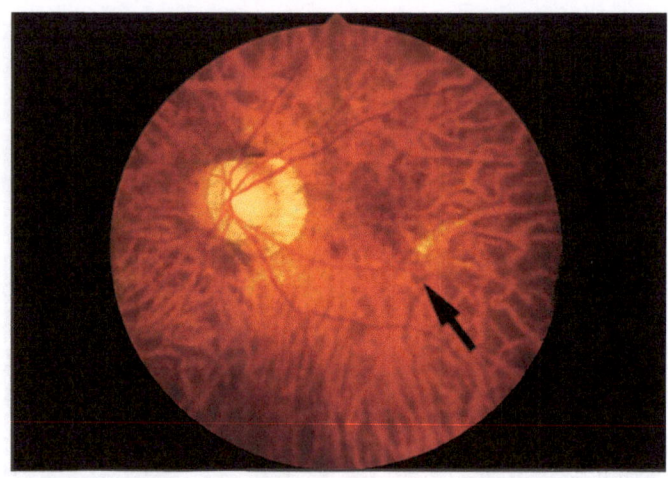

Fig. 8A. Left fundus at the initial examination (May 1986) shows spotty or linear lesions of diffuse atrophy temporal to the macula and inferior to the peripapillary crescent. A pigmented spot is seen inferotemporally to the macula (*arrow*). The optic disc tilts temporally. A temporal peripapillary crescent is seen. No posterior staphyloma is present

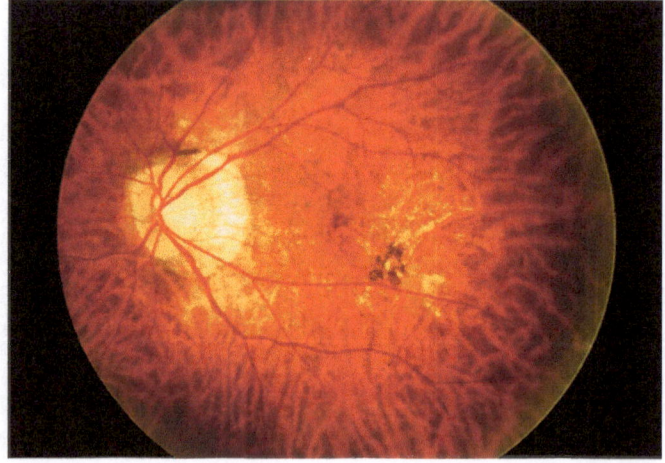

Fig. 8B. Three years after the initial examination (September 1989), spotty or linear lesions of diffuse atrophy have increased temporal to the macula. Pigmentation within the lesion of diffuse atrophy has also enlarged. Visual acuity is 0.9, and the refractive error is −16.50 D

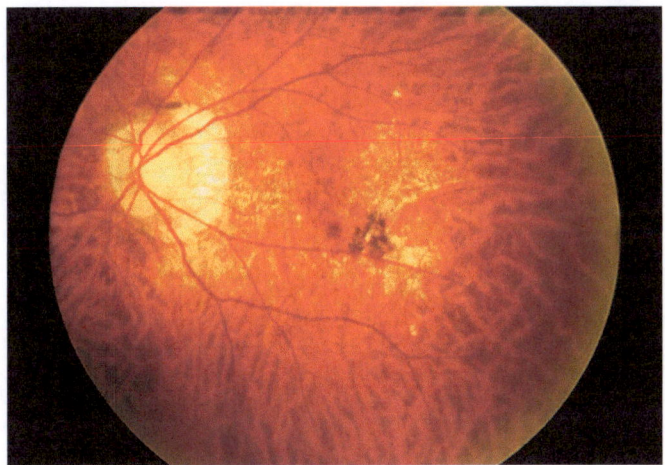

Fig. 8C. Six years after the initial examination (December 1992), spotty or linear lesions of diffuse atrophy have increased around the optic disc and in the macula. Pigmentation has also enlarged. Visual acuity is 1.0, and the refractive error is −16.25 D

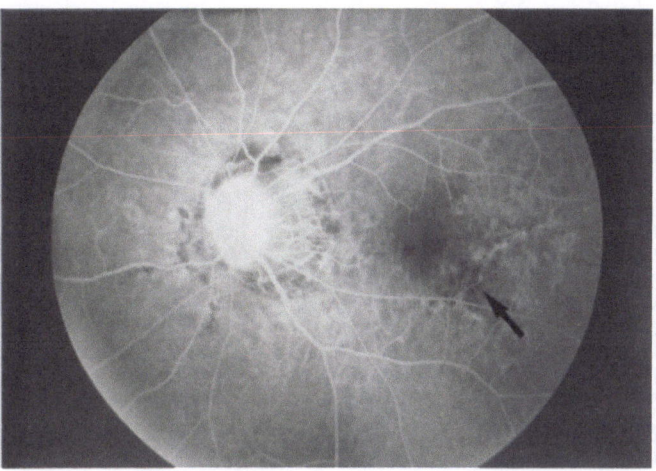

Fig. 8E. Fluorescein fundus angiogram 6 years after the initial examination (December 1992). At 1 min after dye injection, spotty or linear lesions of diffuse atrophy show irregular hyperfluorescence. Pigmentation is seen as blocked fluorescence (*arrow*). The absence of dye leakage fails to suggest the existence of choroidal neovascularization

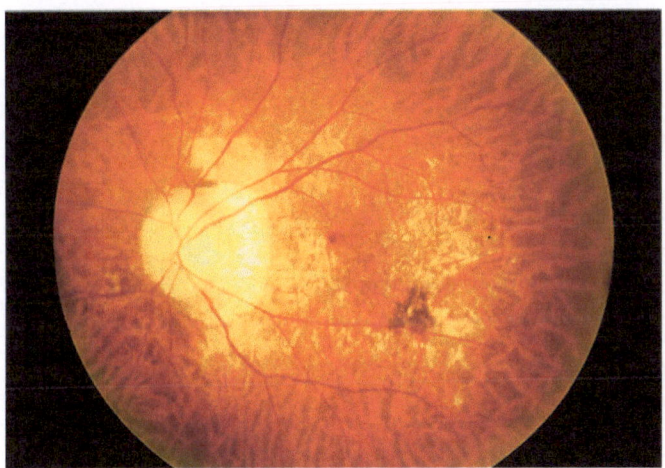

Fig. 8D. Eight years after the initial examination (August 1994), spotty or linear lesions of diffuse atrophy have increased between the optic disc and the macula. Visual acuity is 1.0, and the refractive error is −17.00

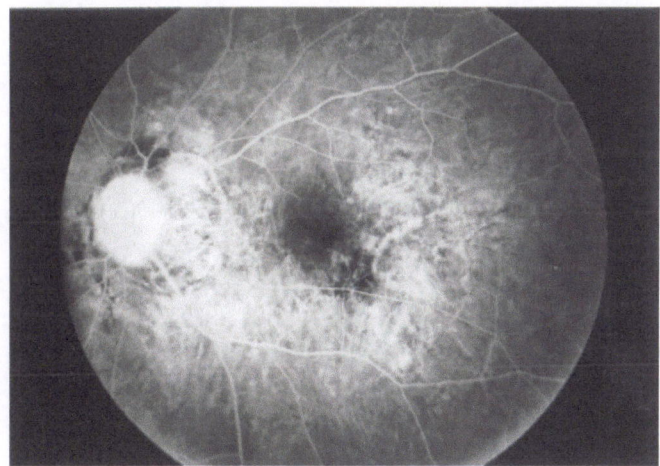

Fig. 8F. Fluorescein fundus angiogram 10 years after the initial examination (August 1996). At 3 min after dye injection, the hyperfluorescent area has enlarged as a result of the increase of spotty or linear lesions of diffuse atrophy

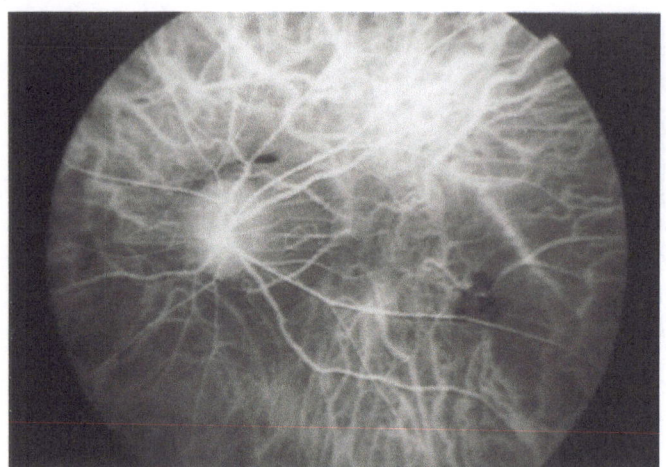

Fig. 8G. Indocyanine green fundus angiogram 8 years after the initial examination (August 1994). The early phase of the angiogram shows only blocked fluorescence corresponding to the pigmentation near the macula

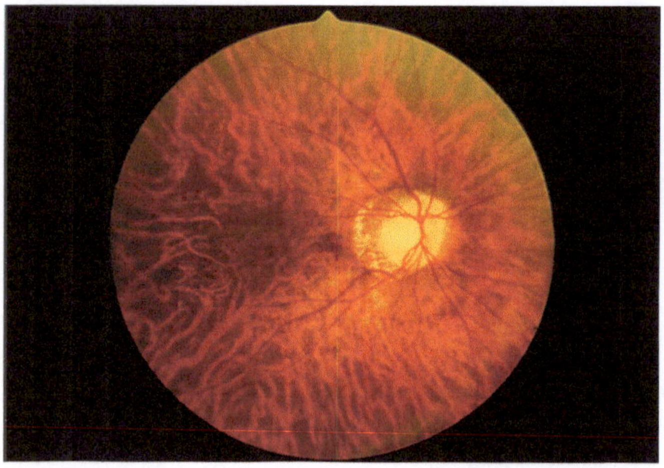

Fig. 8I. Right fundus at the initial examination (May 1986) shows spotty or linear lesions of diffuse atrophy around the optic disc. The optic disc tilts temporally. A temporal peripapillary crescent is seen. No posterior staphyloma is present. In the right eye, visual acuity is 1.0, and the refractive error is −15.50 D. The axial length measurement is 29.4 mm

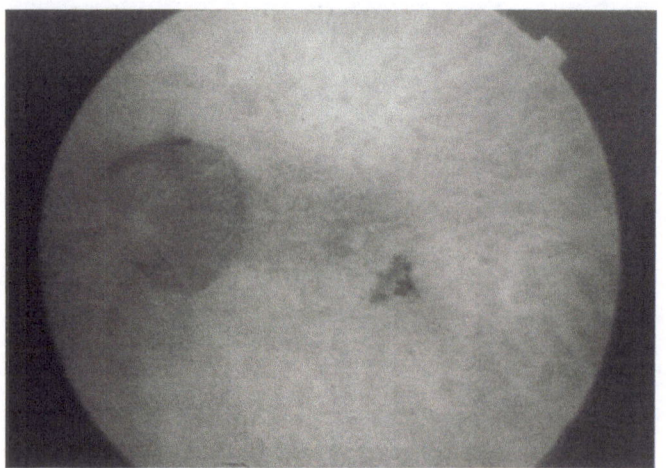

Fig. 8H. Indocyanine green fundus angiogram 8 years after the initial examination (August 1994). The late phase of the angiogram shows blocked fluorescence corresponding to the pigmented spot. The macular area shows slight hypofluorescence in the late phase

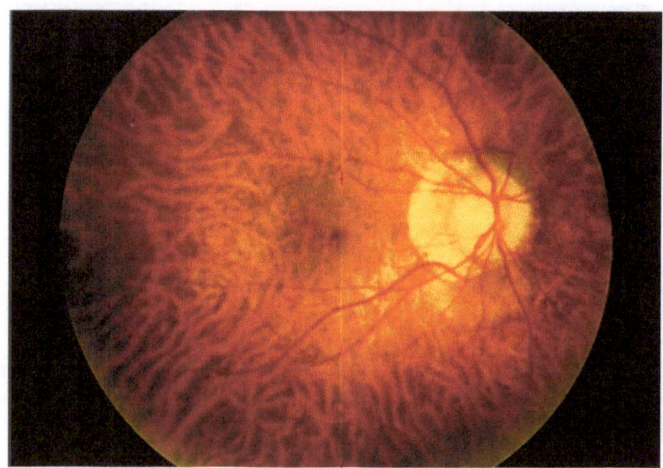

Fig. 8J. Right fundus 8 years after the initial examination (December 1994). Spotty or linear lesions of diffuse atrophy have increased in the posterior fundus, as in his left fundus. Visual acuity is 1.0, and the refractive error is −16.75 D

Case 9

A 58-year-old woman was examined for high myopia in both eyes on November 22, 1976. She had no complaints of visual disturbance as a child. She began wearing glasses in high school. Her medical history was noncontributory. Her father was highly myopic.

In the initial examination, the patient's best corrected visual acuity was 0.7 in the right eye and 0.6 in the left. The refractive error was −13.50 D sphere in the right eye and −12.00 D sphere in the left, and the axial length measurements were 27.0 mm in the right eye and 26.0 mm in the left. Intraocular pressures and anterior segments were normal in both eyes. We show the long-term fundus changes in both her eyes

Summary

This patient had deep posterior staphyloma and diffuse atrophy in both eyes. In highly myopic eyes with sharp margined and deep staphyloma, diffuse atrophy is likely to progress in the posterior fundus. Diffuse atrophy gradually enlarges and finally occupies the entire macular lesion. However, no other lesions appear in the posterior fundus than diffuse atrophy. She retained good visual acuity during the period.

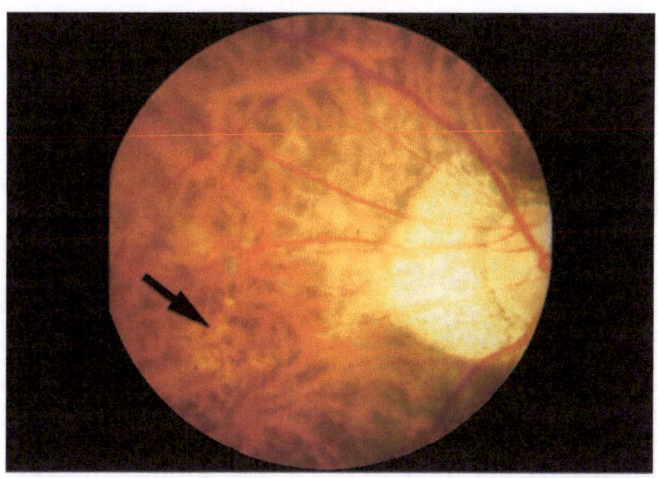

Fig. 9A. Right fundus at the initial examination (November 1976) shows a vertically oriented lacquer crack in the macula (*arrow*). Spotty or linear lesions of diffuse atrophy are observed temporal to the optic disc. The optic disc tilts temporally. A temporal peripapillary crescent is also seen. Type I staphyloma is present

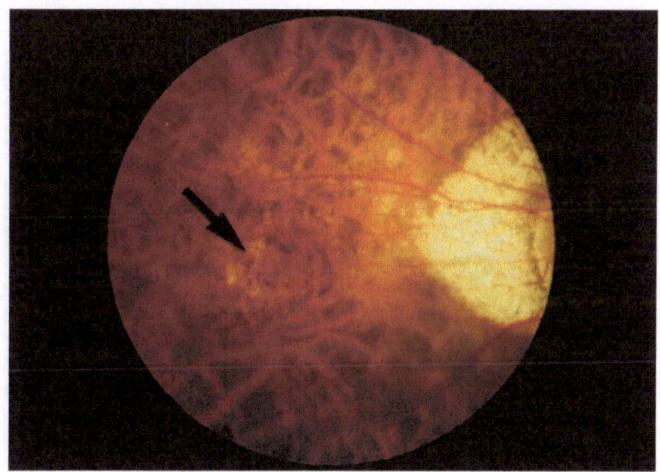

Fig. 9B. Two years later (March 1978), a vertically oriented lacquer crack lesion is seen in the macula (*arrow*). It is surrounded by diffuse atrophy. Visual acuity is 0.7, and the refractive error is −13.50 D

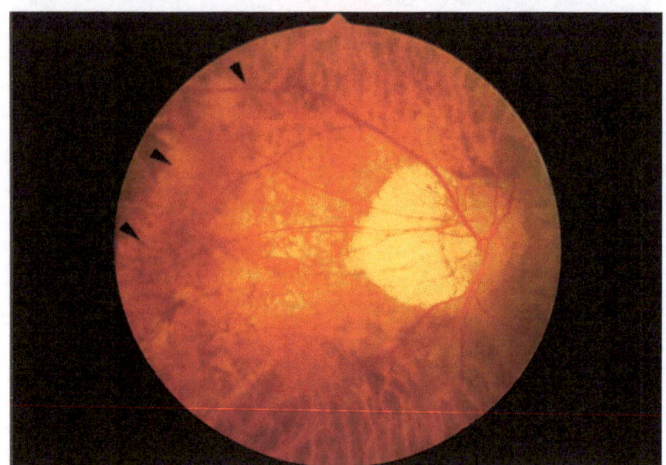

Fig. 9C. Three years after the initial examination (October 1979), spotty or linear lesions of diffuse atrophy have increased. The lacquer crack is obscured by the surrounding diffuse atrophy. The edge of the posterior staphyloma is clear temporal to the macula (*arrowheads*)

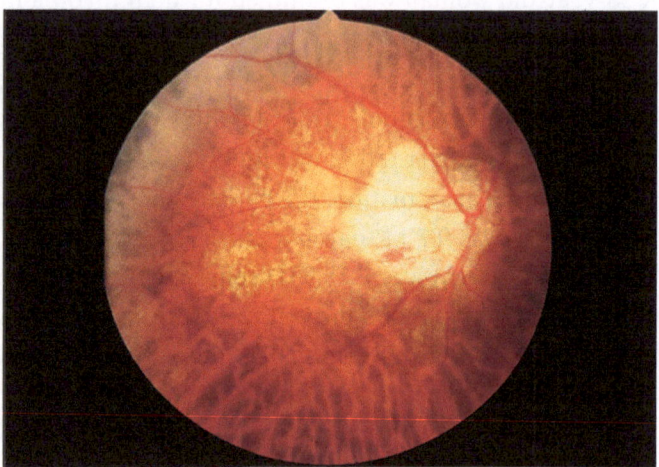

Fig. 9E. Eight years after the initial examination (June 1984), spotty or linear lesions of diffuse atrophy in the macula have enlarged into a lesion of diffuse atrophy

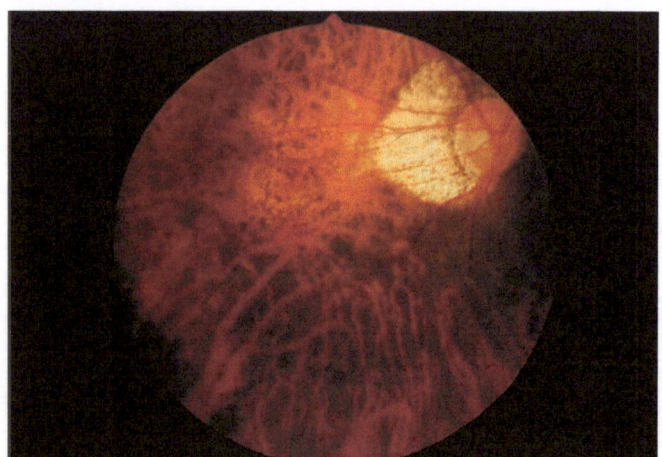

Fig. 9D. Four years after the initial examination (May 1980), spotty or linear lesions of diffuse atrophy around the optic disc have increased further

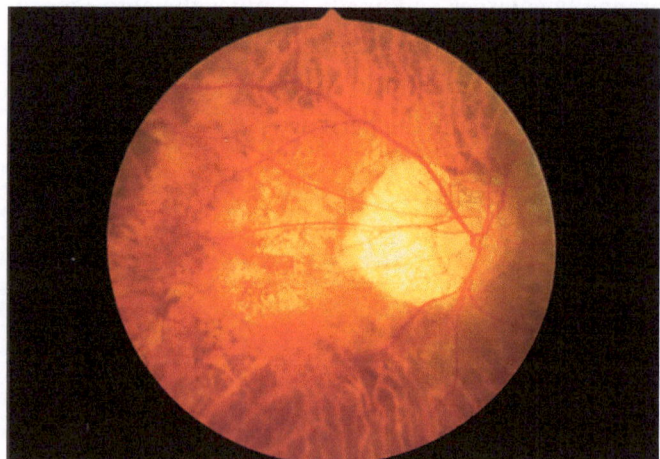

Fig. 9F. Ten years after the initial examination (June 1986), the posterior fundus is covered by an enlarged lesion of diffuse atrophy

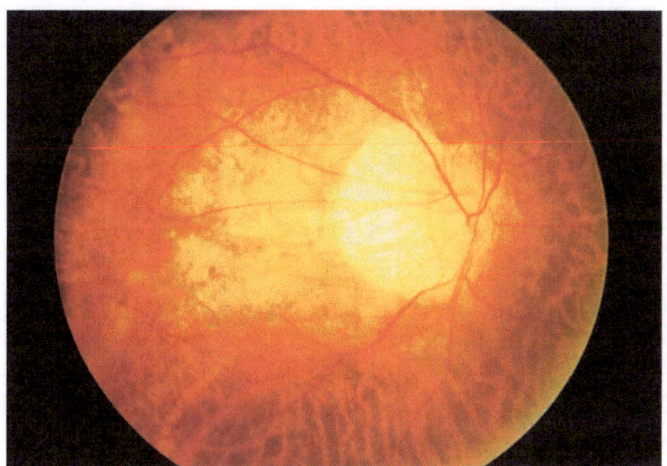

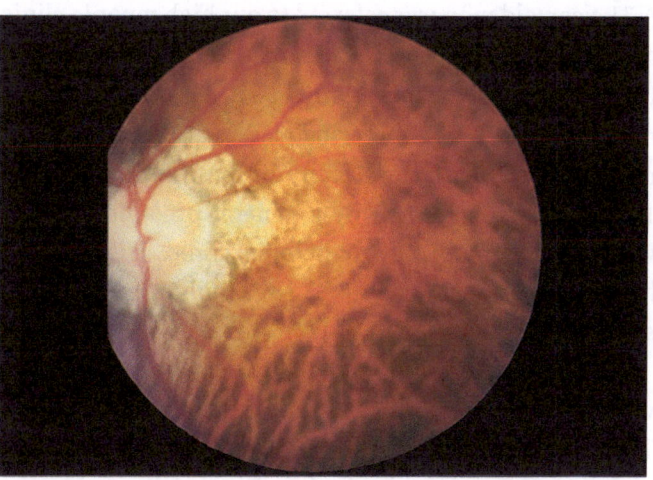

Fig. 9G. Twelve years after the initial examination (May 1988), the enlarged lesion of diffuse atrophy has progressed temporally

Fig. 9I. Left fundus at the initial examination (November 1976) shows spotty or linear lesions of diffuse atrophy temporal to the optic disc, which tilts temporally. A peripapillary crescent and type I staphyloma are present. Visual acuity is 0.6, and the refractive error is −12.00 D. The axial length measurement is 26.0 mm

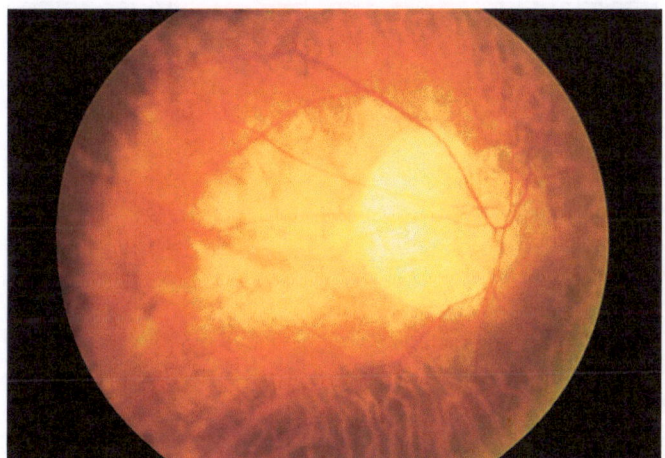

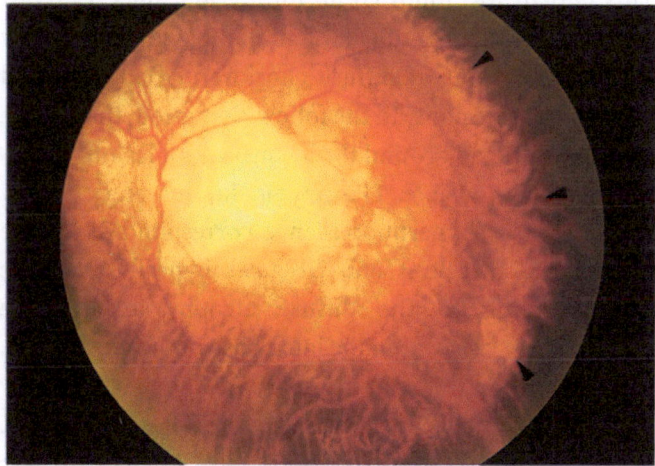

Fig. 9H. Fifteen years after the initial examination (May 1991), the enlarged lesion of diffuse atrophy has become whitish and is progressing into macular atrophy. Visual acuity is 0.4, and the refractive error is −13.50 D

Fig. 9J. Fifteen years after the initial examination (May 1991), the enlarged lesion of diffuse atrophy covers the posterior fundus. The peripapillary crescent has enlarged temporally. The edge of the posterior staphyloma is clean temporal to the macula (*arrowheads*). Visual acuity is 0.3, and the refractive error is −13.00 D

Case 10

A 31-year-old man was referred to our high myopia clinic on January 9, 1987, for macular bleeding in the right eye. He reported disturbances with distance vision in elementary school. He began wearing glasses at age 7 years. He noticed decreased visual acuity in the right eye in May 1983. He was examined by a general practitioner, and was referred to our high myopia clinic. His medical history was noncontributory. No family members had severe myopia.

In the initial examination, the patient's best corrected visual acuity was 0.3 in the right eye and 0.9 in the left. The refractive error was −14.00 D sphere in the right eye and −13.00 D sphere in the left. The axial length measurements were 30.2 mm in the right eye and 30.1 mm in the left. Intraocular pressures and anterior segments were normal in both eyes. We describe the long-term fundus changes in the left eye.

Summary

This patient was followed up for 9 years, since 1987. At the initial examination, his left fundus showed spotty and linear lesions of diffuse chorioretinal atrophy and lacquer crack lesions. In the follow-up period, the diffuse atrophy enlarged around the lacquer crack lesions, making them less visible. Fluorescein fundus angiography showed linear hyperfluorescence corresponding to the lacquer crack lesions and irregular hyperfluorescence corresponding to the diffuse atrophy around the peripapillary crescent in the late phase of the angiogram. Irregular hyperfluorescence around the peripapillary crescent gradually enlarged during the follow-up period. Spotty or linear lesions in this patient will probably progress into an enlarged lesion of diffuse atrophy in the next few years.

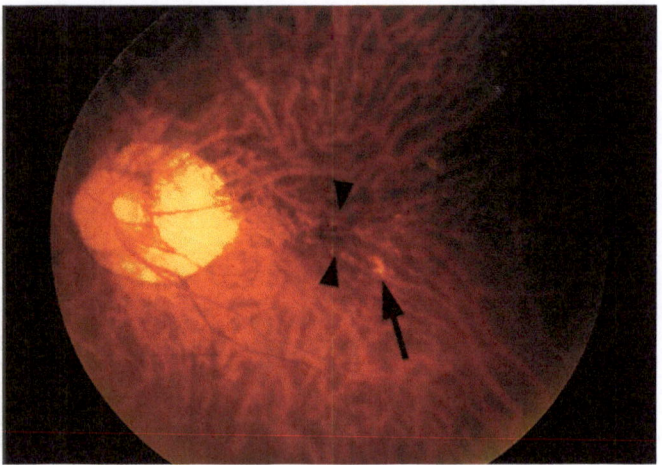

Fig. 10A. Left fundus at the initial examination (January 1987) shows lacquer crack lesions in the macula (*arrowheads*). A small spotty lesion of patchy atrophy is seen at the temporal edge of the lacquer crack lesion (*arrow*). The optic disc tilts temporally. Temporal peripapillary crescent is seen. No posterior staphyloma is present

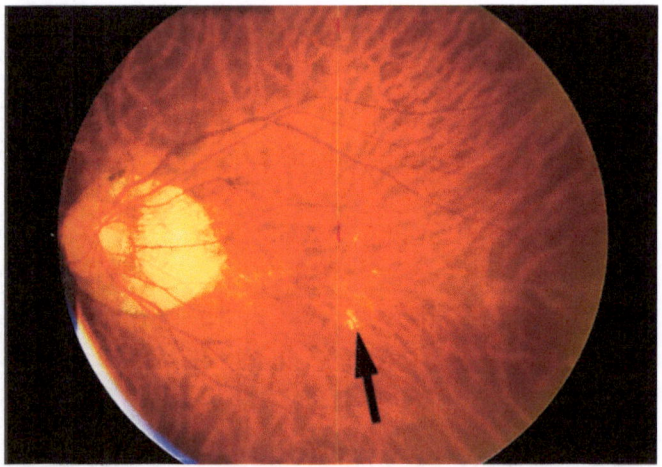

Fig. 10B. One year later (October 1988), lacquer crack lesions have increased. The spotty lesion of patchy atrophy has slightly enlarged (*arrow*). Visual acuity is 0.7, and the refractive error is −13.75 D

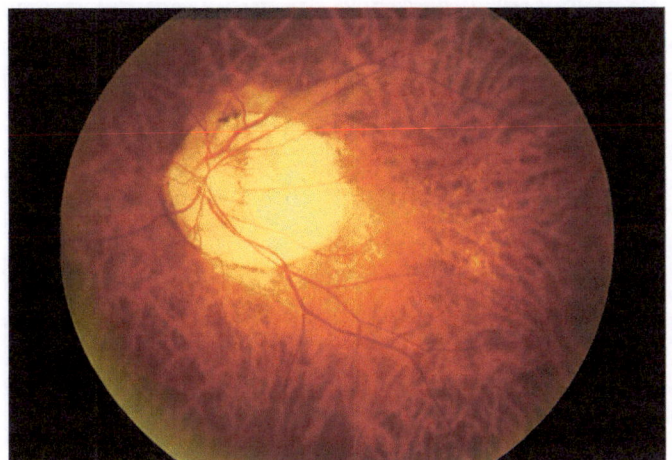

Fig. 10C. Six years after the initial examination (November 1993), spotty or linear lesions of diffuse atrophy have increased temporal to the peripapillary crescent. Lacquer crack lesion is losing clarity as it is surrounded by diffuse atrophy

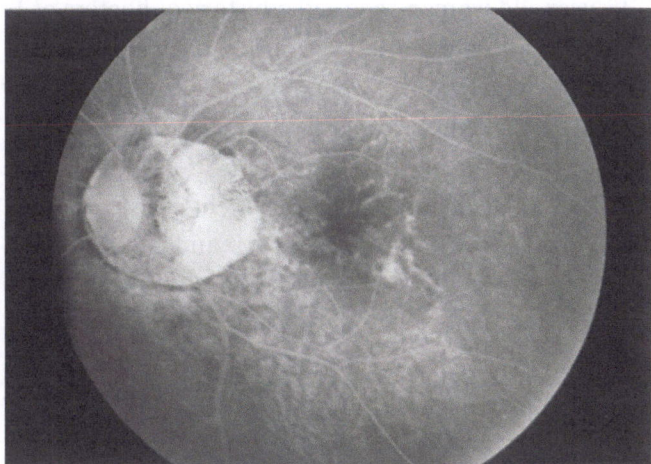

Fig. 10E. Fluorescein fundus angiogram 5 years after the initial examination (June 1992). At 6 min after dye injection, lacquer crack lesions show linear hyperfluorescence in the macula. Irregular hyperfluorescence corresponding to diffuse atrophy is seen temporal to the peripapillary crescent

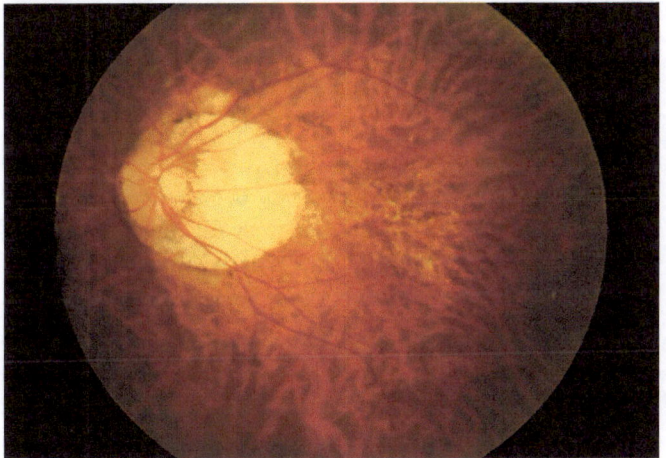

Fig. 10D. Seven years after the initial examination (December 1994), diffuse atrophy covers the entire posterior fundus. The peripapillary crescent has also enlarged. Visual acuity is 0.7, and the refractive error is −14.0 D

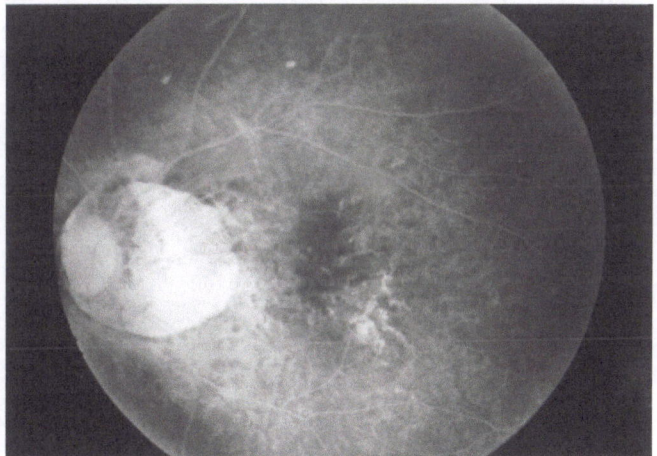

Fig. 10F. Fluorescein fundus angiogram 7 years after the initial examination (December 1994). At 8 min after dye injection, hyperfluorescent lesions have increased around the lacquer crack lesion. Linear hyperfluorescence corresponding to the lacquer crack lesion is becoming less noticeable

Case 11

A 35-year-old woman reported a history of floaters of 1-month duration in her left eye on July 12, 1985. She had no visual disturbance when she was in elementary school. She began wearing glasses at age 12 years. No family members had severe myopia.

In the initial examination, the patient's best corrected visual acuity was 1.0 in the right eye and 0.8 in the left. The refractive error was −14.75 D sphere in the right eye and −17.50 D sphere in the left, and the axial length measurements were 28.8 mm in the right eye and 29.6 mm in the left. Intraocular pressures and anterior segments were normal in both eyes. We describe the long-term fundus changes in her left eye.

Summary

This patient was followed up for 11 years, since 1985. A series of fundus photographs of the left eye showed the progression of linear lesions into an enlarged lesion of diffuse atrophy between the optic disc and macula. The progressive pattern of myopic fundus changes in this patient was from D_1 to D_2. Long-term follow-up (more than 10 years) is necessary to detect progressive changes of linear lesions of diffuse atrophy.

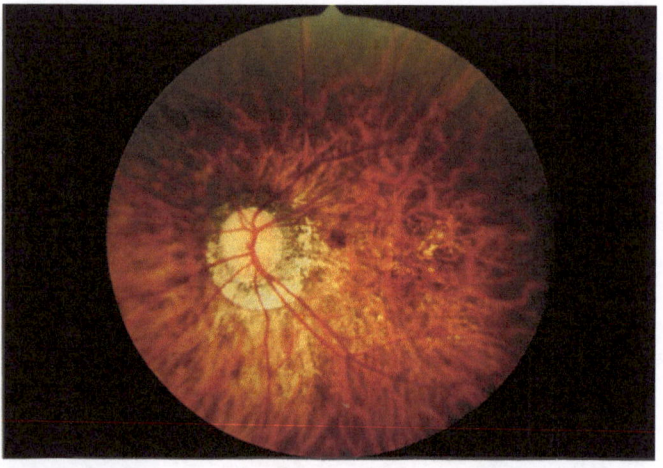

Fig. 11A. Left fundus at the initial examination (July 1985) shows spotty and linear lesions of diffuse atrophy around the optic disc and macula. The optic disc tilts temporally. An annular peripapillary crescent is seen. Type I posterior staphyloma is present

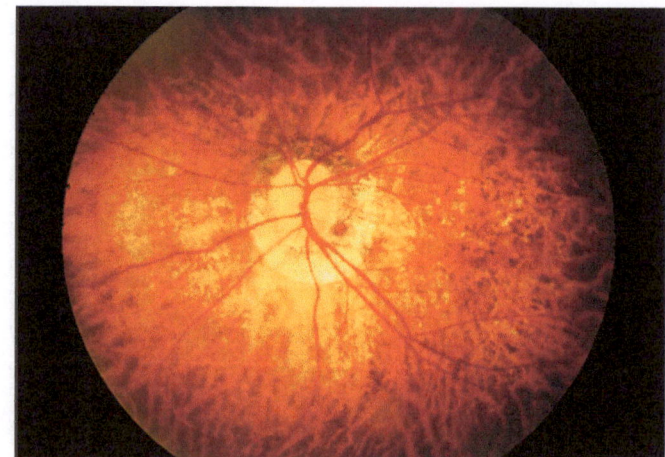

Fig. 11B. Three years after the initial examination (September 1988), linear lesions of diffuse atrophy around the optic disc have progressed into an enlarged lesion of diffuse atrophy

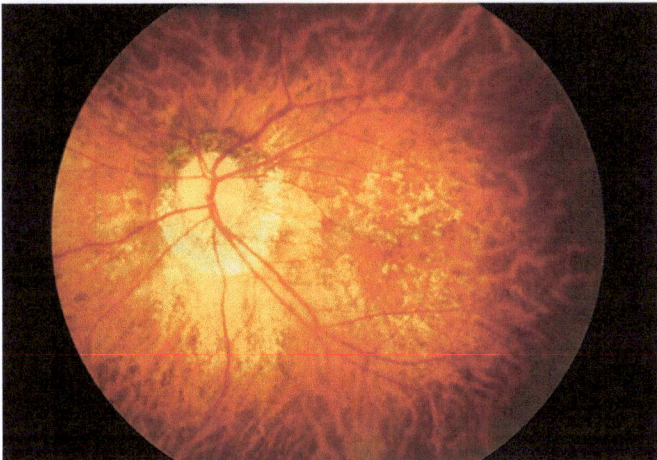

Fig. 11C. Four years later (September 1989), linear lesions of diffuse atrophy have enlarged. Yellowish-white linear lesions similar to lacquer cracks have increased in the macula. Visual acuity is 0.6, and the refractive error is −20.00 D

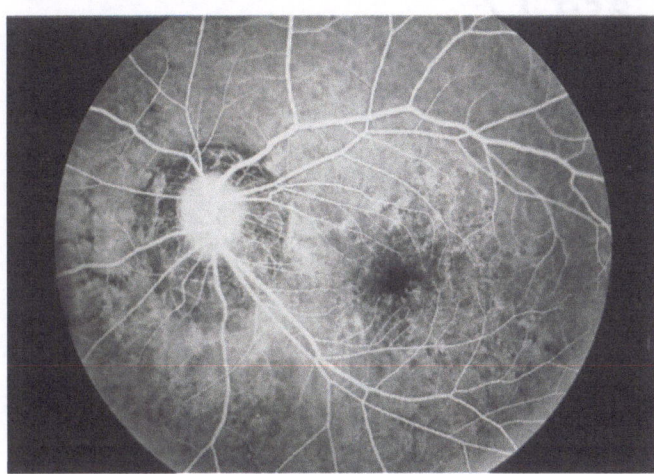

Fig. 11E. Fluorescein fundus angiogram 6 years after the initial examination (November 1991). At 28 sec after dye injection, diffuse chorioretinal atrophy is seen as an irregular hyperfluorescence

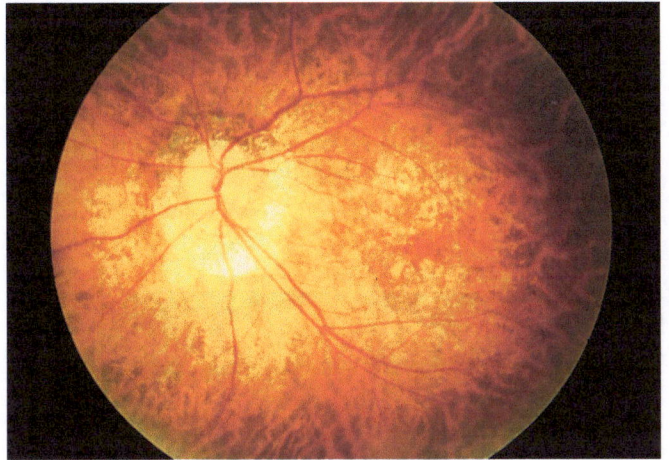

Fig. 11D. Nine years after the initial examination (June 1994), the enlarged lesion of diffuse atrophy has covered the posterior fundus. The peripapillary crescent has also enlarged. Visual acuity is 0.5, and the refractive error is −22.50 D. The myopia in her left eye has become more myopic by −5.00 D in 9 years

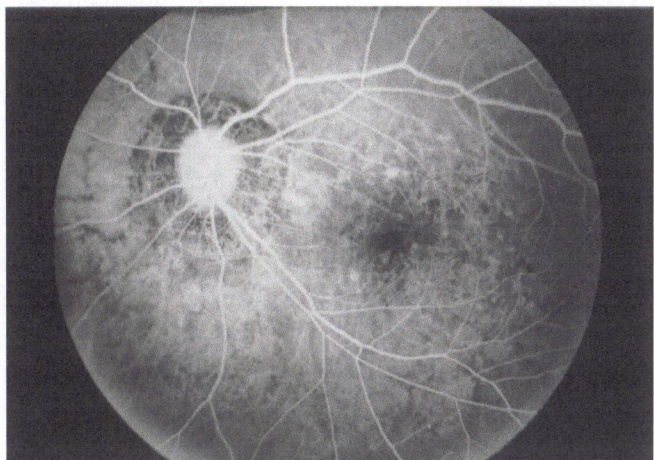

Fig. 11F. Fluorescein fundus angiogram 9 years after the initial examination (June 1994). At 33 sec after dye injection, the irregular hyperfluorescence corresponding to diffuse atrophy has enlarged. Linear hypofluorescent lesions are observed within the enlarged lesion of diffuse atrophy, especially nasal to the optic disc

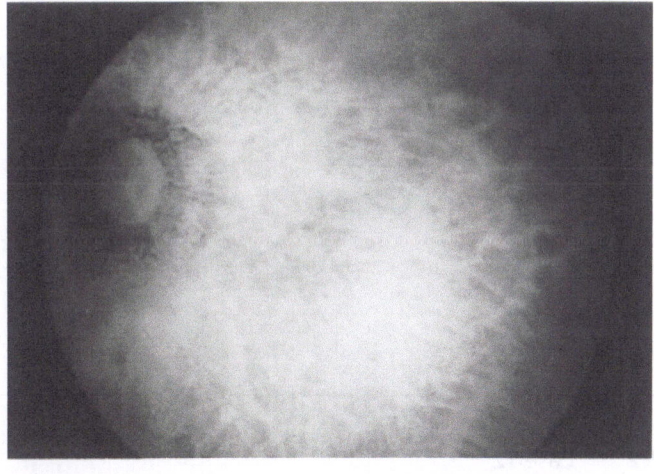

Fig. 11G. The late phase of indocyanine green fundus angiogram taken 11 years after the initial examination (January 1996). Spotty and linear hypofluorescence corresponding to diffuse atrophy is observed in the macula

Case 12

A 49-year-old woman was examined on April 25, 1980, for gradually decreasing visual acuity in her right eye. She reported no visual disturbance as a child. She began to notice visual disturbance at age 12 years. Her left eye became blind in her twenties because of a retinal detachment. Her medical history was noncontributory. No family members had severe myopia.

In the initial examination, the patient's best corrected visual acuity was 0.7 in the right eye and no light perception in the left. The refractive error was −10.50 D sphere and the axial length measurement was 28.8 mm in the right eye. Intraocular pressures and anterior segments were normal in the right eye. We describe the long-term fundus changes in her right eye.

Summary

This patient has been followed up for 16 years, since 1980. In the fundus photographs taken 5 and 8 years after the initial examination, the linear lesions of diffuse atrophy were enlarged. After that, linear lesions of diffuse atrophy gradually progressed into an enlarged lesion of diffuse atrophy. The progression of myopic fundus changes was observed within the posterior staphyloma.

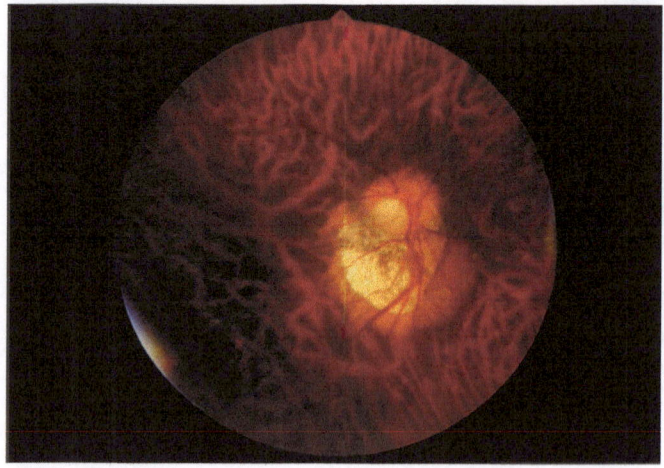

Fig. 12A. Right fundus at the initial examination (April 1980) shows spotty or linear lesions of diffuse atrophy just inferior to the peripapillary crescent. The optic disc tilts inferiorly. Type V posterior staphyloma is present. The edge of the posterior staphyloma crosses the macula obliquely

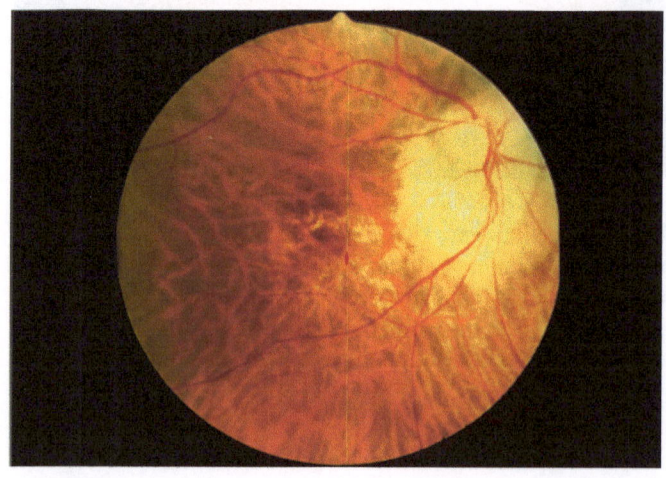

Fig. 12B. Five years later (April 1985), linear lesions of diffuse atrophy have increased inferior to the peripapillary crescent. Visual acuity is 0.5, and the refractive error is −11.50 D

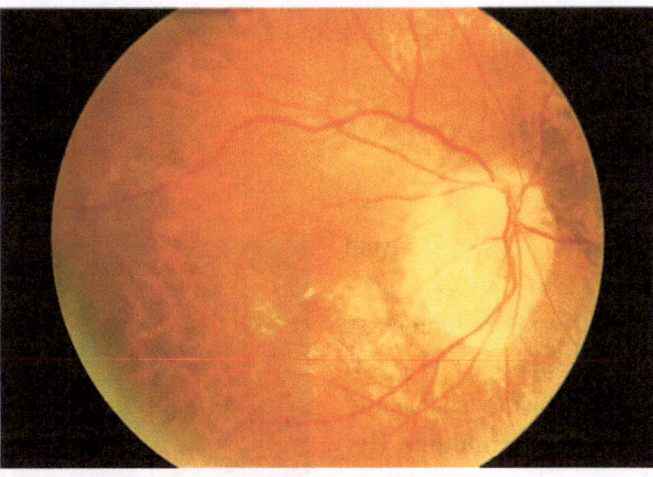

Fig. 12C. Eight years after the initial examination (February 1988), linear lesions of diffuse atrophy inferior to the peripapillary crescent have progressed into an enlarged lesion of diffuse atrophy

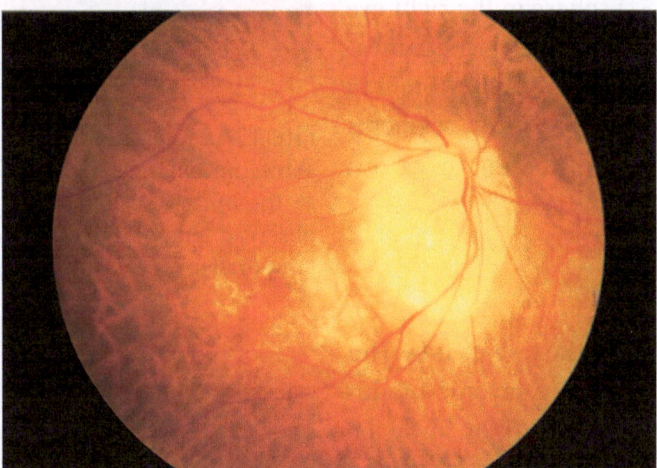

Fig. 12D. Ten years after the initial examination (January 1990), an enlarged lesion of diffuse atrophy temporal and inferior to the peripapillary crescent is noticeable. Diffuse atrophy is progressing rapidly

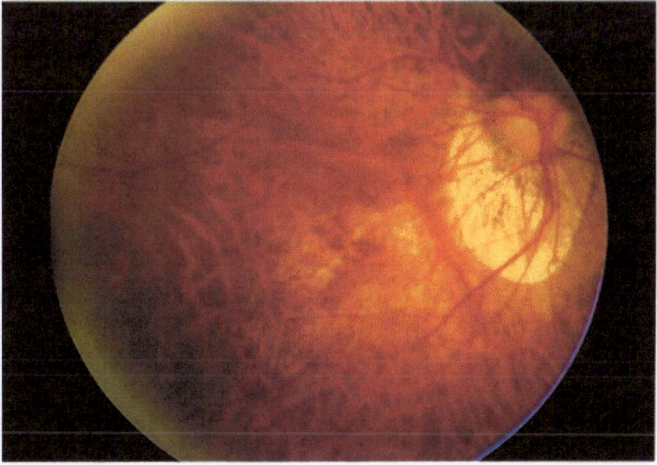

Fig. 12E. Fourteen years after the initial examination (January 1994), the enlarged lesion of diffuse atrophy has been unchanged since 1992. The peripapillary crescent has gradually enlarged inferiorly. Visual acuity is 0.4, and the refractive error is −15.00 D. The degree of myopia has increased by −4.50 D in 14 years

Case 13

A 48-year-old woman presented with decreased visual acuity in both her eyes on July 13, 1984. She was diagnosed as having myopia when she was an elementary school student. She began wearing glasses at age 11 years. She reported a gradual bilateral decrease of visual acuity recently. Her medical history was noncontributory. Her father was highly myopic. None of her five siblings showed high myopia.

In the initial examination, the patient's best corrected visual acuity was 0.7 in the right eye and 0.8 in the left. The refractive error was $-20.5\,D$ sphere in the right eye and $-13.0\,D$ sphere in the left, and the axial length measurements were 31.9 mm in the right eye and 29.1 mm in the left. Intraocular pressures and anterior segments were normal in both eyes. We describe the long-term fundus changes in her right eye.

Summary

This woman was followed up for 12 years, since 1984. Her right fundus already showed advanced myopic fundus changes at the initial examination. Spotty or linear lesions of diffuse atrophy were visible in the macula, and an enlarged lesion of diffuse atrophy was seen around the optic disc. During the follow-up period, an enlarged lesion of diffuse atrophy increased. However, visual function of the right eye was maintained. No other myopic fundus changes, such as patchy atrophy or choroidal neovascularization, occurred.

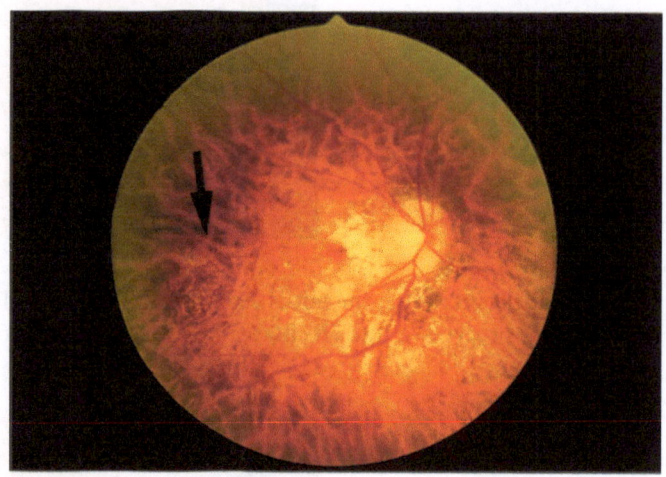

Fig. 13A. Right fundus at the initial examination (July 1984) shows an enlarged lesion of diffuse atrophy inferotemporal to the optic disc. Linear lesions of diffuse atrophy are also observed temporal to the macula (*arrow*). The optic disc tilts temporally. Type II posterior staphyloma is present

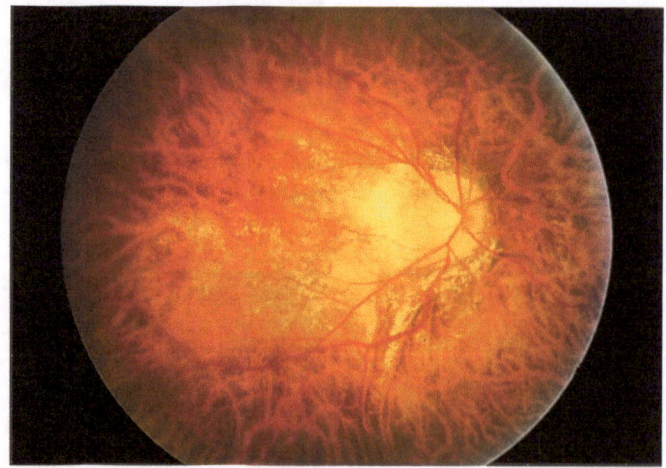

Fig. 13B. Six years later (April 1990), diffuse atrophy has enlarged within the posterior staphyloma. Linear lesions temporal to the macula have progressed into an enlarged lesion of diffuse atrophy. Visual acuity remains 0.7

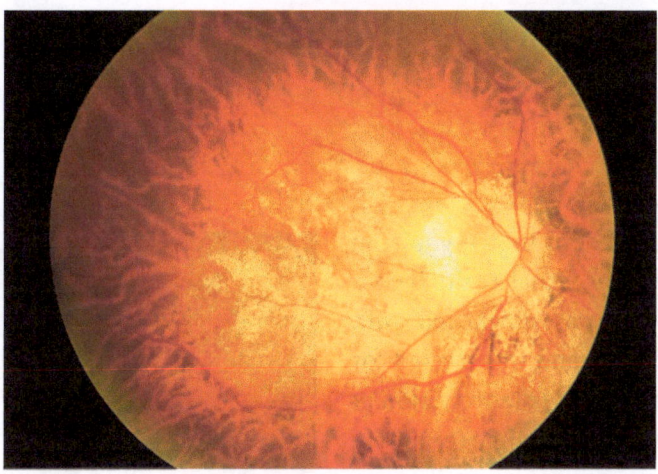

Fig. 13C. Eight years after the initial examination (March 1992), the enlarged lesion of diffuse atrophy has increased further

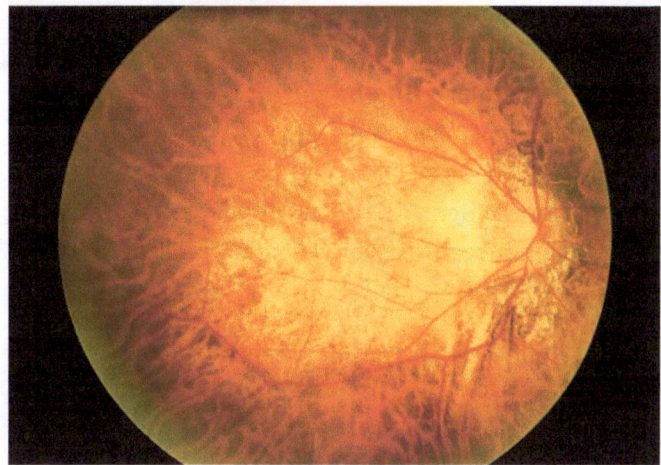

Fig. 13D. Ten years after the initial examination (July 1994), the enlarged lesion of diffuse atrophy has progressed into macular atrophy. Visual acuity is 0.6

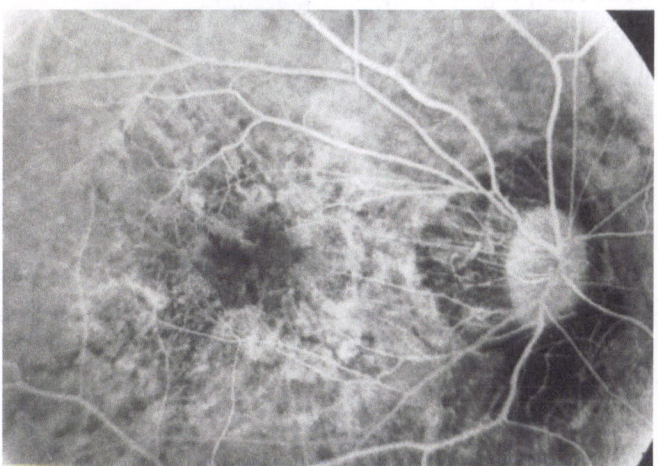

Fig. 13E. Fluorescein fundus angiogram 9 years after the initial examination (May 1993). At 41 sec after dye injection, many lesions of linear hypofluorescence are seen in the posterior fundus. These lesions are not noticeable ophthalmoscopically. An enlarged lesion of diffuse atrophy shows irregular hyperfluorescence

Case 14

A 43-year-old woman was examined for high myopia on June 18, 1976. She noticed decreased visual acuity before entering elementary school. She was diagnosed with amblyopia by a general practitioner and was treated for 4 years. She began wearing glasses for distance vision at age 9 years. She visited our high myopia clinic for severe myopia. Her medical history was noncontributory. One of her nephews has unilateral severe myopia and amblyopia.

In the initial examination, the patient's best corrected visual acuity was 0.1 in the right eye and 0.2 in the left. The refractive error was −23.00 D sphere in the right eye and −23.00 D sphere in the left, and the axial length measurements were 31.3 mm in the right eye and 31.4 mm in the left. Slight cataractous changes were noted. Intraocular pressures and anterior segments were normal in both eyes. We describe the long-term fundus changes in both her eyes.

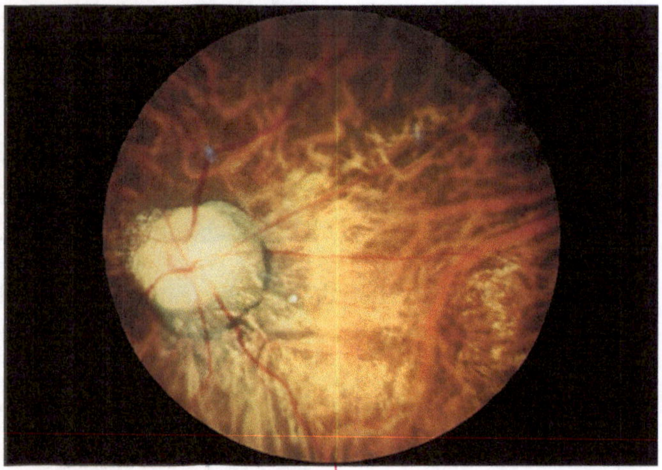

Summary

This woman was followed up for 20 years, since 1976. At the initial examination, linear lesions of diffuse atrophy were observed within the posterior staphyloma. During the follow-up period, an enlarged lesion of diffuse atrophy progressed into macular atrophy (MA). No other myopic fundus changes occurred. The progressive pattern of myopic fundus changes in this patient was from D_2 to MA. No decreased visual acuity was noted during the follow-up period.

Fig. 14A. Left fundus at the initial examination (June 1976) shows an enlarged lesion of diffuse atrophy temporal to the peripapillary crescent. The optic disc tilts temporally. Type I posterior staphyloma is present

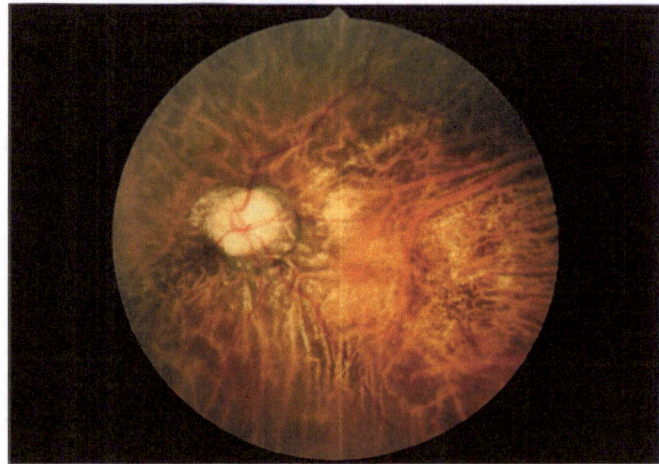

Fig. 14B. Five years later (May 1981), the posterior fundus is covered by an enlarged lesion of diffuse atrophy

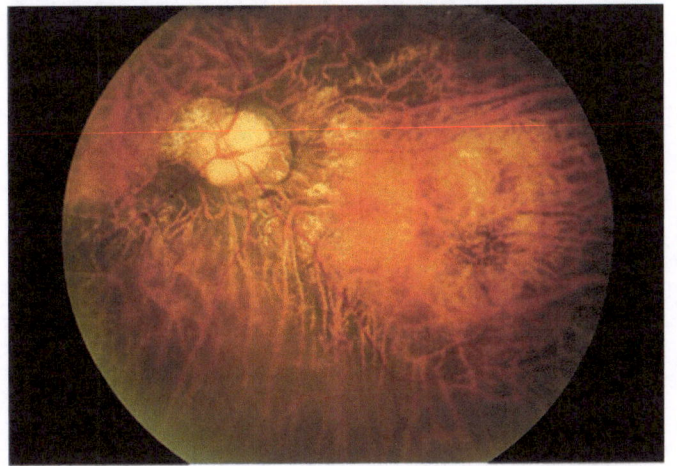

Fig. 14C. Thirteen years after the initial examination (February 1989), an enlarged lesion of diffuse atrophy is found within the posterior staphyloma. The macular lesion has been covered by an enlarged lesion of diffuse atrophy and has become macular atrophy

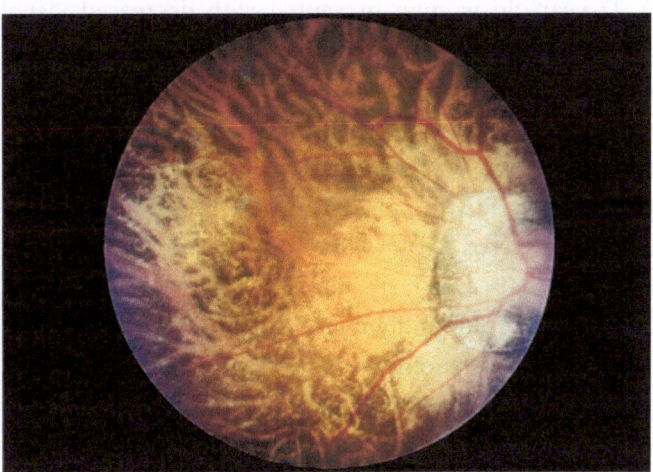

Fig. 14E. Right fundus at the initial examination shows an enlarged lesion of diffuse atrophy temporal to the peripapillary crescent. Sclerotic choroidal vessels are also seen temporal to the macula. The optic disc tilts temporally

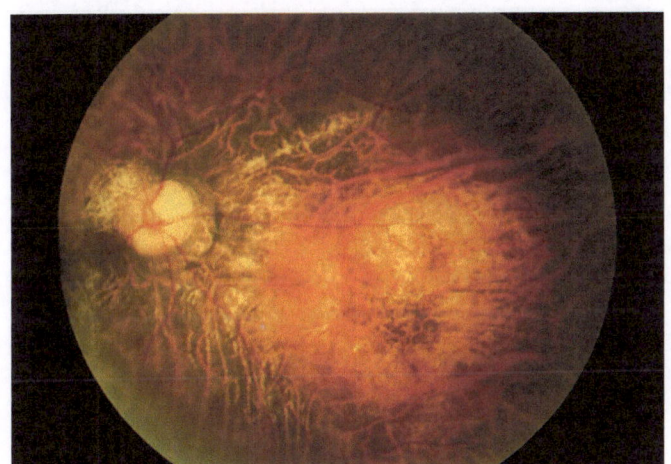

Fig. 14D. Eighteen years after the initial examination (January 1994), the macular lesion is atrophic (MA). Visual acuity is 0.2, and the refractive error is −27.0 D

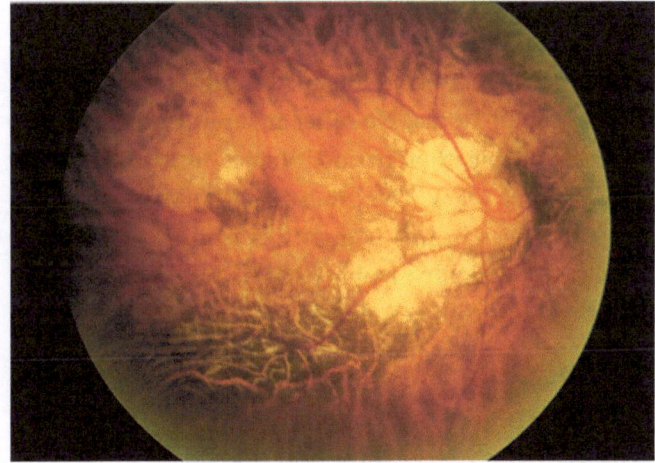

Fig. 14F. Eighteen years later (January 1994), an enlarged lesion of diffuse atrophy covers the entire posterior fundus. The macular lesion is atrophic (MA)

Case 15

A 22-year-old woman presented with decreased visual acuity in both her eyes on October 14, 1983. She was diagnosed with myopia when she entered elementary school and began wearing glasses then. She started wearing contact lenses at age 15 years. Recently, she has reported visual disturbance even with the contact lenses. She was referred to our severe myopia clinic for myopic fundus changes. Her medical history was noncontributory. No family members had severe myopia.

In the initial examination, the patient's best corrected visual acuity was 0.4 in both eyes. The refractive error was −23.00D sphere in the right eye and −22.00D sphere in the left, and the axial length measurements were 31.5mm in the right eye and 31.1mm in the left. Intraocular pressures and anterior segments were normal in both eyes. We describe the long-term fundus changes in her right eye.

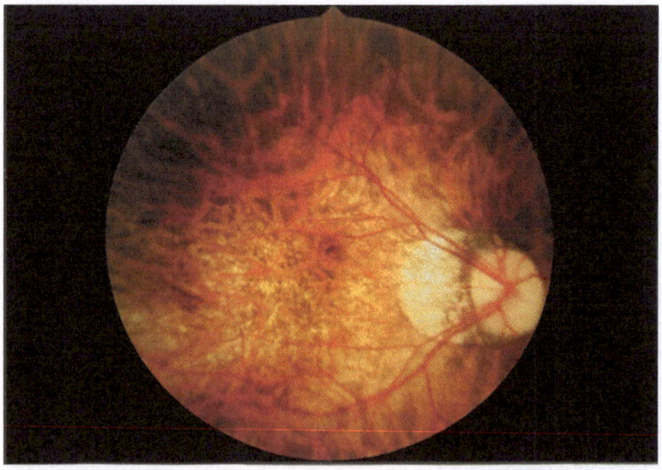

Fig. 15A. Right fundus at the initial examination (October 1983) shows an enlarged lesion of diffuse atrophy in the posterior fundus. The optic disc tilts temporally. Type I posterior staphyloma is present

Summary

This young woman was followed up for 12 years, since 1983. An enlarged lesion of diffuse atrophy gradually enlarged until it covered the posterior fundus within the posterior staphyloma. No other myopic fundus changes occurred during that period. Visual function did not change for 12 years. The progressive pattern of myopic fundus changes in this patient was from D_2 to MA. Although young highly myopic patients rarely show severe myopic fundus changes, diffuse atrophy may progress in extremely myopic young eyes, as in this patient.

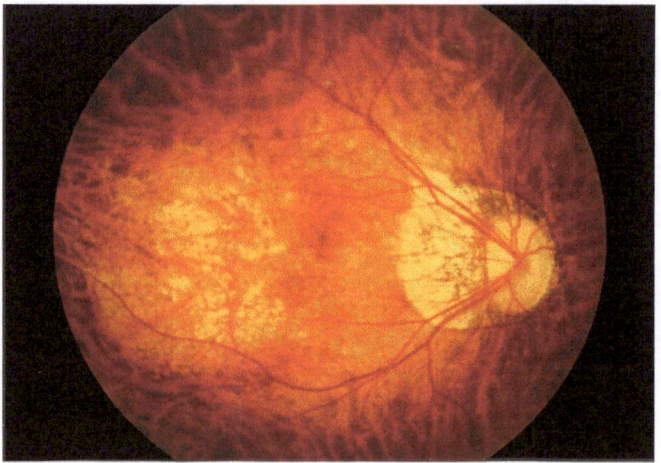

Fig. 15B. Seven years later (April 1991), the enlarged lesion of diffuse atrophy is clear within the posterior staphyloma. Medium- to large-sized choroidal vessels are seen within the lesion of diffuse atrophy. A peripapillary crescent has also enlarged temporally

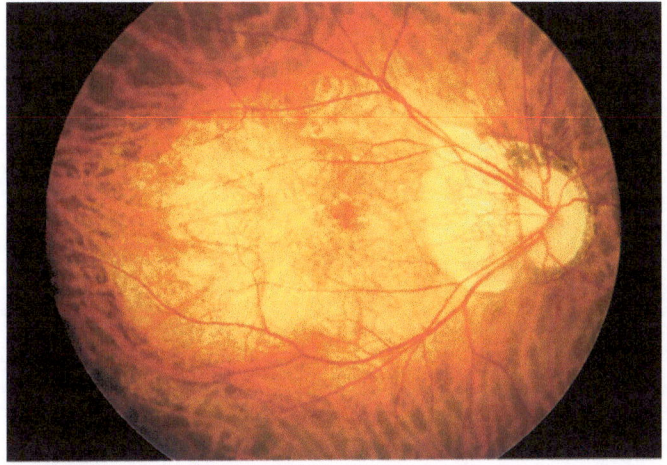

Fig. 15C. Nine years after the initial examination (May 1993), the entire posterior fundus is covered by an enlarged lesion of diffuse atrophy. In the right eye, visual acuity is 0.4, and the refractive error is −23.0 D

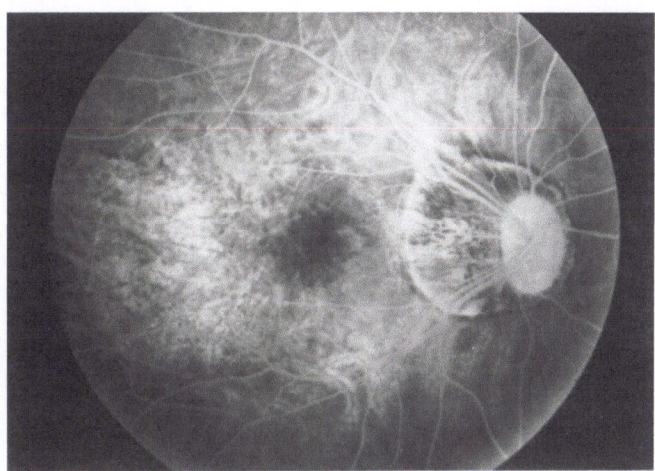

Fig. 15E. Fluorescein fundus angiogram 9 years after the initial examination (May 1993). At 7 min after dye injection, diffuse atrophy shows irregular hyperfluorescence because of tissue staining

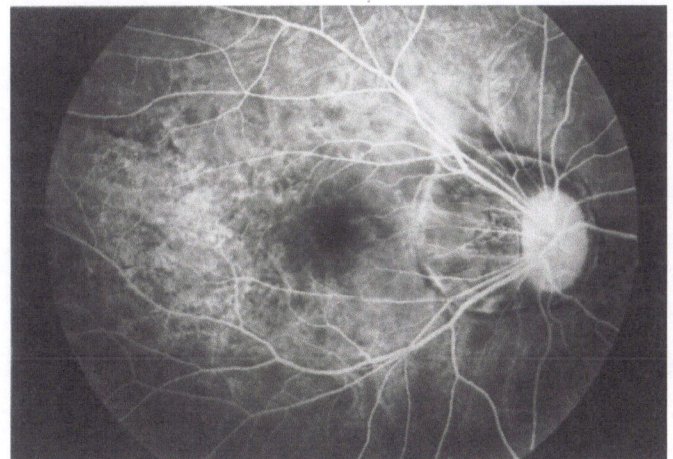

Fig. 15D. Fluorescein fundus angiogram 9 years after the initial examination (May 1993). At 1 min after dye injection, irregular hyperfluorescence is seen temporal to the macula

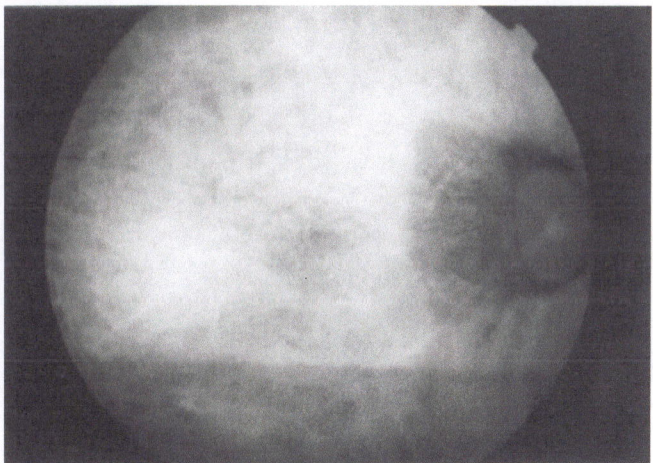

Fig. 15F. Indocyanine green fundus angiogram 10 years after the initial examination (April 1994). At 20 min after dye injection, irregular and linear hypofluorescence is observed in the macular lesion

Lacquer Crack Lesions and Simple Bleeding

Lacquer crack lesions are categorized as D_1, according to the diagnostic guide to myopic chorioretinal atrophy of the Ministry of Health and Welfare, Japan. These lesions commonly run in a crossed fashion against the choroidal vessels, unlike other linear lesions in diffuse atrophy. Lacquer crack lesions first appear around the macular lesion. The progression of lacquer crack lesions is gradual; they gradually increase and widen with time. Fluorescein fundus angiography clearly reveals lacquer crack lesions as linear hyperfluorescence and is very useful in evaluating the progression of lacquer crack lesions.

Lacquer crack lesions show several different progressive patterns. It is well known that lacquer crack lesions are precursors of myopic choroidal neovascularization. However, we have experienced only a few cases in which choroidal neovascularization later developed from lacquer crack lesions. Although choroidal neovascularization is a significant pathological condition accompanying lacquer crack lesions, the rate of the occurrence of choroidal neovascularization is considered to be low.

Diffuse chorioretinal atrophy sometimes enlarges around the lacquer crack lesions and may obscure the lesions and prevent their clear observation. This progressive pattern is noted most frequently. In other cases, the lacquer crack lesions gradually widen with time, and a part of the lesions become atrophic, similar to a spotty lesion of patchy atrophy. Spotty lesions of patchy atrophy sometimes develop within lacquer crack lesions. These show ophthalmoscopic and angiographic findings similar to typical patchy atrophy. Patchy atrophy developed within the lacquer crack lesions is slowly progressive and usually does not impair vision.

Macular bleeding without choroidal neovascularization, called simple bleeding, is caused by the mechanical rupture of Bruch's membrane and choriocapillaris complex because of axial elongation of the eyeball. After the bleeding is absorbed, lacquer crack lesions or spotty lesions of diffuse atrophy may appear at the site of the previous bleeding. Simple bleeding is usually asymptomatic, unless it occurs near the fovea and creates a scotoma in the central visual field. Most simple bleeding occurs besides the macula lesion and is absorbed quickly, making it difficult to detect in highly myopic eyes. The significance of simple bleeding is that it might be a precursor of lacquer crack lesions. Sometimes, other lesions of diffuse atrophy and choroidal sclerosis progress after absorption of simple bleeding. Careful observation is necessary in patients with simple bleeding.

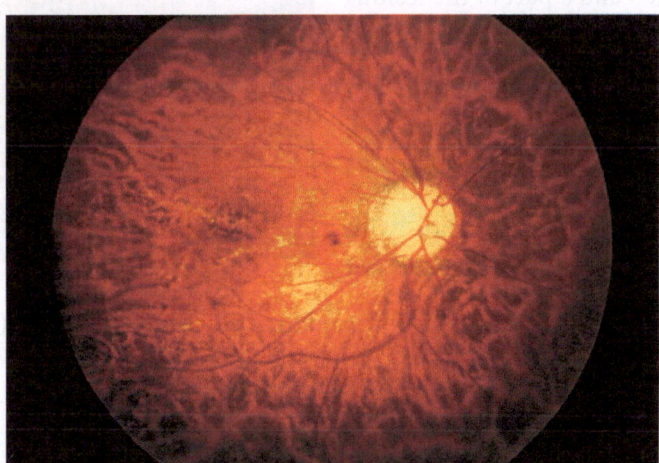

Fig. 18D. *(see page 111)*

Cases 16–23 ▶

Abbreviations *T*: Tessellated fundus; *D*: Diffuse chorioretinal atrophy; *Lc*: Lacquer crack lesion; *P*: Patchy atrophy; *NS*: Simple macular hemorrhage; *HN*: Neovascular macular hemorrhage; *MA*: Chorioretinal atrophy of the macula. For details, refer to Table 3.1 and Fig. 7.1.

Case 16

A 14-year-old girl presented on December 15, 1981, with a history of metamorphopsia in the right eye. She was first examined by a general practitioner when she was 3 years old, and began wearing glasses for severe myopia at that time. The glasses did not improve her visual acuity very much. She was referred to our severe myopia clinic for further examination. Her medical history was noncontributory. No family members had severe myopia.

In the initial examination, the patient's best corrected visual acuity was 1.0 in both eyes. The refractive error was $-20.75\,D$ sphere in both eyes, and her axial length measurements were 29.3 mm in the right eye and 29.4 mm in the left. Intraocular pressures and anterior segments were normal bilaterally. We describe the long-term changes in both her eyes.

Summary

In this patient, lacquer crack lesions appeared and progressed in both eyes during the follow-up period. Before the development of lacquer crack lesions, her left fundus showed only slight diffuse atrophy (D_1) around the optic disc. In the left eye, the lacquer crack lesion developed after absorption of subretinal bleeding. Later, lacquer crack lesions gradually enlarged and a part of the lesions became atrophic, similar to a spotty lesion of patchy atrophy. This pattern of change (from D_1 to $D_1 + Lc$) sometimes occurs in young highly myopic patients who have eyes with relatively long axial length. The lacquer cracks seen in these patients usually first appear temporal to the macula, because this area stretches most with posterior staphyloma. However, this patient did not show evidence of posterior staphyloma.

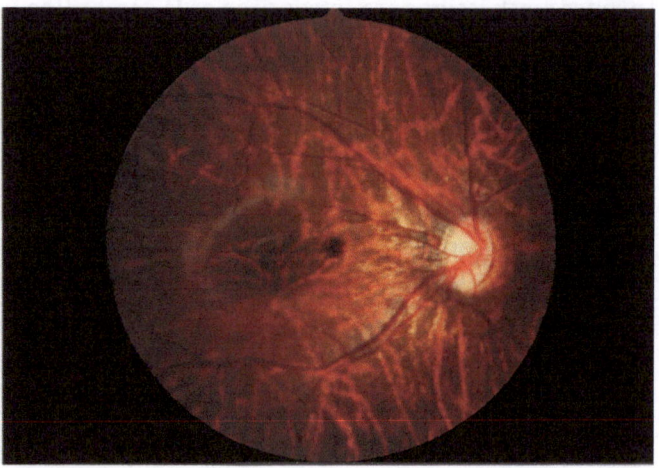

Fig. 16A. Right fundus at the initial examination (December 1981) shows spotty or linear lesions of diffuse atrophy temporal to the optic disc. The optic disc tilts temporally. No posterior staphyloma is present

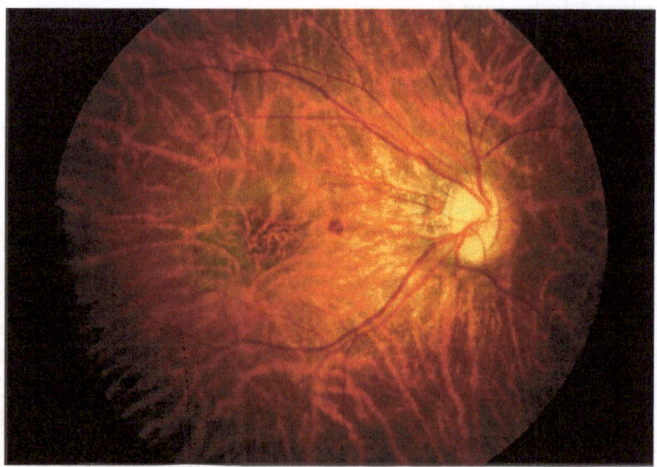

Fig. 16B. Nine years later (September 1992), linear lesions around the optic disc have increased

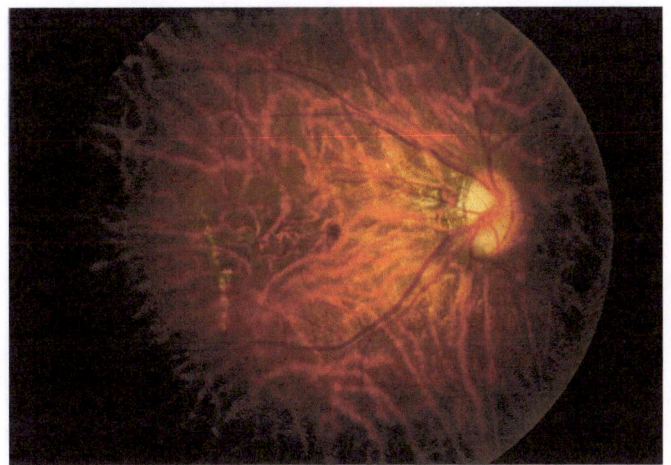

Fig. 16C. Ten years after the initial examination (September 1992), a vertically oriented lacquer crack lesion appears temporal to the macula. No simple bleeding is detected

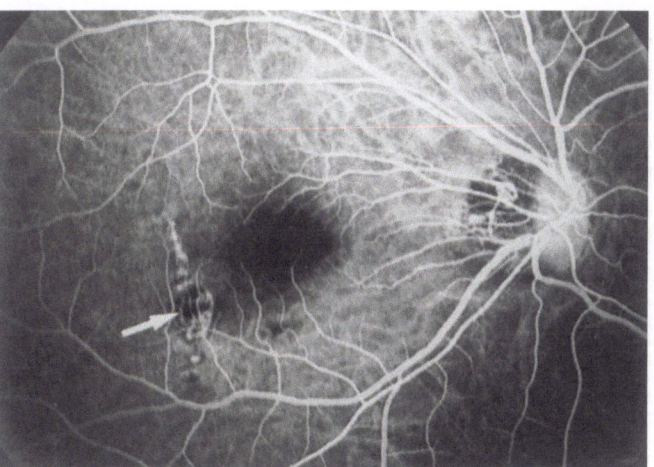

Fig. 16E. Fluorescein fundus angiogram of Fig. 16D. At 34 sec after dye injection, the lacquer crack lesion appears as linear hyperfluorescence because of a window defect. The central part of the lesion is hypofluorescent (*arrow*)

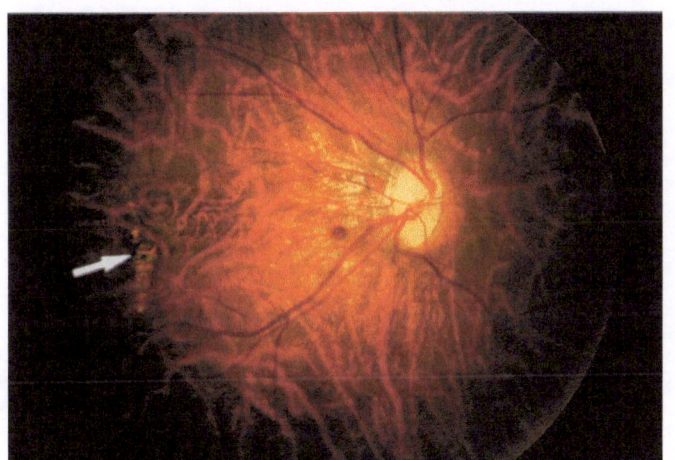

Fig. 16D. Twelve years after the initial examination (March 1994), the lacquer crack lesion has enlarged. The central part of the lacquer crack lesion is pigmented and is beginning to progress to small patchy atrophy (*arrow*)

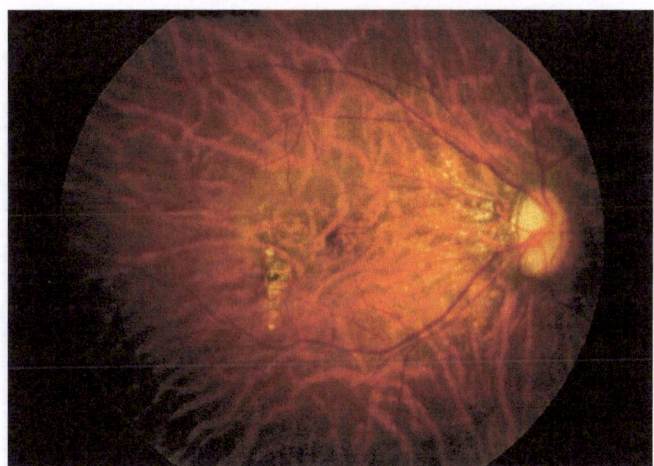

Fig. 16F. Twelve years after the initial examination (December 1994), the lacquer crack lesion has slightly widened. Visual acuity is 1.0, and the refractive error is −20.0 D

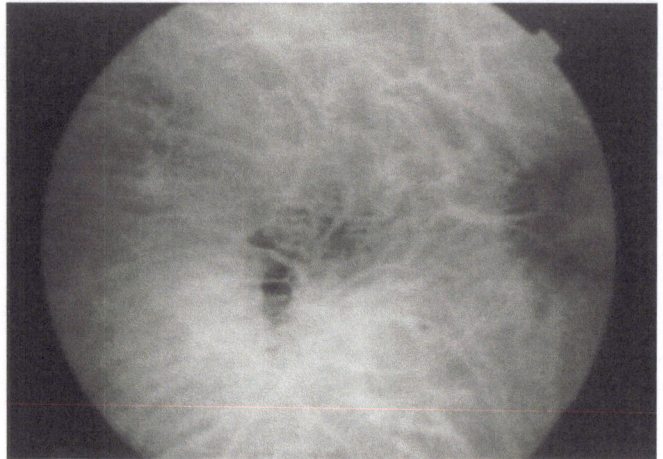

Fig. 16G. Indocyanine green fundus angiogram 13 years after the initial examination (March 1995) shows linear hypofluorescence corresponding to the lacquer crack lesion in the late angiographic phase

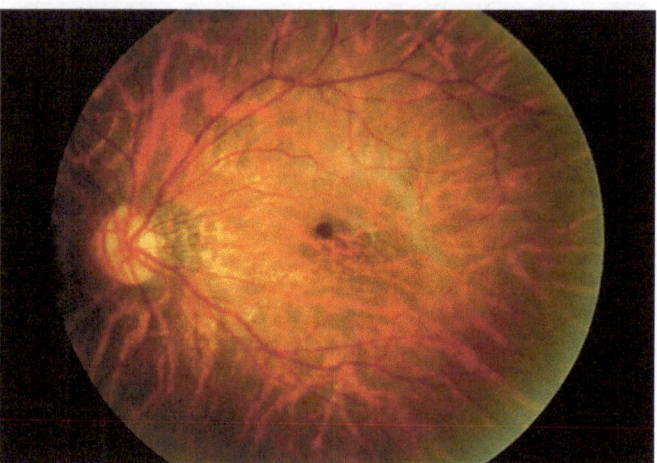

Fig. 16I. Five years later (August 1987), spotty and linear lesions of diffuse atrophy have increased temporal to the optic disc. A red dot in the center is a photographic artifact

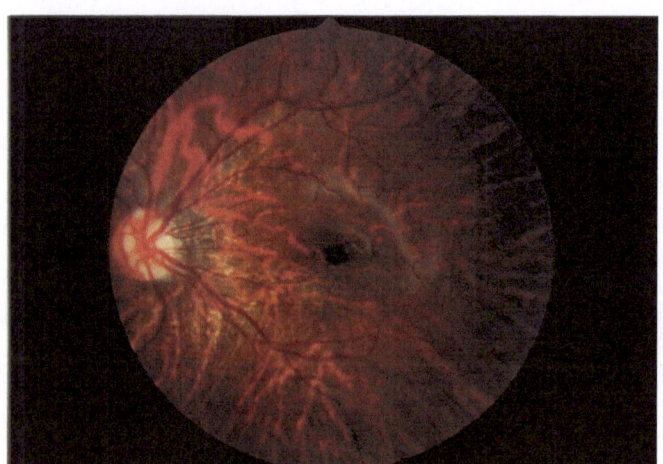

Fig. 16H. Left fundus at the initial examination (December 1981) shows a slight diffuse atrophy around the optic disc. The optic disc tilts temporally. No posterior staphyloma is present

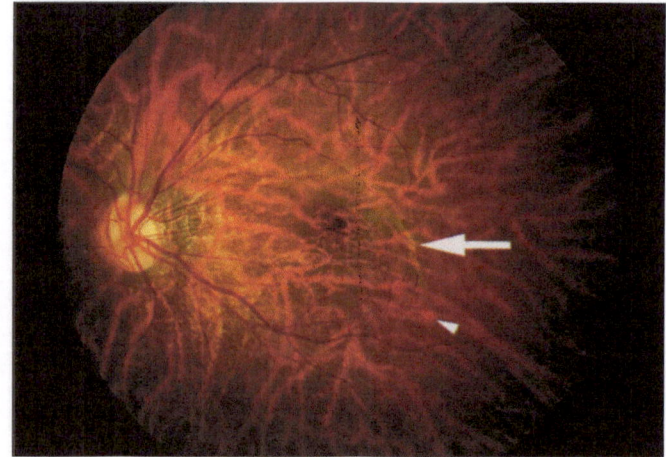

Fig. 16J. Ten years after the initial examination (September 1992), a short and vertically oriented lacquer crack lesion is noted temporal to the macula (*arrow*). A small retinal bleeding is seen inferior to the lacquer crack lesion (*arrowhead*). Visual acuity is 1.0, and the refractive error is −21.0 D

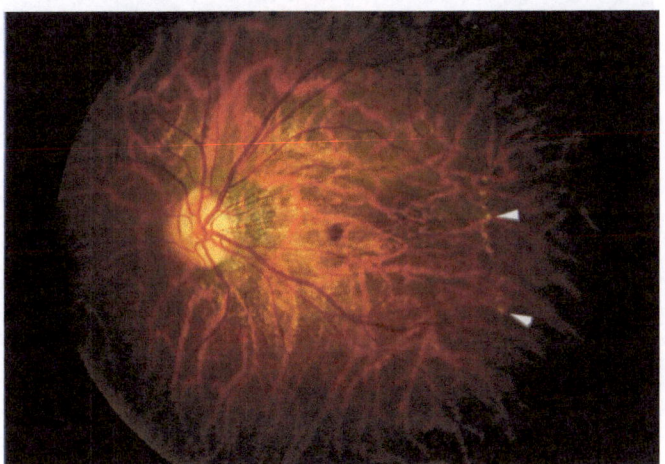

Fig. 16K. Eleven years after the initial examination (September 1993), the lacquer crack has elongated. Some areas within the lacquer crack have progressed to spotty lesions of patchy atrophy (*arrowheads*)

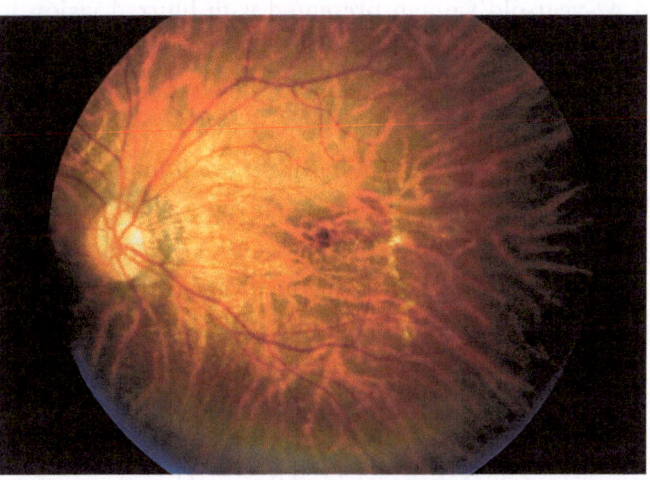

Fig. 16M. Twelve years after the initial examination (December 1994), subretinal bleeding has occurred next to the earlier lacquer crack lesion. Visual acuity is 1.0, and the refractive error is −21.0 D. Patient reported no visual disturbance as a result of the bleeding

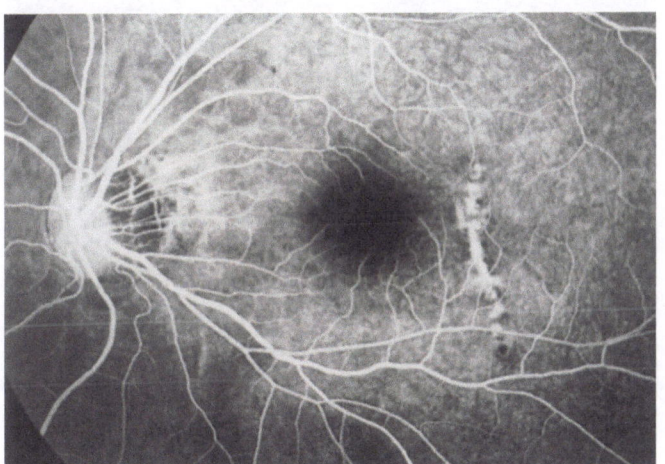

Fig. 16L. Fluorescein angiogram 12 years after the initial examination (March 1994). At 54 sec after dye injection, the lacquer crack lesion shows linear hyperfluorescence because of a window defect

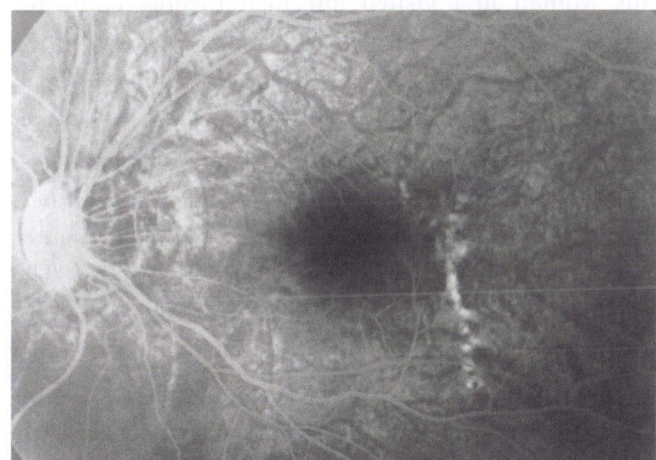

Fig. 16N. Fluorescein angiogram 13 years after the initial examination (March 1995). Subretinal bleeding has spontaneously absorbed in 2 months. At 8 min after dye injection, a new lacquer crack lesion is observed branching from the original lacquer crack lesion at the corresponding site of the previous hemorrhage. Dye leakage suggesting the existence of choroidal neovascularization is not seen

Case 17

A 42-year-old woman presented with blurred vision in her right eye on June 22, 1977. She noticed decreased visual acuity after entering junior high school. She began wearing glasses for distance vision at age 18 years. She noticed blurred vision in her right eye 3 months before her first examination in our high myopia clinic. A general practitioner had diagnosed the cause as macular bleeding in the right fundus. Her medical history was noncontributory. No family members had severe myopia.

In the initial examination, the patient's best corrected visual acuity was 0.7 in the right eye and 1.0 in the left eye. The refractive error was −13.50 D sphere in the right eye and −6.25 D in the left, and the axial length measurements were 28.4 mm in the right eye and 25.3 mm in the left. Intraocular pressures and anterior segments were normal in both eyes. We describe the long-term fundus changes in her right eye.

Summary

This woman first visited our high myopia clinic for further examination of myopic macular bleeding in the right eye. At the initial examination, the bleeding had already absorbed, and lacquer crack lesions had developed in the macula. The lacquer crack lesions increased with time and finally showed a reticular appearance. Their margins gradually became less clear as a result of an enlargement of surrounding diffuse atrophy. The cause of a sudden visual decrease in 1990 was not obvious. A small macular hole could have caused it, but a myopic macular hole without retinal detachment is difficult to find because of the chorioretinal atrophy in highly myopic eyes.

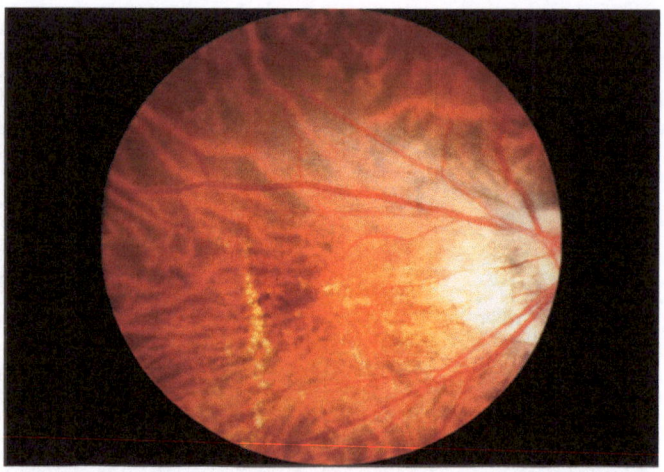

Fig. 17A. Right fundus at the initial examination (June 1977) shows a vertically oriented lacquer crack lesion temporal to the macula. Macular bleeding has already absorbed. Spotty or linear lesions of diffuse atrophy are visible temporal to the optic disc. The optic disc tilts temporally. A temporal peripapillary crescent is observed

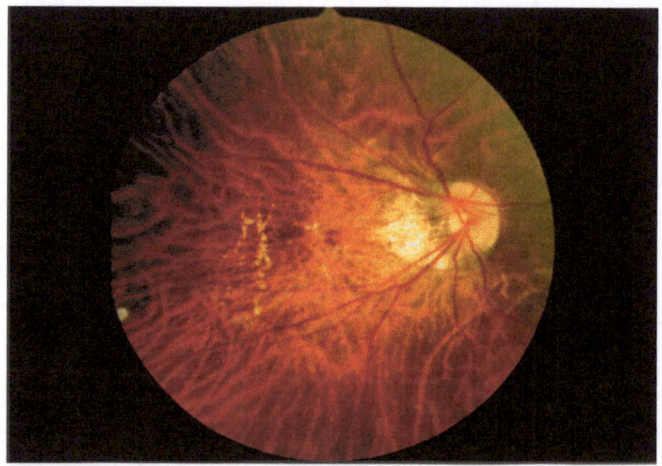

Fig. 17B. One year later (July 1978), lacquer crack lesions have increased. Diffuse atrophy has also enlarged temporal to the optic disc. Visual acuity is 0.7, and the refractive error is −13.50 D

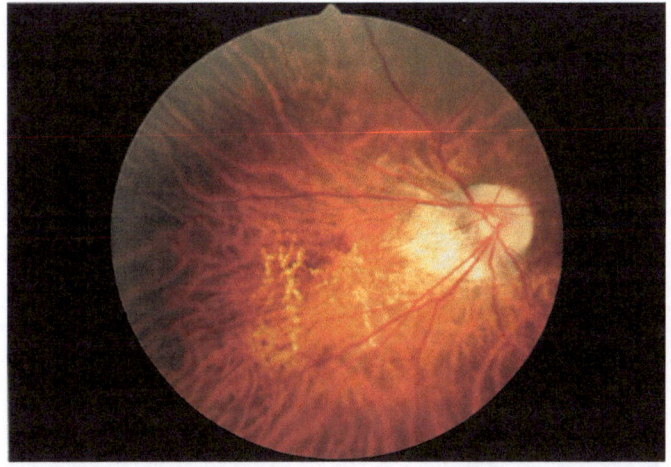

Fig. 17C. Four years after the initial examination (November 1981), lacquer crack lesions have branched off and increased. Diffuse atrophy has also enlarged, covering the lacquer crack lesion nasal to the macula

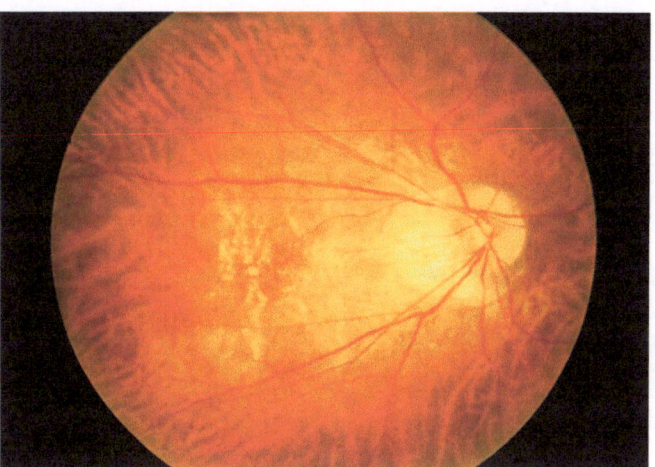

Fig. 17E. Eleven years after the initial examination (July 1988), the margin of lacquer crack lesions is becoming less clear, as it is surrounded by an enlarged lesion of diffuse atrophy

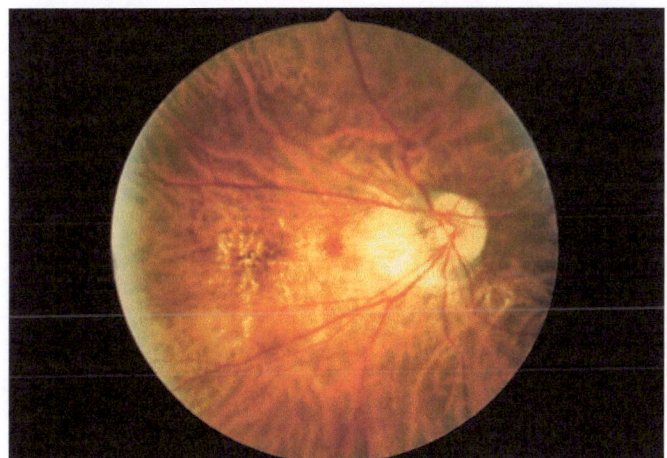

Fig. 17D. Eight years after the initial examination (October 1985), lacquer crack lesions have further increased. An enlarged lesion of diffuse atrophy is observed temporal to the optic disc

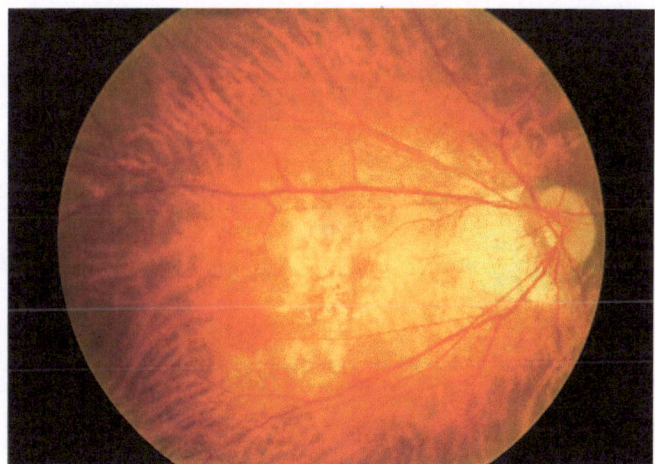

Fig. 17F. Thirteen years after the initial examination (June 1990), lacquer crack lesions have widened and appear reticular. The peripapillary crescent has also enlarged. A small macular hole is observed. Visual acuity has decreased to 0.2, and the refractive error is −15.00 D. No retinal bleeding or choroidal neovascularization is detected

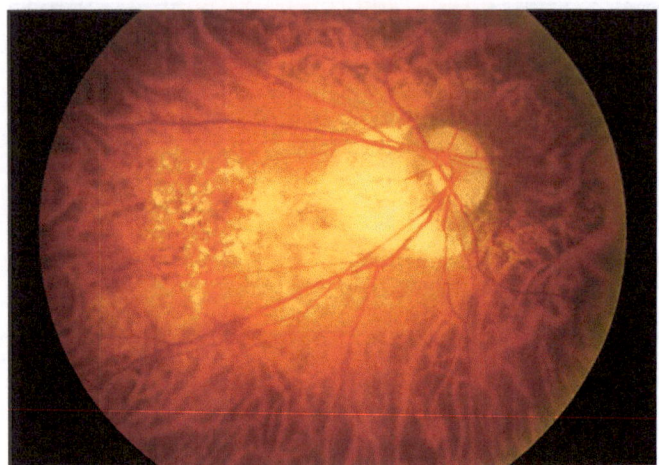

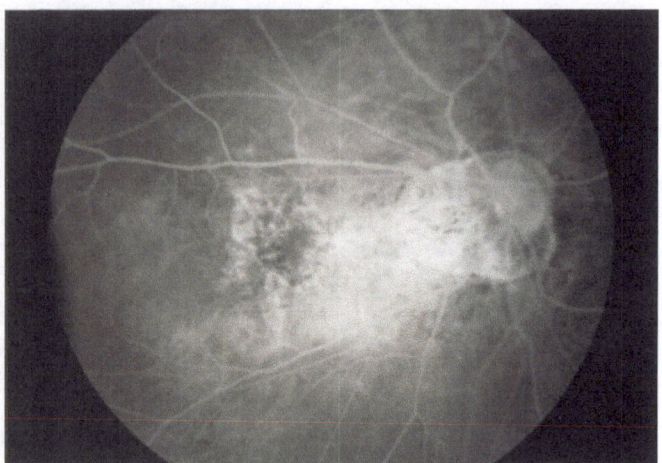

Fig. 17G. Sixteen years after the initial examination (January 1993), lacquer crack lesions are not obvious and are surrounded by an enlarged lesion of diffuse atrophy. The macular lesion is atrophic. Visual acuity remains 0.2, and the refractive error is −15.00 D

Fig. 17I. Fluorescein fundus angiogram 16 years after the initial examination (January 1993). At 8 min after dye injection, irregular hyperfluorescence corresponding to diffuse atrophy is still visible in the late phase. Lacquer crack lesions do not show typical hyperfluorescence. No choroidal neovascularization is observed

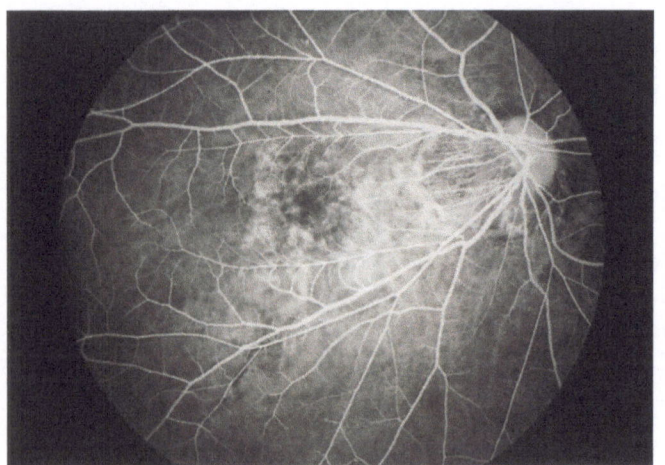

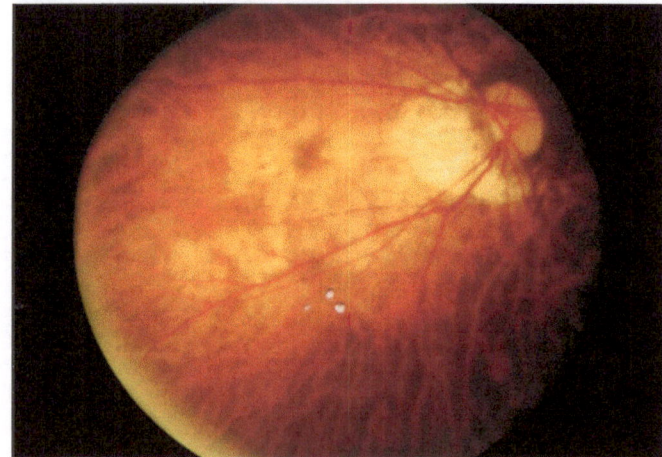

Fig. 17H. Fluorescein fundus angiogram 16 years after the initial examination (January 1993). At 29 sec after dye injection, lacquer crack lesions do not show typical linear hyperfluorescence. Irregular hyperfluorescence is seen, corresponding to the diffuse atrophy in the posterior fundus

Fig. 17J. Eighteen years after the initial examination (January 1995), a shallow retinal detachment caused by a myopic macular hole has occurred. Visual acuity remains 0.1, and the refractive error is −14.00 D

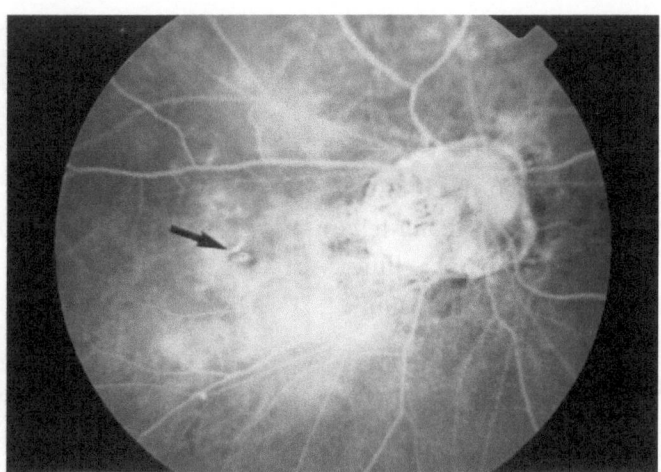

Fig. 17K. Fluorescein fundus angiogram 18 years after the initial examination (January 1995). At 7 min after dye injection, a macular hole shows hyperfluorescence (*arrow*). Pooling of the dye is visible in the subretinal space of the detached retina

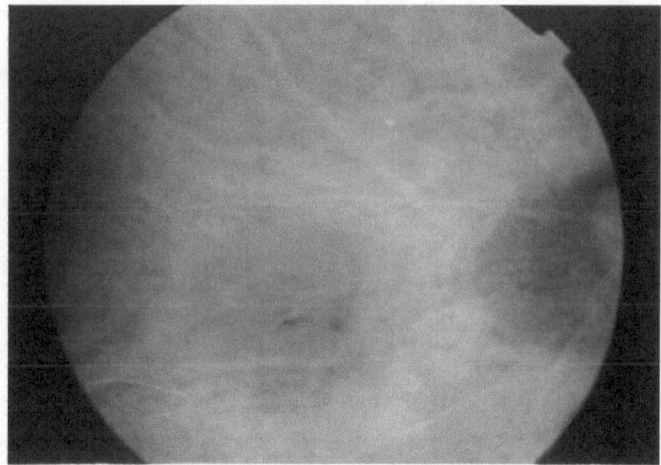

Fig. 17L. Indocyanine green fundus angiogram 18 years after the initial examination (January 1995). In the late phase of the angiogram, the macular lesion is hypofluorescent and corresponds to the area of retinal detachment

Case 18

A 24-year-old woman was examined for retinal bleedings in both her eyes on April 13, 1990. She was diagnosed with myopia as an infant. She began wearing glasses for distance vision at age 5 years and began wearing contact lenses at age 14. A general practitioner reported fundus bleeding in her right eye in 1982 and 1985 and in her left eye in 1983. She was referred to our high myopia clinic for further examination. Her medical history was non-contributory. No family members had severe myopia.

In the initial examination, the patient's best corrected visual acuity was 0.8 in the right eye and 0.8 in the left. The refractive error was −16.25 D sphere in the right eye and −18.25 D sphere in the left, and the axial length measurements were 30.1 mm in the right eye and 30.7 mm in the left. Intraocular pressures and anterior segments were normal in both eyes. We describe the long-term fundus changes in both her eyes.

Summary

This woman was followed up for 5 years, since 1990. Both fundi showed typical lacquer crack lesions at the initial examination. Simple macular bleeding was observed in both fundi. After the absorption of the simple bleeding, new lacquer crack lesions have developed at the site of the previous bleeding. The progression of lacquer crack lesions in this patient is typical of that in highly myopic eyes. In the left eye, although the lacquer crack lesions are not obvious ophthalmoscopically, they are clear with fluorescein fundus angiography. The lacquer crack lesions gradually widened with time, and a part of the lesions became atrophic, similar to a spotty lesion of patchy atrophy.

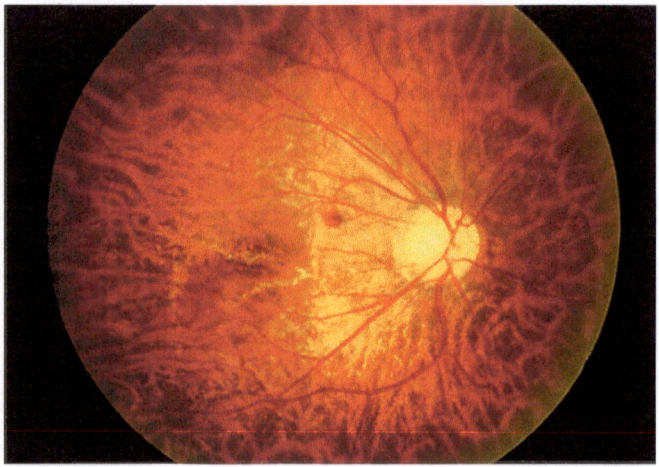

Fig. 18A. Right fundus at the initial examination (April 1990) shows vertical and horizontal lacquer crack lesions in the macula. Simple bleeding is seen inferotemporal to the macula. Spotty or linear lesions of diffuse atrophy are observed temporal to the optic disc. The optic disc tilts temporally. No posterior staphyloma is present

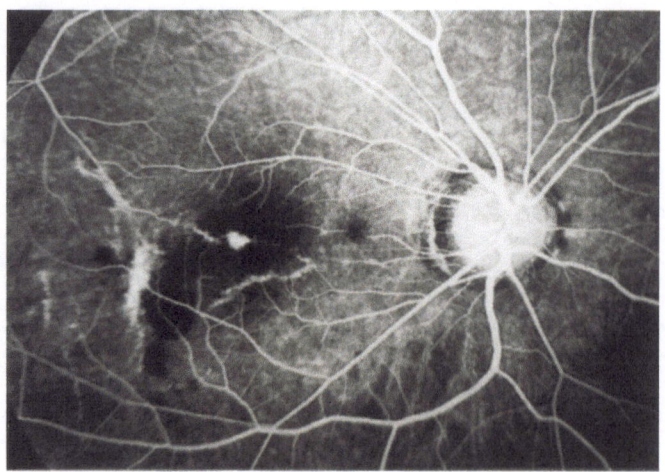

Fig. 18B. Fluorescein angiogram 1 month after the initial examination (May 1990). At 1 min after dye injection, lacquer crack lesions show linear hyperfluorescence. Simple bleeding shows blocked fluorescence. The hyperfluorescent spot, similar to myopic choroidal neovascularization, is seen in the fovea

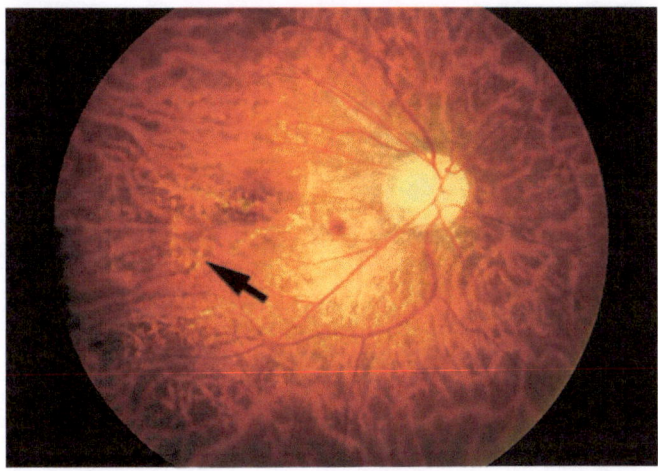

Fig. 18C. Six months later (September 1990), the bleeding has absorbed, and lacquer crack lesions have newly appeared at the site of the previous bleeding (*arrow*)

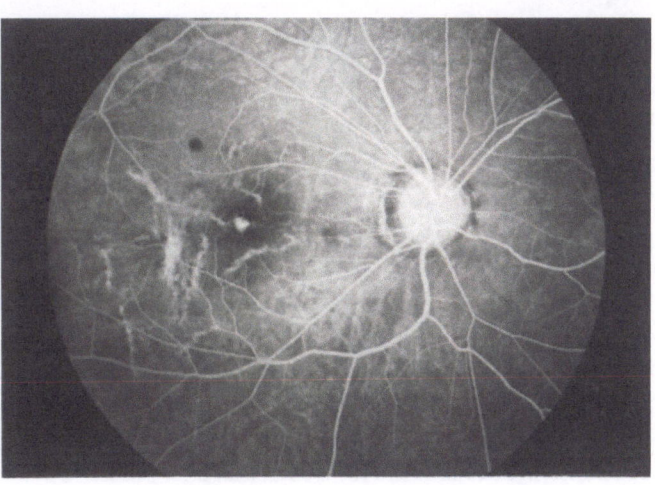

Fig. 18E. Fluorescein fundus angiogram 1 year after the initial examination (July 1991). At 3 min after dye injection, lacquer crack lesions are seen to have increased inferior to the macula. They are clearly visible as linear hyperfluorescence angiographically

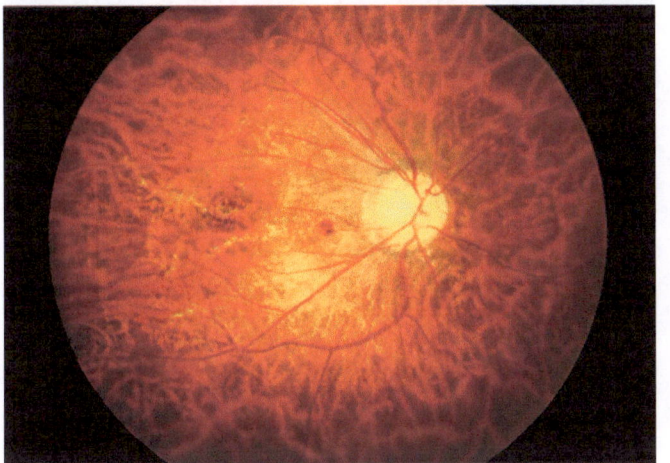

Fig. 18D. One year after the initial examination (June 1991), lacquer crack lesions show no remarkable progression. Visual acuity is 0.7, and the refractive error is −19.75 D

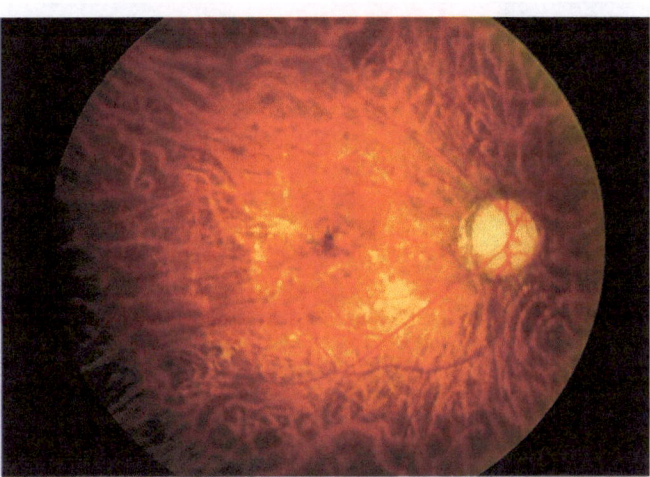

Fig. 18F. Two years after the initial examination (October 1992), lacquer crack lesions have widened and increased. Spotty or linear lesions of diffuse atrophy have also enlarged. Visual acuity is 0.7, and the refractive error is −19.75 D

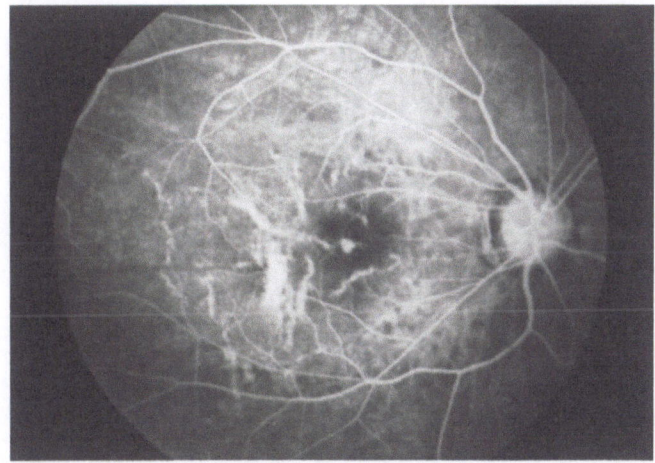

Fig. 18G. Fluorescein fundus angiogram 3 years after the initial examination (December 1993). At 2 min after dye injection, linear hyperfluorescence corresponding to the lacquer crack lesions have increased and widened

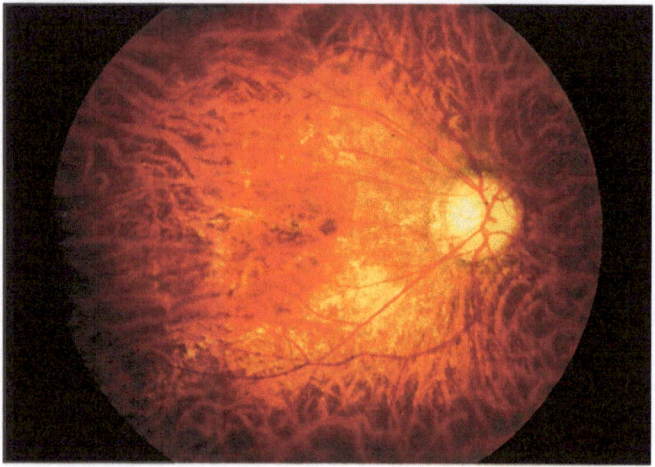

Fig. 18H. Four years after the initial examination (May 1994), the lacquer crack lesions have further increased. Spotty or linear lesions of diffuse atrophy have also enlarged. Visual acuity is 0.7, and the refractive error is −20.00 D

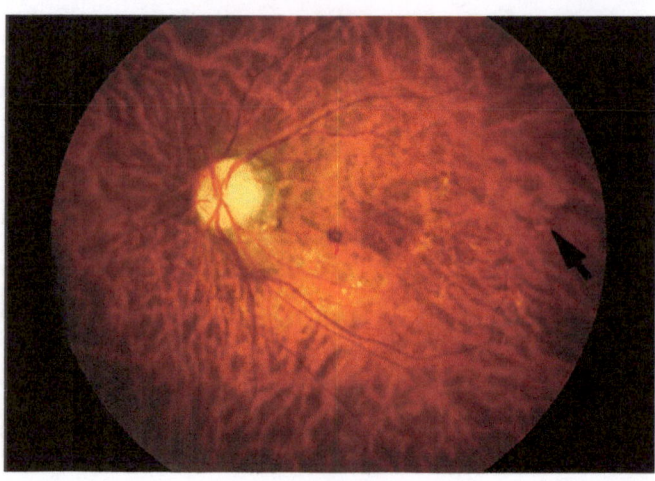

Fig. 18K. Six months later (September 1990), the bleeding is absorbed. A new lacquer crack lesion has appeared at the site of the previous bleeding (*arrow*)

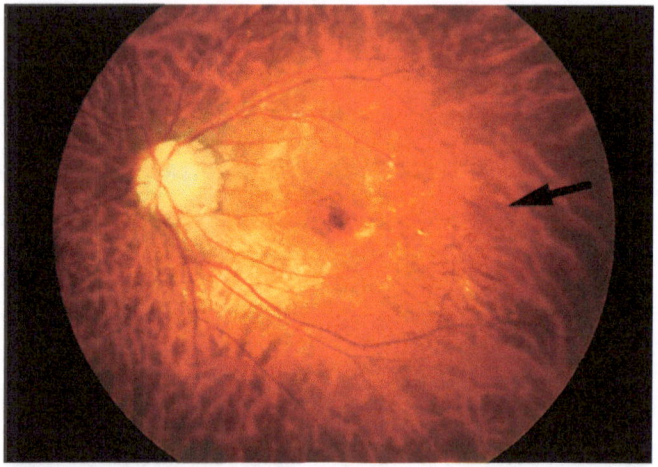

Fig. 18I. Left fundus at the initial examination (April 1990) shows vertically oriented lacquer crack lesions temporal to the macula. Round bleeding is seen temporal to the lacquer crack lesions (*arrow*). Linear lesions of diffuse atrophy are observed temporal to the optic disc. The optic disc tilts temporally. No posterior staphyloma is present

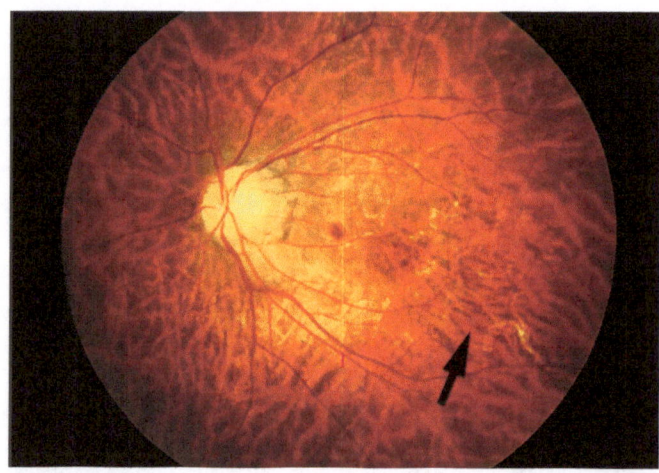

Fig. 18L. One year after the initial examination (June 1991), new bleeding appears inferotemporal to the macula (*arrow*). Diffuse atrophy temporal to the optic disc has enlarged

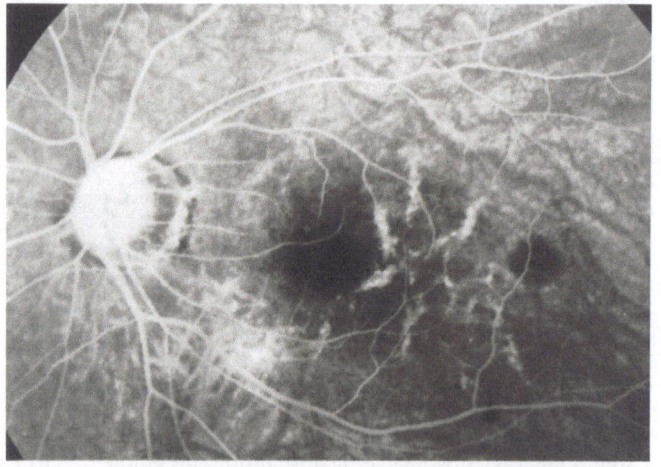

Fig. 18J. Fluorescein fundus angiogram at the initial examination (April 1990). At 513 sec after dye injection, lacquer crack lesions show linear hyperfluorescence. The round bleeding shows blocked fluorescence. No choroidal neovascularization is detected. Linear lesions of diffuse atrophy show irregular hyperfluorescence inferotemporal to the optic disc

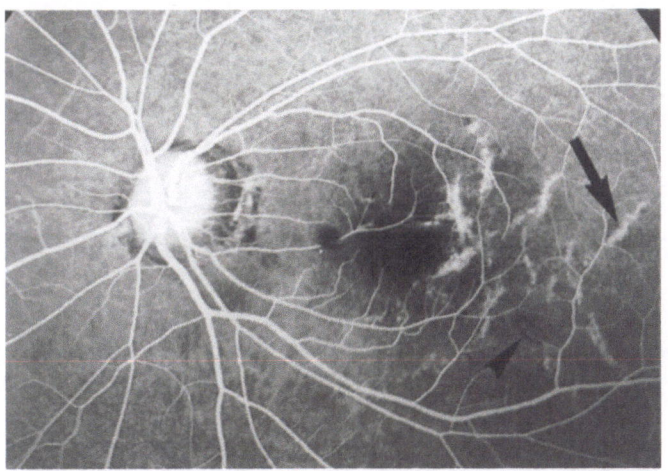

Fig. 18M. Fluorescein fundus angiogram 1 year after the initial examination (July 1991). At 45 sec after dye injection, a new lacquer crack lesion at the site of the previous bleeding shows linear hyperfluorescence (*arrow*). Simple bleeding shows blocked fluorescence (*arrowhead*)

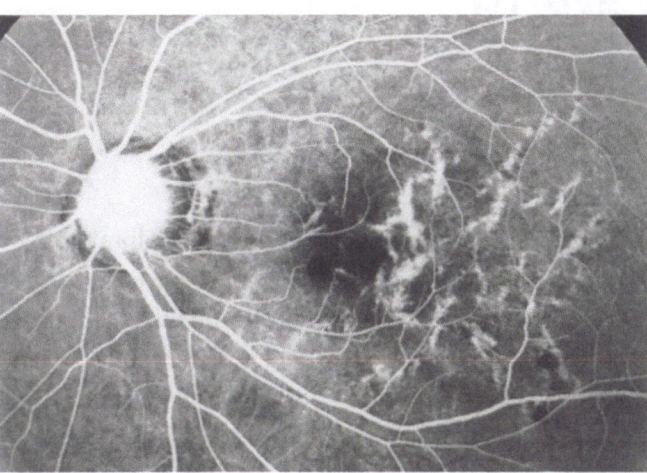

Fig. 18O. Fluorescein fundus angiogram 3 years after the initial examination (December 1993). At 47 sec after dye injection, it is noticeable that the lacquer crack lesions have increased. They are reticular in appearance. Spotty lesions of patchy atrophy are hypofluorescent in the early phase

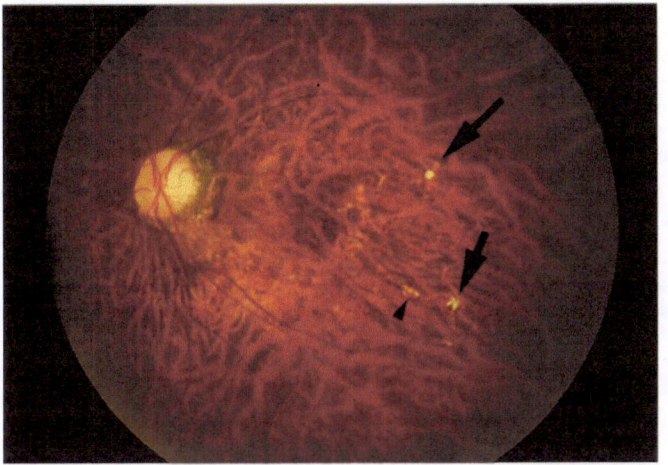

Fig. 18N. Two years after the initial examination (October 1992), two spotty lesions of patchy atrophy have appeared temporal to the macula (*arrows*). A new lacquer crack lesion is found at the corresponding site of the previous bleeding (*arrowhead*)

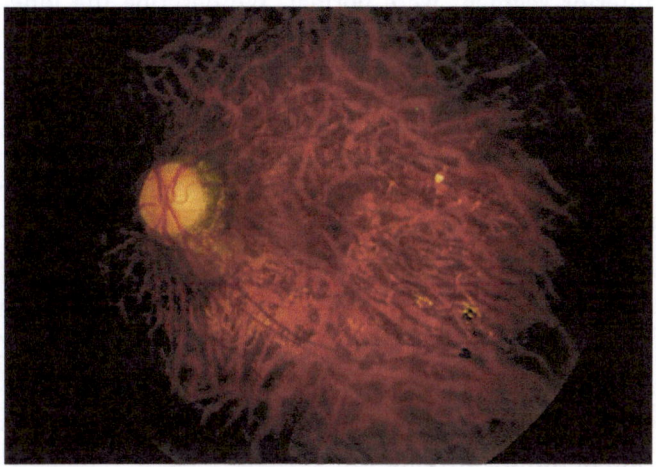

Fig. 18P. Four years after the initial examination (May 1994), lacquer crack lesions and spotty lesions of patchy atrophy have not progressed. Pigmentation is observed within the patchy atrophy

Fig. 18Q. Indocyanine green fundus angiogram 3 years after the initial examination (December 1993). In the early phase of the angiogram, spotty lesions of patchy atrophy show hypofluorescence. Lacquer crack lesions show mild hypofluorescence (*arrowheads*)

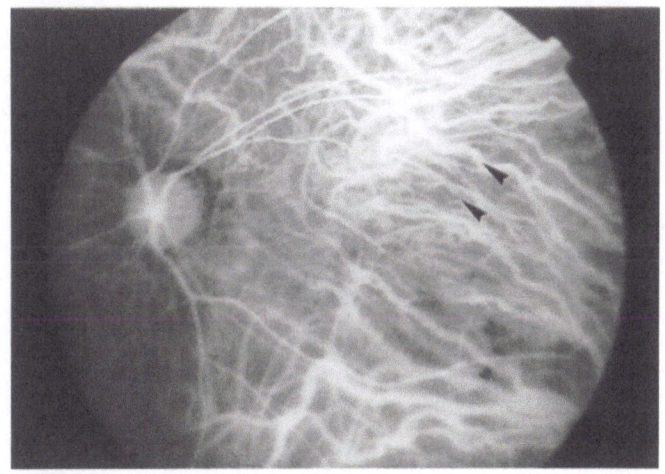

Case 19

A 27-year-old woman was examined for high myopia on March 1, 1983. Her right eye was enucleated because of retinoblastoma at age 1 year. The uncorrected visual acuity of her left eye was 0.3 when she entered elementary school. She began wearing glasses at age 11 years, and began wearing contact lenses at age 21. Her medical history was noncontributory. One of her siblings was highly myopic.

In the initial examination, the patient's best corrected visual acuity was 1.0 in the left eye. The refractive error was −15.25 D sphere, and the axial length measurement was 28.9 mm in the left eye. Intraocular pressure and anterior segment were normal. We describe the long-term fundus changes in her left eye.

Summary

This woman was followed up for 10 years, since 1983. Her left fundus showed the progression of spotty and linear lesions of diffuse atrophy and the occurrence of lacquer crack lesions during the follow-up period. Simple macular bleeding also appeared with the progression of diffuse atrophy. These findings show the close relationship between simple macular bleeding and the progression of diffuse atrophy.

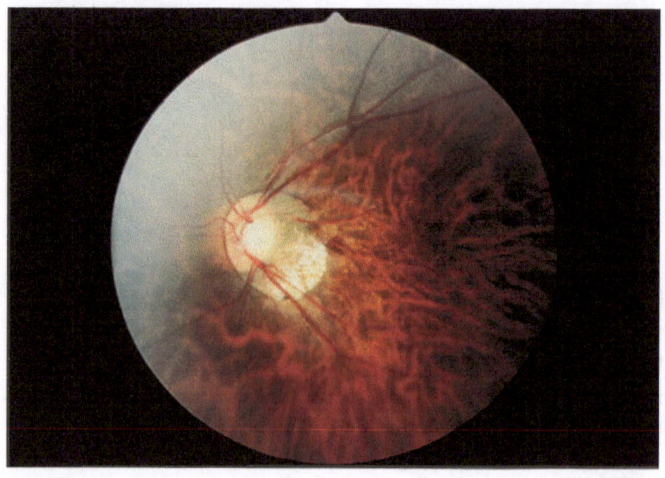

Fig. 19A. Left fundus at the initial examination (March 1983) shows only a tessellated fundus. The optic disc tilts temporally. Temporal peripapillary crescent is seen. No posterior staphyloma is present

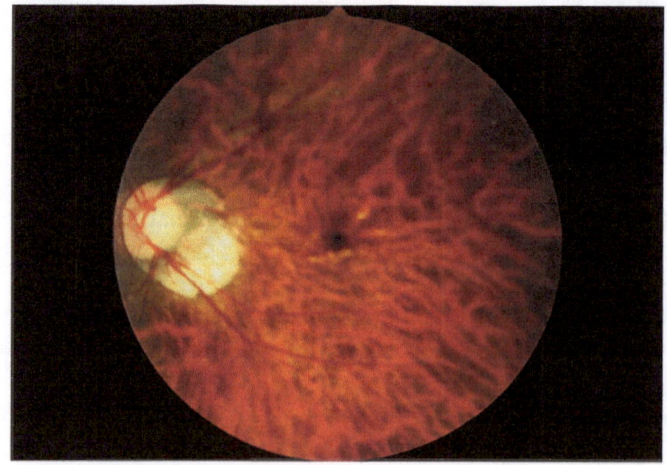

Fig. 19B. Two years later (October 1985), lacquer crack lesions and linear lesions of diffuse atrophy appear in the macular lesion. In the left eye, visual acuity is 0.9, and the refractive error is −18.00 D

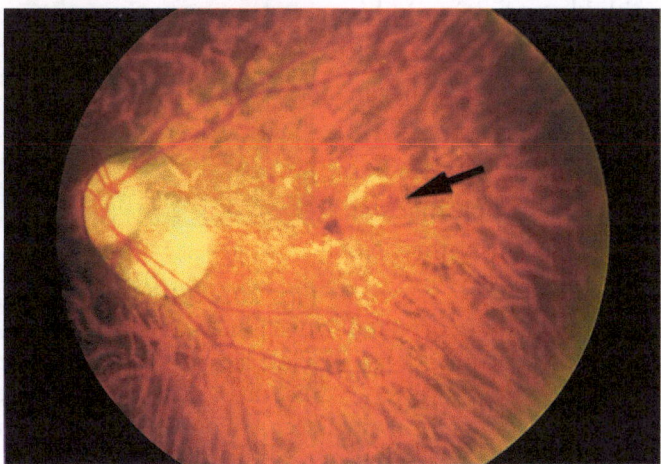

Fig. 19C. Five years after the initial examination (April 1988), lacquer crack lesions have increased. Spotty and linear lesions of diffuse atrophy have also increased around the lacquer crack lesions. Retinal bleeding appears temporal to the macula (*arrow*)

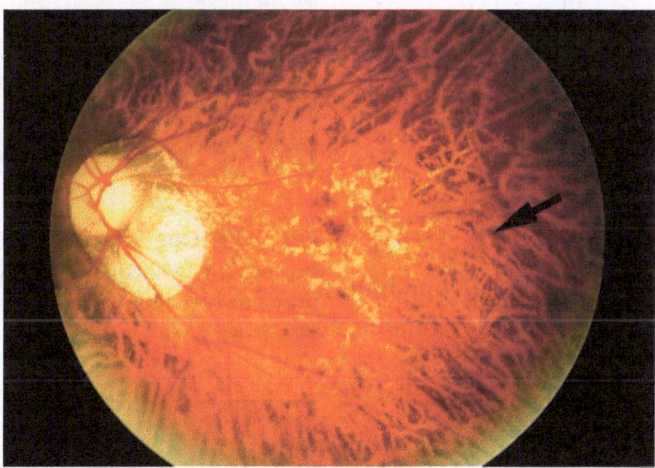

Fig. 19D. Seven years after the initial examination (March 1990), lacquer crack lesions are becoming unclear with the enlargement of surrounding diffuse atrophy. The peripapillary crescent has enlarged inferotemporally. A new retinal bleeding appears temporal to the macula (*arrow*)

Case 20

A 31-year-old man presented with blurred vision in his right eye on January 9, 1987. He was diagnosed with myopia on entering elementary school. He began wearing glasses for distance vision at age 8 years. He noticed a central scotoma in his right eye in 1983. He was diagnosed in a nearby hospital as having myopic macular bleeding. His medical history was noncontributory. No family members had severe myopia.

In the initial examination, the patient's best corrected visual acuity was 0.7 in the right eye and 1.0 in the left. The refractive error was −14.00 D sphere in the right eye and −13.00 D sphere in the left, and the axial length measurements were 30.2 mm in the right eye and 30.1 mm in the left. Intraocular pressures and anterior segments were normal in both eyes. We describe the long-term fundus changes in his right eye.

Summary

This man was followed up for 9 years, since 1987. He presented with blurred vision caused by simple macular bleeding. After the bleeding absorbed, his vision gradually recovered, diffuse atrophy progressed, and lacquer crack lesions appeared. A spotty lesion of patchy atrophy later appeared at the temporal edge of the lacquer crack lesion and gradually enlarged. The progressive pattern of myopic fundus changes in this patient was from Lc to P_1. With the appearance of patchy atrophy, surrounding diffuse atrophy also enlarged in the posterior fundus, suggesting sclerotic changes of the choroidal vessels.

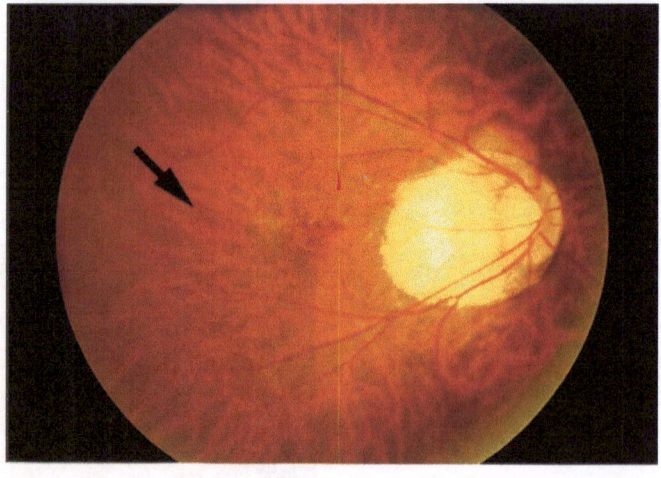

Fig. 20A. Right fundus at the initial examination (January 1987) shows a retinal bleeding temporal to the macula (*arrow*). Short lacquer crack lesions are seen in the macula. The optic disc tilts temporally. A large temporal peripapillary crescent is seen. No posterior staphyloma is present

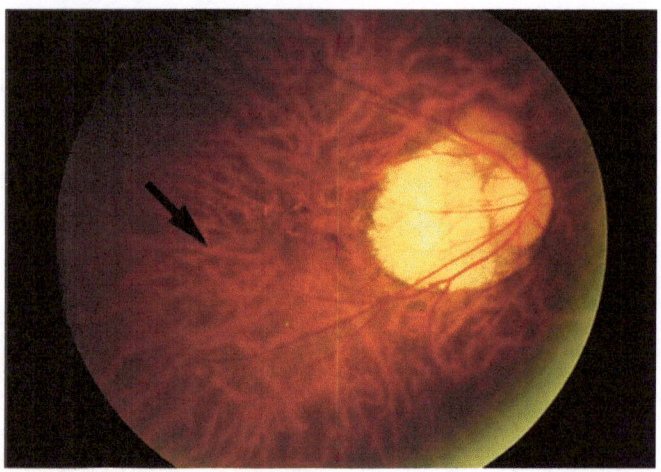

Fig. 20B. One year later (March 1988), the bleeding is absorbed. A new lacquer crack lesion is formed at the site of the previous bleeding (*arrow*). Visual acuity is 0.6, and the refractive error is −14.00 D

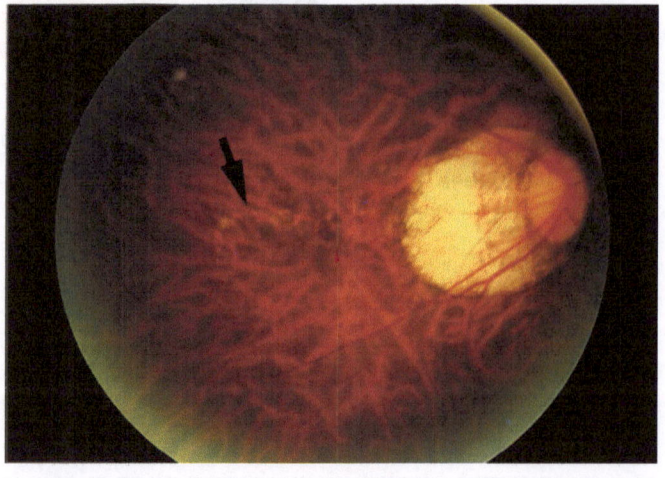

Fig. 20C. Two years after the initial examination (April 1989), lacquer crack lesions have increased. A new lacquer crack lesion is observed as a horizontal yellowish line in the macula (*arrow*)

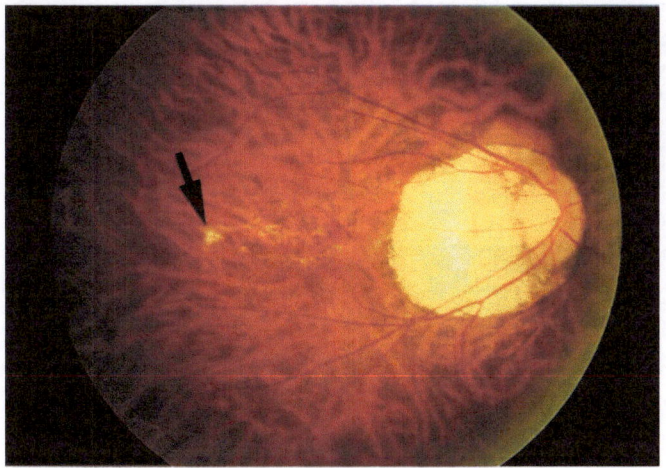

Fig. 20D. Five years after the initial examination (June 1992), linear lesions of diffuse atrophy are seen just temporal to the peripapillary crescent. The lacquer crack lesions have increased, and the temporal end of the lacquer crack lesion has widened and become whitish, resembling a spotty lesion of patchy atrophy (*arrow*). Visual acuity is 0.6, and the refractive error is −14.00 D

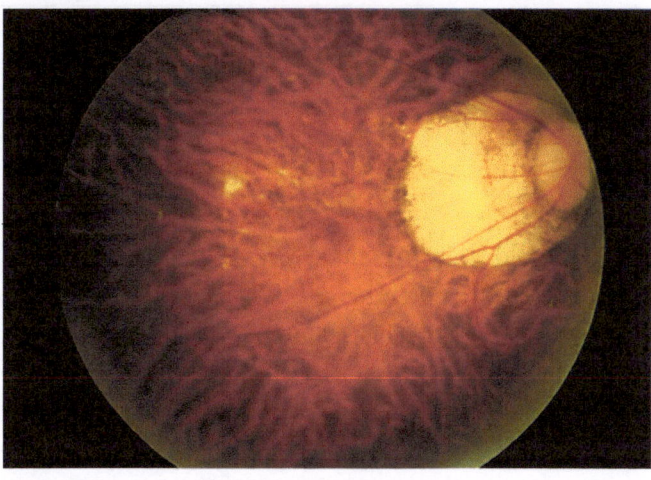

Fig. 20F. Seven years after the initial examination (December 1994), the white spotty lesion at the temporal end of the lacquer crack lesion has enlarged and progressed into a spotty lesion of patchy atrophy. Spotty and linear lesions of diffuse atrophy have increased in the macula. The lacquer crack lesions have widened

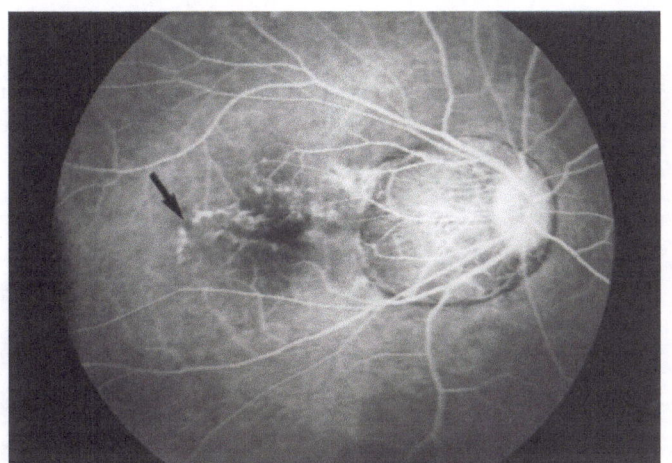

Fig. 20E. Fluorescein fundus angiogram 5 years after the initial examination (June 1992). At 70 sec after dye injection, the lacquer crack lesions are clearly visible and show linear hyperfluorescence. The end of the lacquer crack lesions is hypofluorescent (*arrow*). No choroidal neovascularization is apparent

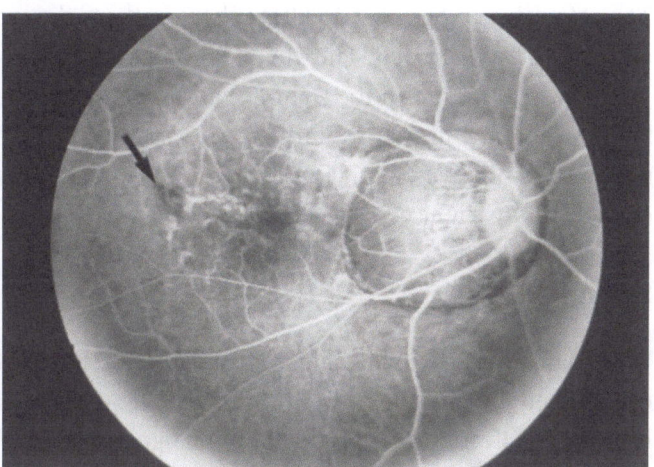

Fig. 20G. Fluorescein fundus angiogram 7 years after the initial examination (December 1994). At 30 sec after dye injection, many lacquer crack lesions show a reticular hyperfluorescent pattern. The spotty lesion of patchy atrophy at the temporal end of the lacquer crack lesion is hypofluorescent in the early phase (*arrow*)

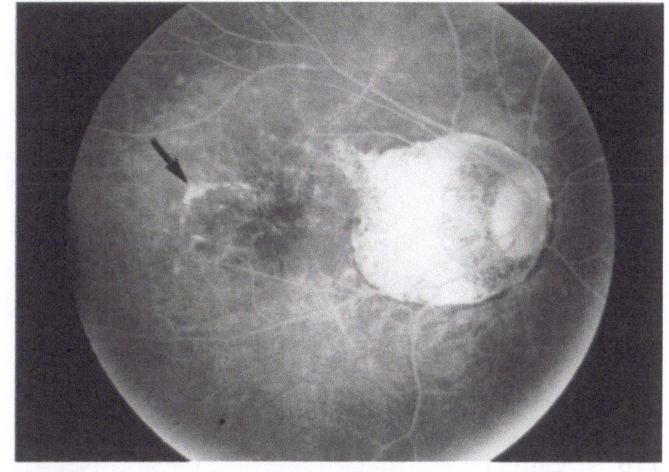

Fig. 20H. Fluorescein fundus angiogram 7 years after the initial examination (December 1994). At 472 sec after dye injection, the spotty lesion of patchy atrophy at the temporal end of the lacquer crack lesions turns hyperfluorescent in the late phase (*arrow*)

Case 21

A 37-year-old man presented with metamorphopsia in his right eye on September 29, 1989. He was diagnosed with myopia on entering elementary school. He began wearing glasses for distance vision at age 12 years. He noticed a sudden decrease in visual acuity in the left eye in 1985. Macular bleeding in his left eye was reported by a general practitioner. Drug treatment did not improve the vision in his left eye. He noticed metamorphopsia in the right eye 3 months before his first visit to our high myopia clinic. His medical history was noncontributory. No family members had severe myopia.

In the initial examination, the patient's best corrected visual acuity was 0.6 in the right eye and 0.1 in the left. The refractive error was −15.00 D sphere in the right eye and −7.75 D in the left, and the axial length measurements were 30.7 mm in the right eye and 27.7 mm in the left. Intraocular pressures and anterior segments were normal in both eyes. We describe the long-term fundus changes in his right eye.

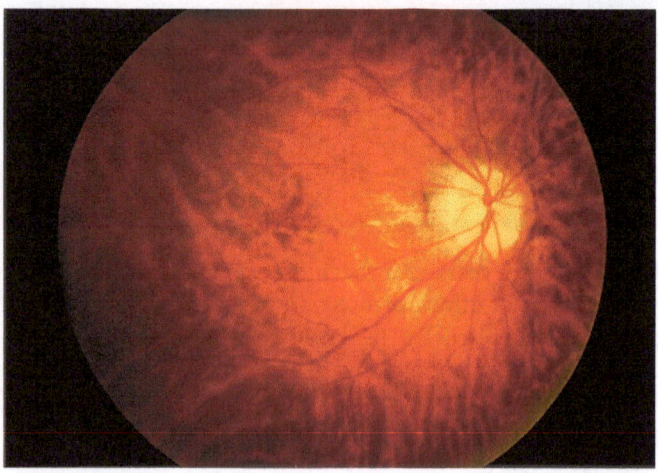

Fig. 21A. Right fundus at the initial examination (September 1989) shows a horizontal lacquer crack lesion just inferior to the fovea. A red central dot is a photographic artifact. Spotty or linear lesions of diffuse atrophy are observed temporal to the peripapillary crescent. No posterior staphyloma is present

Summary

This man presented with metamorphopsia in the right eye caused by macular bleeding and a lacquer crack lesion. His left fundus (not shown in the figures) showed myopic choroidal neovascularization at the initial examination. His right fundus has shown no findings suggestive of choroidal neovascularization so far. Lacquer crack lesions in the right eye did not increase for 3 years after the initial examination. However, 4 years after the initial visit, two lacquer crack lesions newly appeared. The progression of lacquer crack lesions is usually gradual, as seen in this patient.

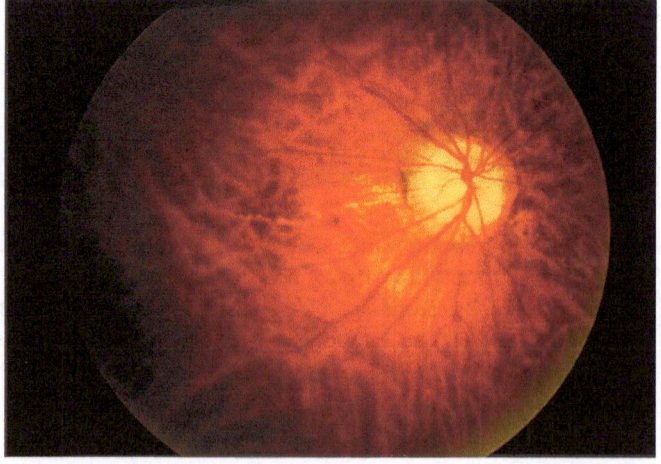

Fig. 21B. One year later (January 1990), the lacquer crack lesion has elongated temporally. Visual acuity is 0.6, and the refractive error is −15.50 D

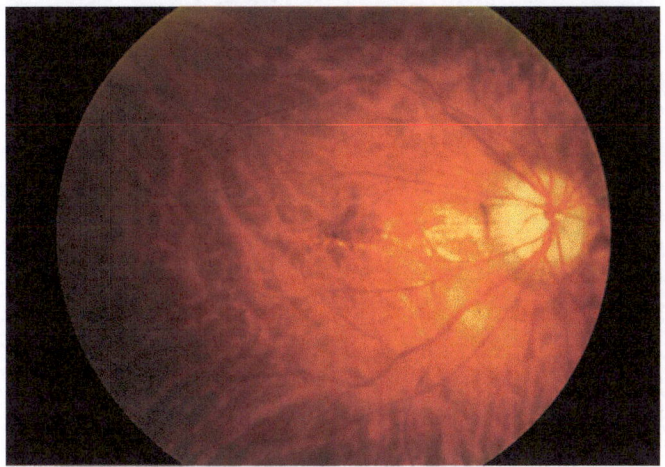

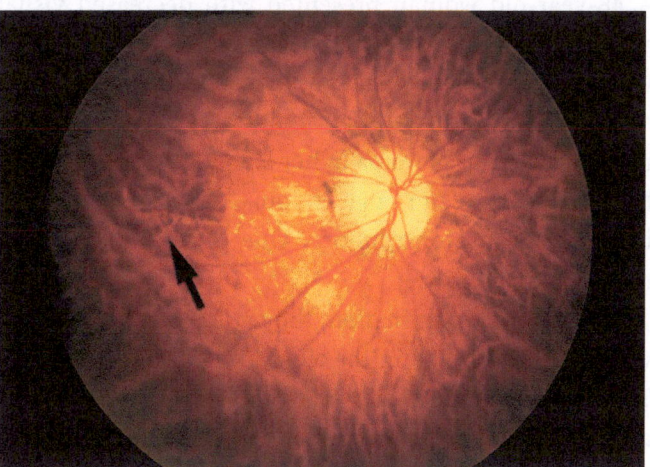

Fig. 21C. Two years after the initial examination (November 1991), the lacquer crack lesion is clearly seen as a yellowish linear lesion. Diffuse atrophy has enlarged inferotemporal to the optic disc

Fig. 21E. Four years after the initial examination (November 1993), a new lacquer crack lesion appears to branch from the original lesion (*arrow*). Diffuse atrophy has slightly enlarged inferotemporal to the optic disc

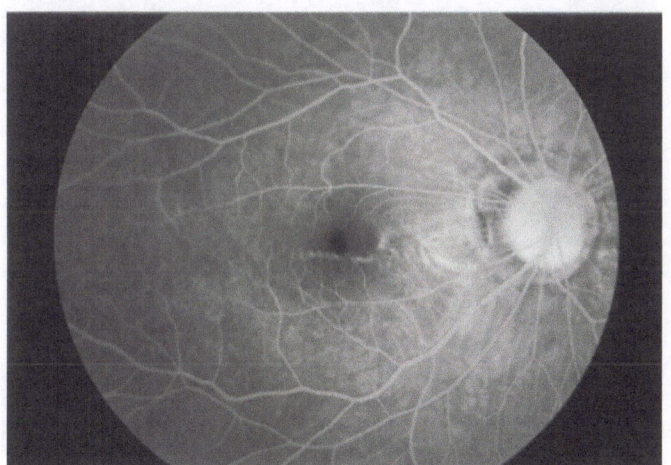

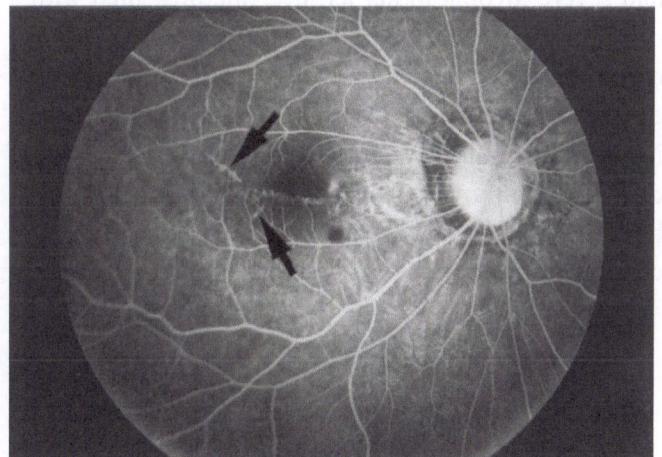

Fig. 21D. Fluorescein fundus angiogram 2 years after the initial examination (May 1991). At 6 min after dye injection, the lacquer crack lesion shows linear hyperfluorescence inferior to the macula. Diffuse atrophy temporal to the optic disc also appears hyperfluorescent

Fig. 21F. Fluorescein fundus angiogram 4 years after the initial examination (April 1993). Two new lacquer crack lesions branched from the original lesion are clearly visible as linear hyperfluorescence (*arrows*)

Case 22

A 48-year-old woman presented with decreased visual acuity in her left eye on June 21, 1985. She reported no visual difficulties until age 18 years. She noticed a gradual decrease in her left visual acuity at age 19. She also noticed a central scotoma in her left eye 2 months before her first visit to our high myopia clinic. Her medical history was noncontributory. One of her siblings was highly myopic.

In the initial examination, the patient's best corrected visual acuity was 0.8 in the right eye and 0.1 in the left. The refractive error was $-3.00\,D$ sphere in the right eye and $-17.00\,D$ sphere in the left, and the axial length measurements were 24.5 mm in the right eye and 29.3 mm in the left. Intraocular pressures and anterior segments were normal in both eyes. We describe the long-term fundus changes in her left eye.

Summary

This woman was followed up for 6 years, since 1985. She had severe myopia in her left eye. She presented with a central scotoma caused by macular bleeding in her left eye in 1985. No choroidal neovascular membrane was detected after absorption of the bleeding. After the bleeding is absorbed, lacquer crack lesions or spotty lesions of diffuse atrophy may appear at the site of the previous bleeding. The progressive pattern of myopic fundus changes in this patient was from Hs_1 to D_1.

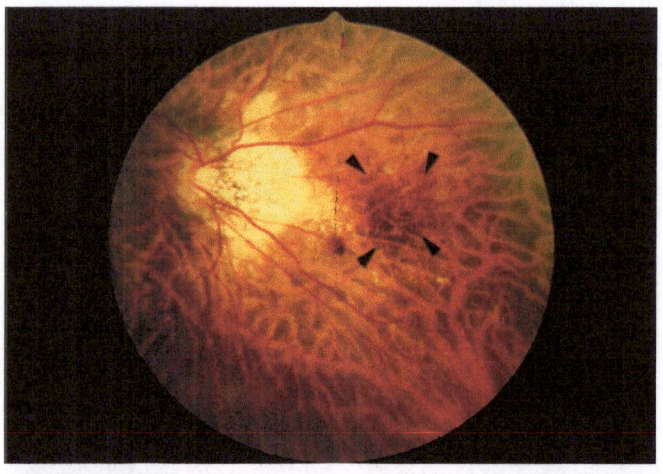

Fig. 22A. Left fundus at the initial examination (June 1985) shows large subretinal bleeding in the macula (*arrowheads*). Spotty or linear lesions of diffuse atrophy are observed temporal to the optic disc. The optic disc tilts temporally. A temporal peripapillary crescent is seen. Type II posterior staphyloma is present

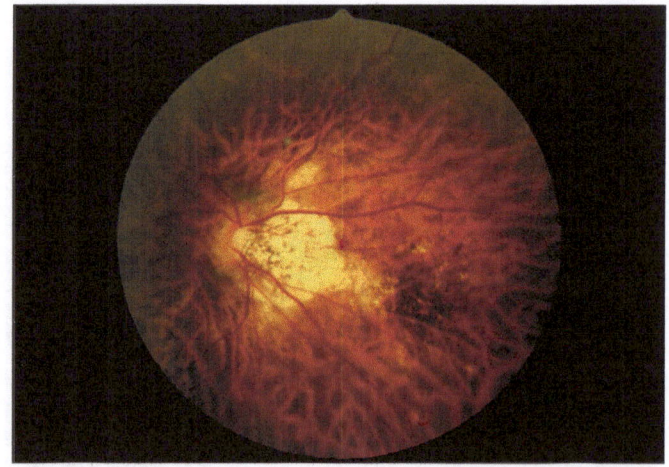

Fig. 22B. One year later (March 1986), macular bleeding is absorbed. Pigmentation is observed at the site of the previous bleeding. Spotty or linear lesions of diffuse atrophy are clearly visible around the macula after the absorption of the bleeding. No choroidal neovascular membrane is obvious

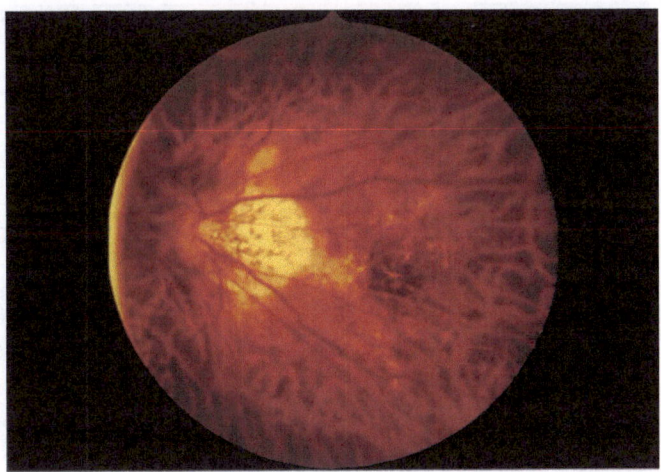

Fig. 22C. Two years after the initial examination (February 1987), several lacquer crack lesions are seen. Visual acuity is 0.1, and the refractive error is −16.00 D

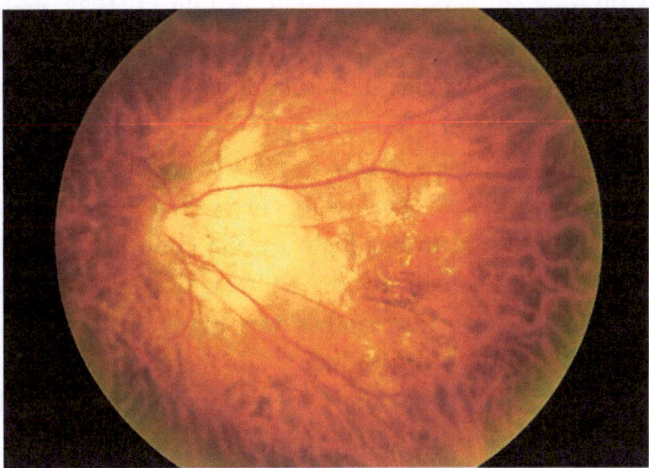

Fig. 22E. Four years after the initial examination (September 1989), the linear lesions in the macula have widened, the spotty lesions of diffuse atrophy have increased, and the peripapillary crescent has enlarged

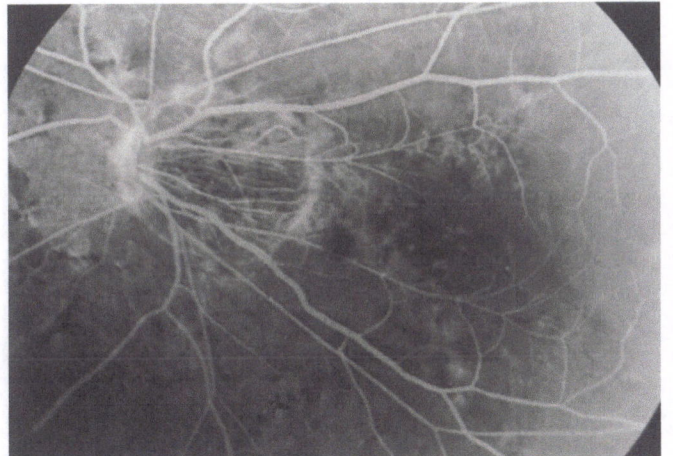

Fig. 22D. Fluorescein fundus angiogram 2 years after the initial examination (February 1987). At 53 sec after dye injection, irregular hyperfluorescence is seen corresponding to the spotty or linear lesions of diffuse atrophy. Lacquer crack lesions show no typical linear hyperfluorescence. No dye leakage suggestive of choroidal neovascularization is apparent

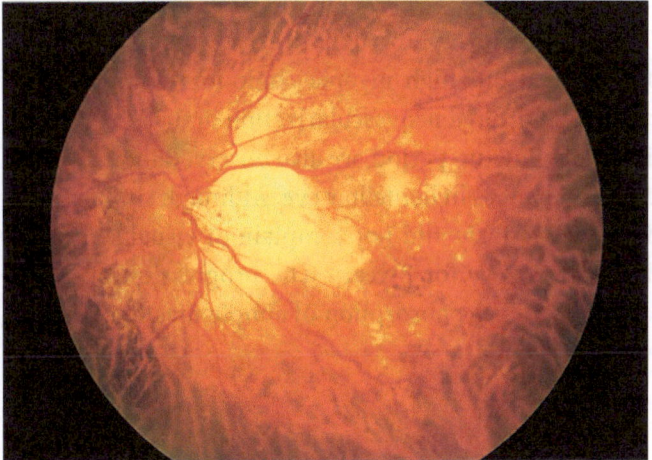

Fig. 22F. Six years after the initial examination (September 1991), spotty or linear lesions of diffuse atrophy have increased further. The peripapillary crescent is continuous with an enlarged lesion of diffuse atrophy

Case 23

A 29-year-old woman presented on July 13, 1988, with decreased visual acuity in her left eye. She was diagnosed with myopia in elementary school. She began wearing glasses for distance vision at age 10 years. At that time, her corrected visual acuity was 1.0 in the left eye. She noticed decreased visual acuity in her left eye in 1978. She was referred to our high myopia clinic for further examination of high myopia. Her medical history was noncontributory. Her mother was highly myopic and had myopic macular bleeding.

In the initial examination, the patient's best corrected visual acuity was 1.2 in the right eye and 0.1 in the left. The refractive error was −14.50 D sphere in the right eye and −16.00 D sphere in the left, and the axial length measurements were 28.8 mm in the right eye and 29.3 mm in the left. Intraocular pressures and anterior segments were normal in both eyes. We describe the long-term fundus changes in her right eye.

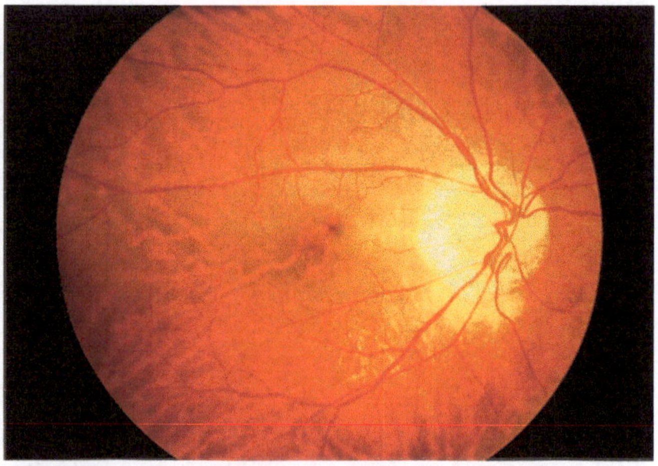

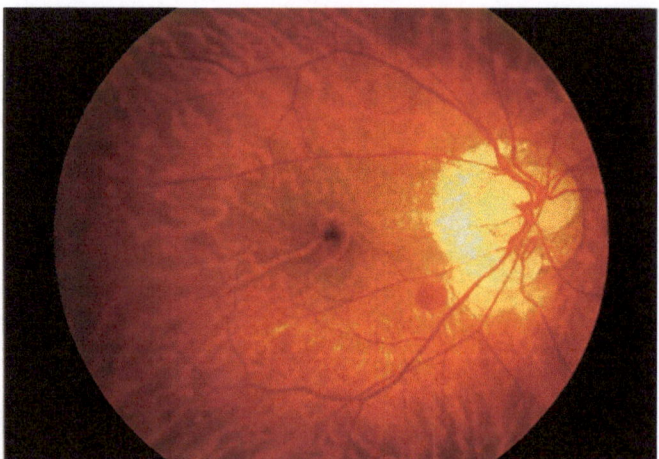

Fig. 23A. Right fundus at the initial examination (July 1988) shows linear lesions of diffuse atrophy along the inferotemporal retinal vessel. The optic disc tilts temporally. An annular peripapillary crescent is seen. No posterior staphyloma is present

Summary

This woman was followed up for 8 years, since 1988. She first visited our high myopia clinic for examination of myopic choroidal neovascularization in the left eye. During the follow-up period, we also observed the long-term fundus changes in her fellow eye. Although simple bleeding occurred, she did not complain of visual symptoms in the right eye for 8 years. The progression of diffuse atrophy after the absorption of simple macular bleeding was not obvious.

Fig. 23B. Three years later (November 1991), a round retinal hemorrhage appears within the linear lesions along the inferotemporal retinal vessel

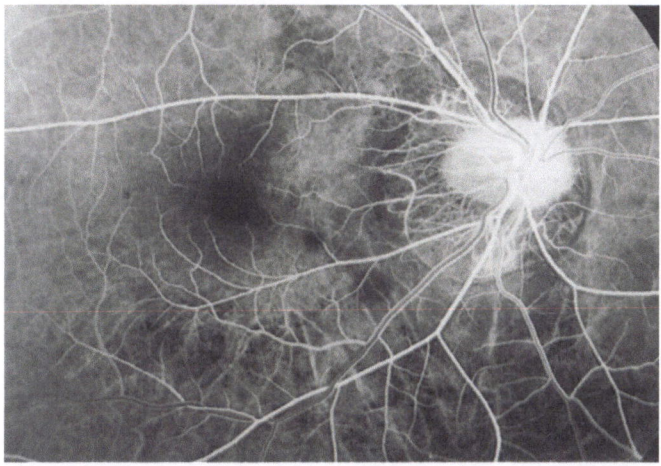

Fig. 23C. Fluorescein fundus angiogram 3 years after the initial examination (November 1991). At 18 sec after dye injection, choroidal filling is slightly delayed within the area of linear lesions of diffuse atrophy

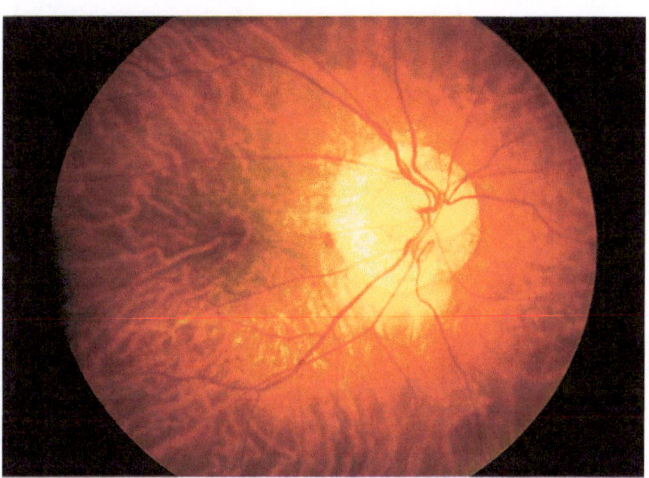

Fig. 23E. Four years after the initial examination (February 1992), the round retinal bleeding is absorbed. Many linear lesions are seen at the site of the previous bleeding. It is unclear whether new linear lesions developed after the bleeding absorbed

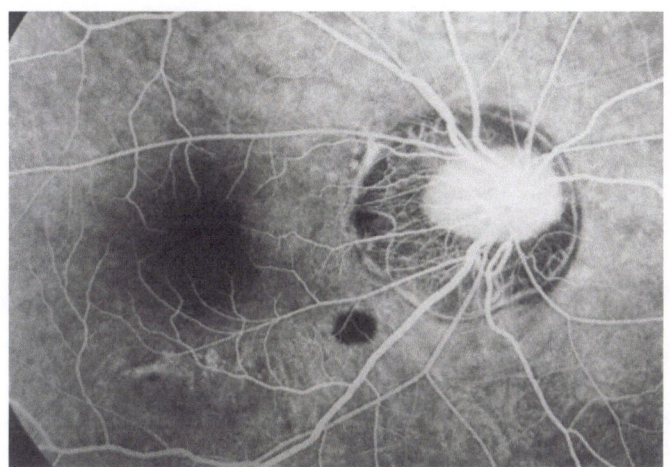

Fig. 23D. Fluorescein fundus angiogram 3 years after the initial examination (November 1991). At 55 sec after dye injection, the retinal bleeding shows blocked fluorescence. No dye leakage suggestive of choroidal neovascularization is seen. The linear lesions inferior to the macula show mild hyperfluorescence

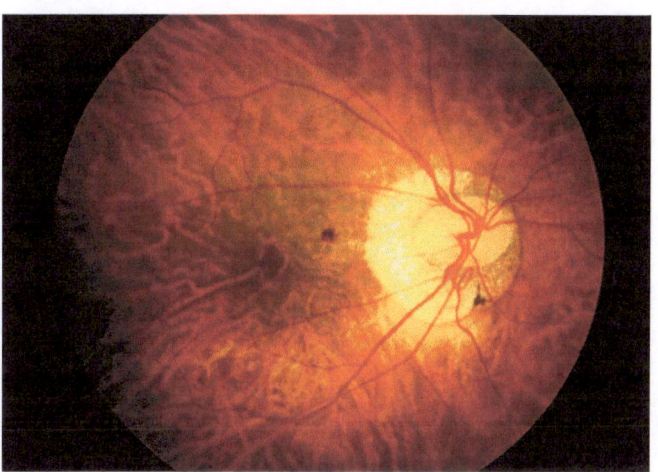

Fig. 23F. Six years after the initial examination (June 1994), the diffuse atrophy has not enlarged ophthalmoscopically

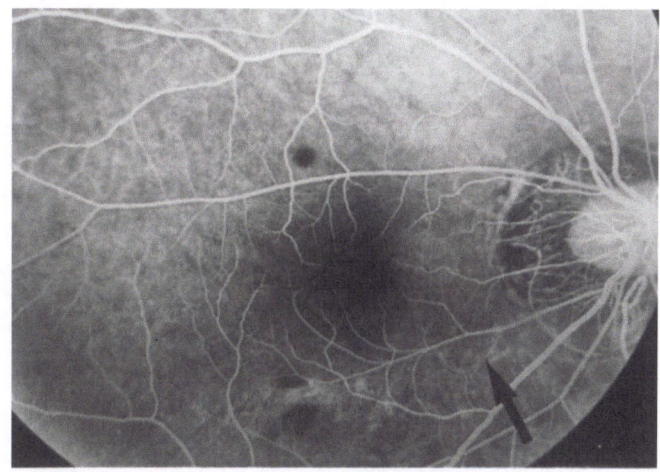

Fig. 23G. Fluorescein fundus angiogram 7 years after the initial examination (February 1995). At 57 sec after dye injection, mild hyperfluorescence is visible at the site of the previous bleeding (*arrow*)

Patchy Chorioretinal Atrophy

Patchy atrophy usually develops around the macula within the lesion of diffuse atrophy in highly myopic eyes with a deep staphyloma. Although the progression of patchy atrophy is relatively slow, it sometimes tends to progress rapidly, especially in the eyes with deep staphyloma of elderly patients. Patchy atrophy gradually enlarges and coalesces with the expansion of the posterior fundus. The lesions sometimes coalesce with the peripapillary crescent and form a large atrophic lesion in the posterior fundus of highly myopic eyes. The progression of surrounding diffuse atrophy is seen with the progression of patchy atrophy. The progression of patchy atrophy and diffuse atrophy is noted only within the posterior staphyloma and not beyond it. With the enlargement of patchy atrophy, axial length elongation or dislocation of retinal vessels is sometimes noted. These findings suggest that the enlargement of patchy atrophy could be caused by the continuous expansion of the posterior fundus.

Vision is not impaired unless the macula is involved with the enlargement of patchy atrophy. Also, patchy atrophy usually does not involve the macula in highly myopic eyes. Although patchy atrophy usually appears and progresses in the fundus of elderly highly myopic patients, it is sometimes seen in young highly myopic patients as well. In young patients, patchy atrophy may progress with the occurrence of simple macular hemorrhage or lacquer crack lesions. However, patchy atrophy in young patients does not enlarge so rapidly. The lesions remain the same size for a long period.

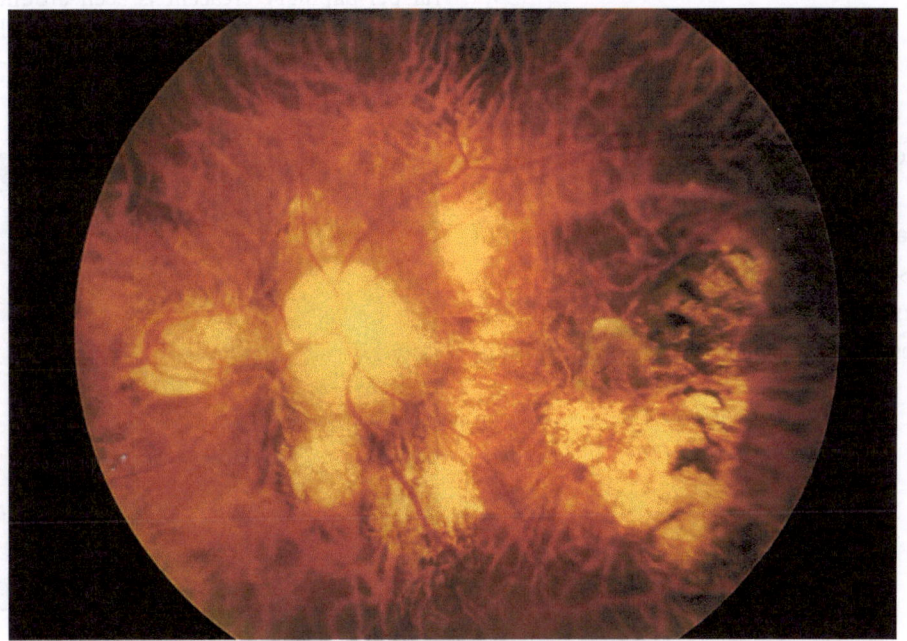

Fig. 37E. *(see page 159)*

Cases 24–37 ▶

Abbreviations *T:* Tessellated fundus; *D:* Diffuse chorioretinal atrophy; *Lc:* Lacquer crack lesion; *P:* Patchy atrophy; *NS:* Simple macular hemorrhage; *HN:* Neovascular macular hemorrhage; *MA:* Chorioretinal atrophy of the macula. For details, refer to Table 3.1 and Fig. 7.1.

Case 24

A 38-year-old woman was examined for high myopia on June 11, 1982. She was diagnosed as having high myopia and amblyopia when she was in infancy. She began wearing glasses for distance vision when she entered elementary school. Her visual acuity did not improve much with the glasses. She currently wears contact lenses and glasses. No severe myopia was reported in her parents or siblings. Two of her three sons are highly myopic.

In the initial examination, the patient's best corrected visual acuity was 0.3 in the right eye and 0.4 in the left eye. The refractive error was −15.5 D sphere in the right eye and −16.0 D in the left, and the axial length measurements were 28.3 mm in the right eye and 28.1 mm in the left. Intraocular pressures and anterior segments were normal bilaterally. We describe the long-term fundus changes in her right eye.

Summary

This patient's right fundus showed slight diffuse atrophy and a spotty lesion of patchy atrophy at the initial examination. During the follow-up period of 14 years, patchy atrophy increased and enlarged with the progression of spotty or linear lesions of diffuse atrophy in her right fundus. Peripapillary crescent also enlarged during the period. The progression of patchy atrophy was slow in this patient.

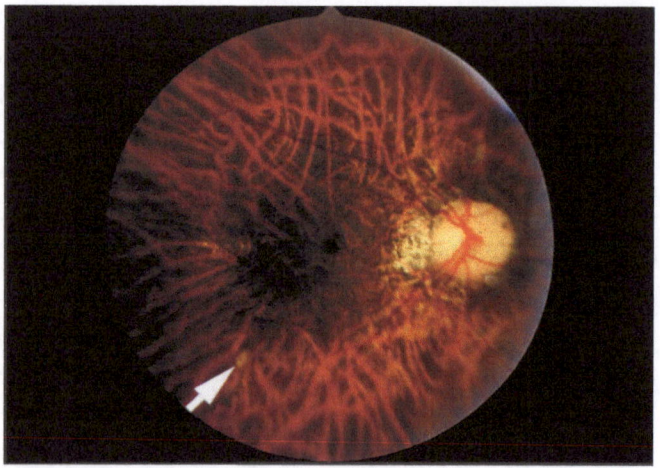

Fig. 24A. Right fundus at the initial examination (June 1982) shows a small spotty lesion of patchy atrophy inferotemporal to the macula (*arrow*). The optic disc tilts temporally. Temporal peripapillary crescent is seen around the optic disc. No posterior staphyloma is present. A linear lesion of diffuse atrophy is seen temporal to the macula

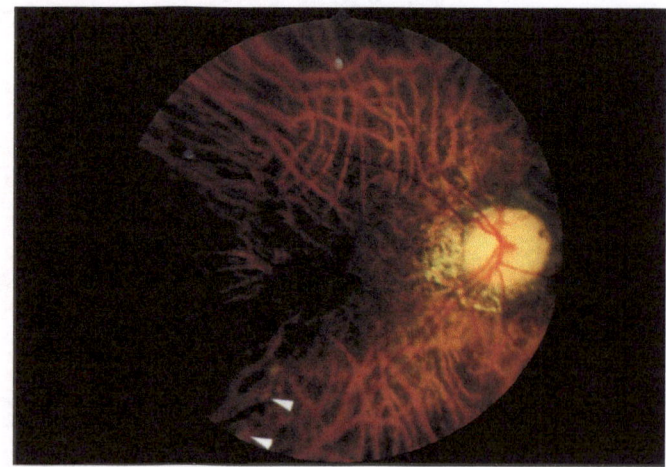

Fig. 24B. One year later (June 1983), two small spotty lesions of patchy atrophy newly appear inferotemporal to the macula (*arrowheads*). Diffuse atrophy is unchanged. Visual acuity is 0.3, and the refractive error is −15.5 D

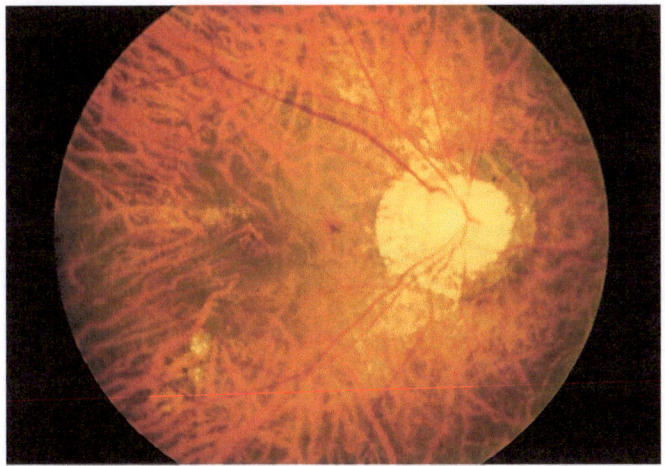

Fig. 24C. Seven years after the initial examination (November 1989), spotty lesions of patchy atrophy have enlarged. Linear lesions of diffuse atrophy have widened temporal to the macula

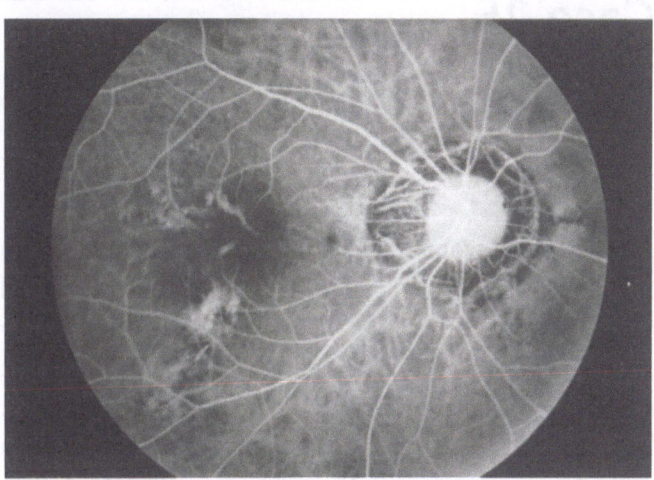

Fig. 24E. Fluorescein angiogram 9 years after the initial examination (December 1991). At 53 sec after dye injection, linear lesions of diffuse atrophy, similar to lacquer crack lesions, show linear hyperfluorescence from a window defect superotemporal to the macula. Spotty lesions of patchy atrophy show hypofluorescence in the early phase of the angiogram because of a choroidal filling defect

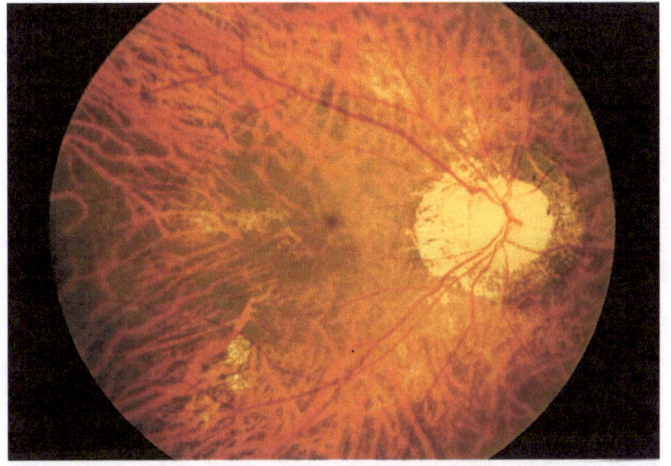

Fig. 24D. Ten years after the initial examination (July 1992), spotty lesions of patchy atrophy have continued to enlarge. Spotty or linear lesions of diffuse atrophy have increased around the optic disc. Visual acuity is 0.4, and the refractive error is −17.0 D

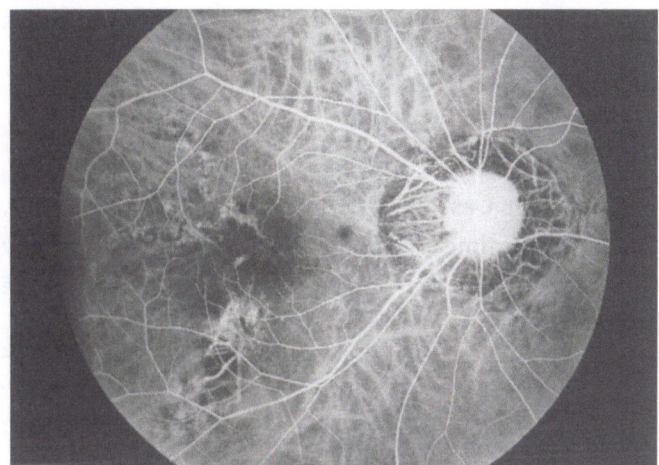

Fig. 24F. Fluorescein angiogram 14 years after the initial examination (September 1996). At 43 sec after dye injection, hypofluorescence corresponding to the spotty lesions of patchy atrophy has enlarged

Fig. 24G. Indocyanine green angiogram 14 years after the initial examination (September 1996). In the late phase of the angiogram, both linear lesions of diffuse atrophy and patchy atrophy are hypofluorescent

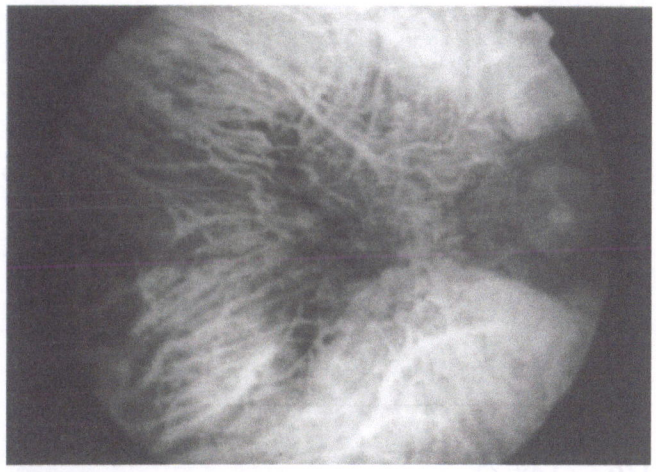

Case 25

A 52-year-old woman presented on April 17, 1992, with myodesopsia in the right eye. She noticed decreased visual acuity in that eye when she was in elementary school. She began wearing glasses at age 12 years. She first reported myodesopsia in the right eye in 1987, and it had worsened since then. She visited our high myopia clinic for myodesopsia in the right eye in 1992. No family members had severe myopia.

In the initial examination, the patient's best corrected visual acuity was 1.0 in both eyes. The refractive error was −13.50 D sphere in the right eye and −2.50 D sphere in the left, and the axial length measurements were 28.3 mm in the right eye and 24.6 mm in the left. Intraocular pressures and anterior segments were normal in both eyes. We describe the long-term fundus changes in her right eye.

Summary

This woman was followed up for 4 years, since 1992. During that time, a spotty lesion of patchy atrophy appeared within the diffuse atrophy temporal to the macula. The patchy atrophy gradually enlarged and coalesced with the expansion of the posterior fundus.

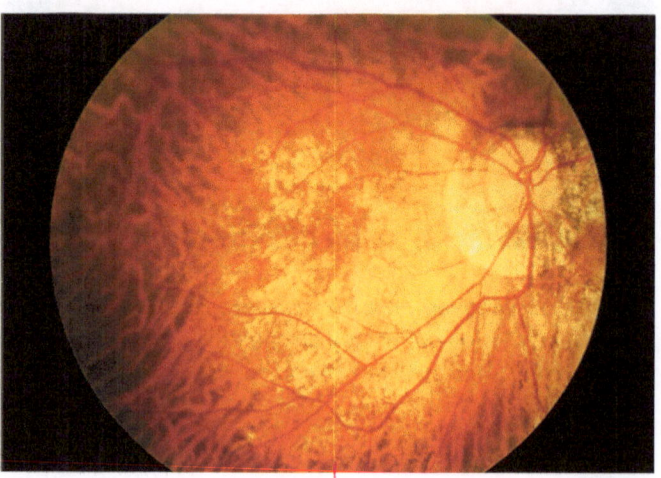

Fig. 25A. Right fundus at the initial examination (April 1992) shows an enlarged lesion of diffuse atrophy in the posterior fundus. An annular peripapillary crescent is seen. Type I posterior staphyloma is present

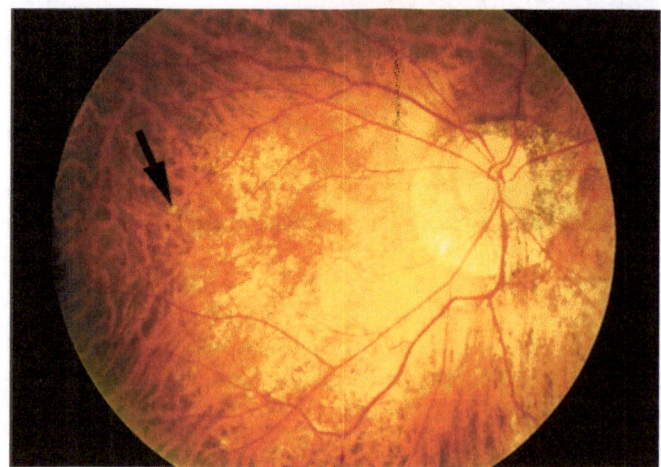

Fig. 25B. One year later (October 1993), a spotty lesion of patchy atrophy has appeared temporal to the macula (*arrow*)

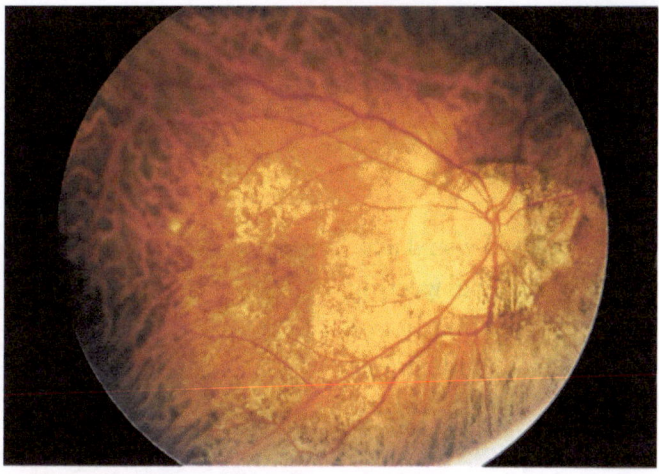

Fig. 25C. Two years after the initial examination (November 1994), the spotty lesion of patchy atrophy has slightly enlarged

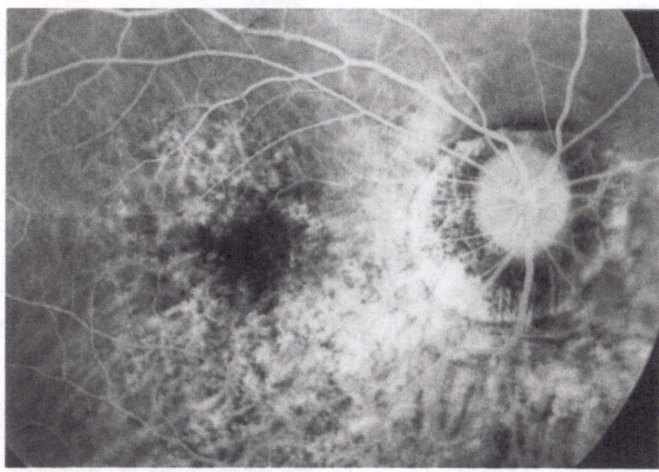

Fig. 25D. Fluorescein fundus angiogram at the initial examination (April 1992). At 8 min after dye injection, an enlarged lesion of diffuse atrophy shows mixed hyperfluorescence and hypofluorescence

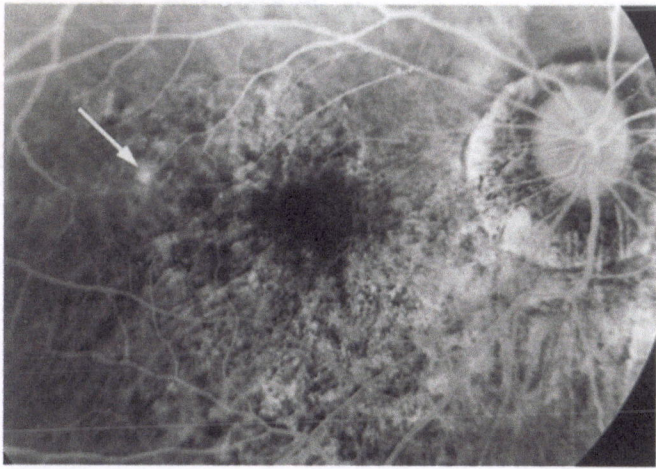

Fig. 25E. Fluorescein fundus angiogram 2 years after the initial examination (November 1994). At 6 min after dye injection, the spotty lesion of patchy atrophy is hyperfluorescent (*arrow*)

Case 26

A 21-year-old man presented with decreased visual acuity in the left eye on November 4, 1988. He began wearing glasses at age 7 years. At the initial examination in our high myopia clinic, lacquer crack lesion and simple macular hemorrhage were found to cause the visual decrease in the left fundus. His medical history was noncontributory. His mother and one brother are highly myopic.

In the initial examination, the patient's best corrected visual acuity was 0.5 in the right eye and 0.1 in the left. The refractive error was −22.75 D sphere in the right eye and −20.00 D sphere in the left, and the axial length measurements were 31.3 mm in the right eye and 29.8 mm in the left. Intraocular pressures and anterior segments were normal in both eyes. During the follow-up, we also observed the fundus changes in the right eye. We describe the long-term fundus changes in his right eye.

Summary

This young man was followed up for 7 years, since 1988. Spotty lesions of patchy atrophy increased and enlarged with the progression of surrounding diffuse atrophy during the period. In this patient, lacquer crack lesions and simple macular hemorrhage were observed before the patchy atrophy enlarged. It remains unclear if patchy atrophy may be caused secondary to the enlargement of lacquer crack lesions. Some spotty lesions of patchy atrophy appeared distant from the previous hemorrhage and lacquer crack lesions.

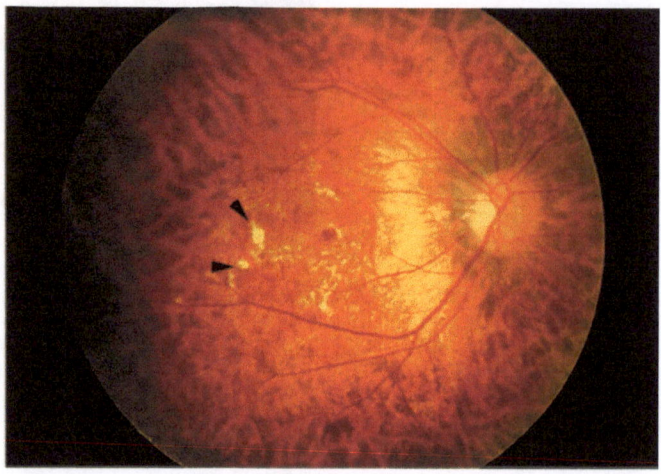

Fig. 26A. Right fundus at the initial examination (November 1988) shows two spotty lesions of patchy atrophy temporal to the macula (*arrowheads*). Spotty or linear lesions of diffuse atrophy are visible around the patchy atrophy. Lacquer crack lesions are also seen. An enlarged lesion of diffuse atrophy is observed temporal to the optic disc. The optic disc tilts temporally. A peripapillary crescent is seen. Type I posterior staphyloma is present

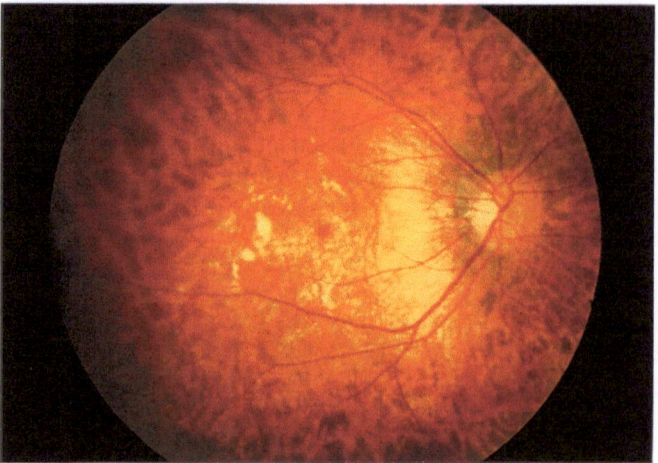

Fig. 26B. Six months later (January 1989), spotty lesions of patchy atrophy have enlarged slightly. Chorioretinal atrophy is limited within the posterior staphyloma

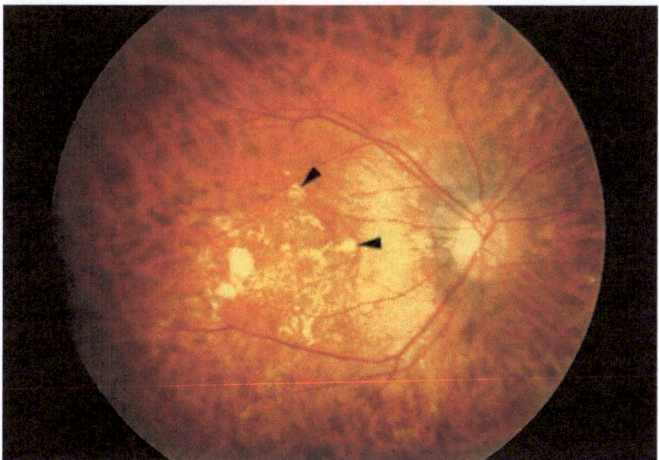

Fig. 26C. Two years after the initial examination (January 1990), spotty lesions of patchy atrophy have enlarged. New spotty lesions of patchy atrophy appear around the macula (*arrowheads*)

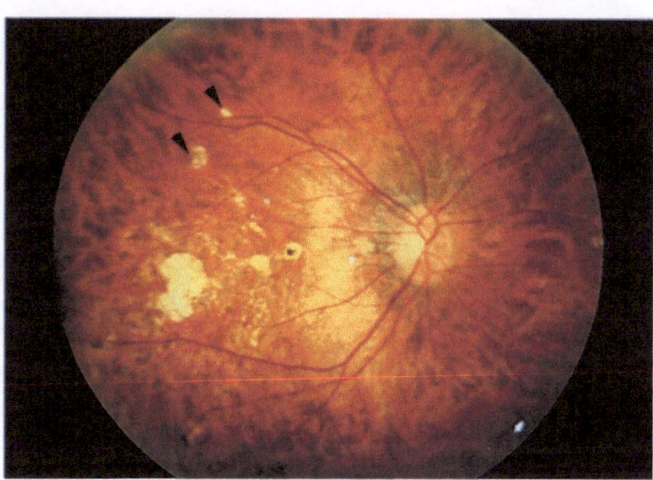

Fig. 26E. Four years after the initial examination (February 1992), patchy atrophy has enlarged further. New spotty lesions have appeared superior to the macula (*arrowheads*). The macula is not involved with the lesions of patchy atrophy. Visual acuity is 0.3, and the refractive error is −25.75 D

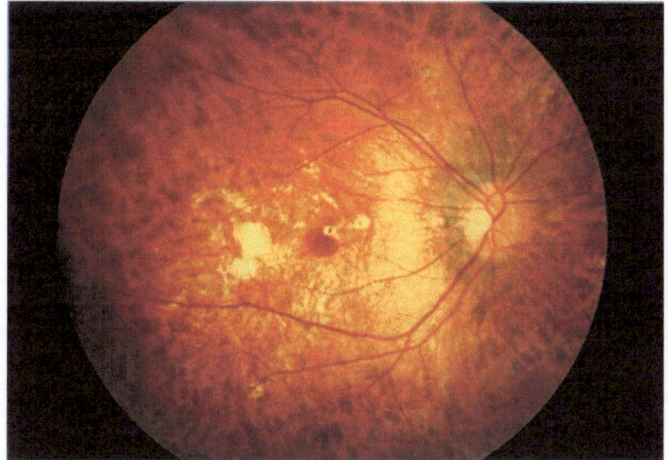

Fig. 26D. Three years after the initial examination (May 1991), simple macular hemorrhage has appeared in the macula. Spotty lesions of patchy atrophy have coalesced temporal to the macula

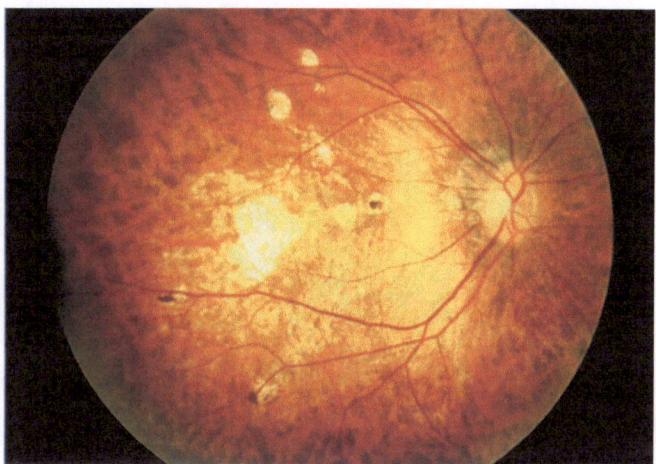

Fig. 26F. Five years after the initial examination (July 1993), all lesions of patchy atrophy have continued to enlarge

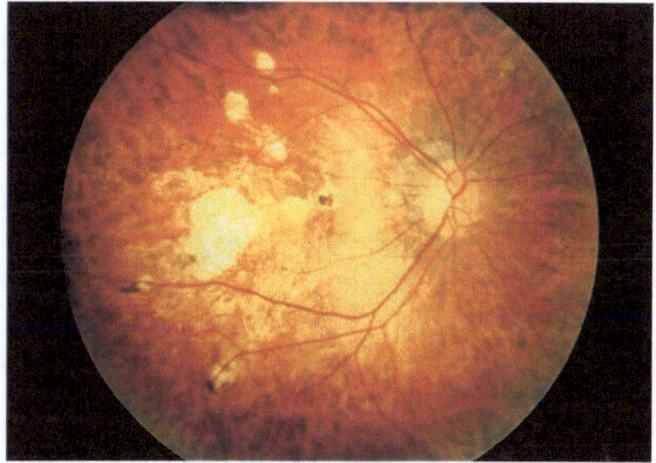

Fig. 26G. Six years after the initial examination (September 1994), all lesions of patchy atrophy have enlarged further. Visual acuity is 0.3, and the refractive error is −28.75 D

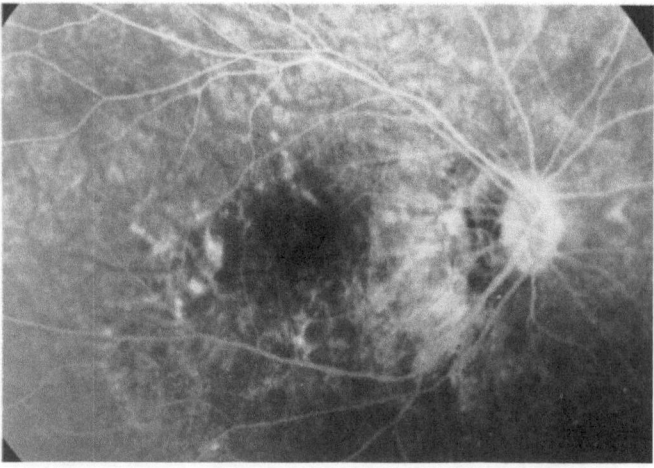

Fig. 26H. Fluorescein fundus angiogram at the initial examination (November 1988). At 5 min after dye injection, spotty lesions of patchy atrophy show late hyperfluorescence. Lacquer crack lesions show linear hyperfluorescence. An enlarged lesion of diffuse atrophy appears hyperfluorescent temporal to the optic disc

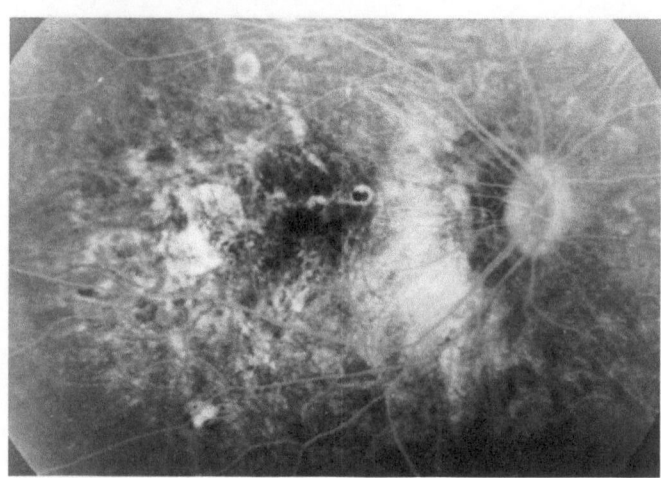

Fig. 26K. Fluorescein fundus angiogram 5 years after the initial examination (March 1993). At 8 min after dye injection, late hyperfluorescence corresponding to the patchy atrophy has enlarged

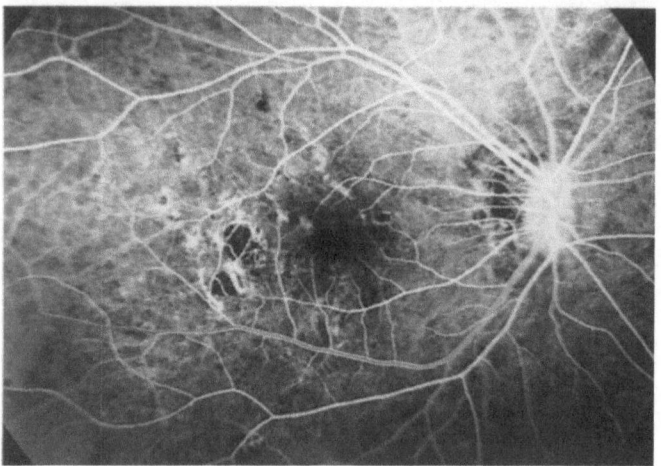

Fig. 26I. Fluorescein fundus angiogram 3 years after the initial examination (May 1991). At 26 sec after dye injection, two spotty lesions of patchy atrophy temporal to the macula show a choroidal filling delay in the early phase

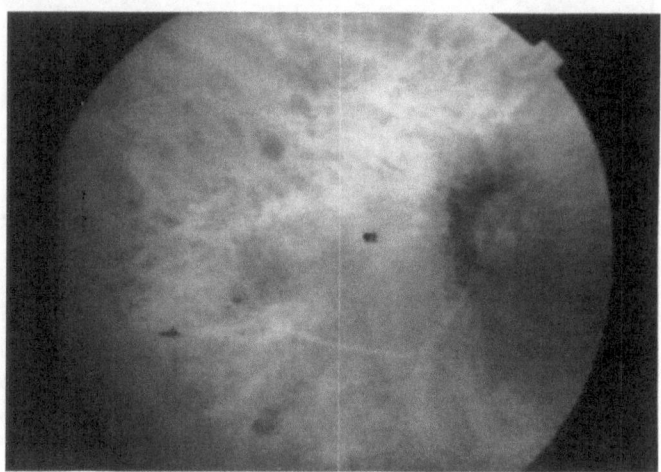

Fig. 26L. Indocyanine green fundus angiogram 5 years after the initial examination (October 1993). Many lesions of patchy atrophy show hypofluorescence in the late phase

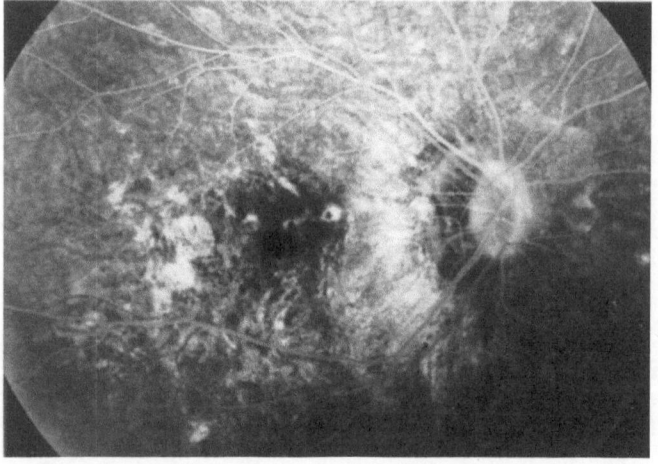

Fig. 26J. Fluorescein fundus angiogram 3 years after the initial examination (May 1991). At 8 min after dye injection, two spotty lesions of patchy atrophy show late hyperfluorescence. Linear hyperfluorescence corresponding to the lacquer crack lesions has slightly enlarged

Case 27

A 43-year-old-woman presented with decreased visual acuity in her right eye on July 20, 1990. She was diagnosed as having myopia as an infant. Her vision did not improve much, even with glasses. She noticed decreased visual acuity, particularly in her right eye, 1 month before the initial examination. Her medical history was noncontributory. Her two siblings are highly myopic.

In the initial examination, the patient's best corrected visual acuity was 0.3 in the right eye and 0.7 in the left. The refractive error was −13.00 D sphere in the right eye and −12.50 D in the left. The axial length measurements were 29.2 mm in the right eye and 28.7 mm in the left. Intraocular pressures and anterior segments were normal in both eyes. We describe the long-term fundus changes in her right eye.

Summary

This woman was followed up for 6 years, since 1990. Her right fundus showed no remarkable progression of patchy atrophy until 3 years after the initial examination. However, patchy atrophy rapidly enlarged and new lesions also appeared in the following year. Since then, all patchy lesions have gradually enlarged. In this patient, patchy atrophy appeared within the lesion of advanced diffuse atrophy in eyes with a deep staphyloma. All patchy lesions continued to enlarge within the staphyloma. Her right fundus showed a typical progressive pattern of patchy atrophy.

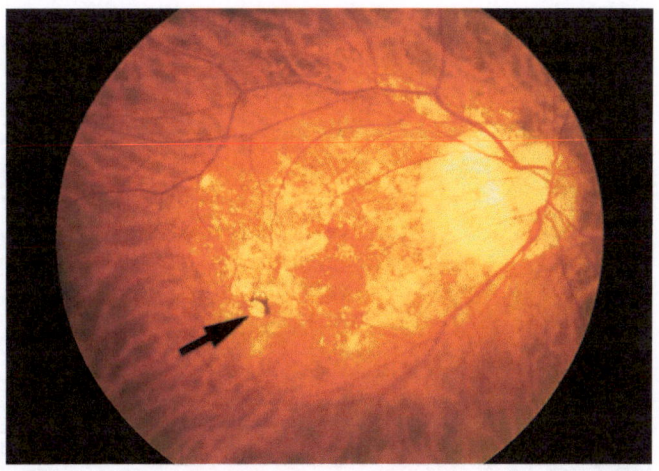

Fig. 27A. Right fundus at the initial examination (July 1990) shows an enlarged lesion of diffuse atrophy in the posterior fundus. A spotty lesion of patchy atrophy is seen inferotemporal to the macula (*arrow*). The optic disc tilts temporally. A temporal peripapillary crescent is seen. Type II posterior staphyloma is present

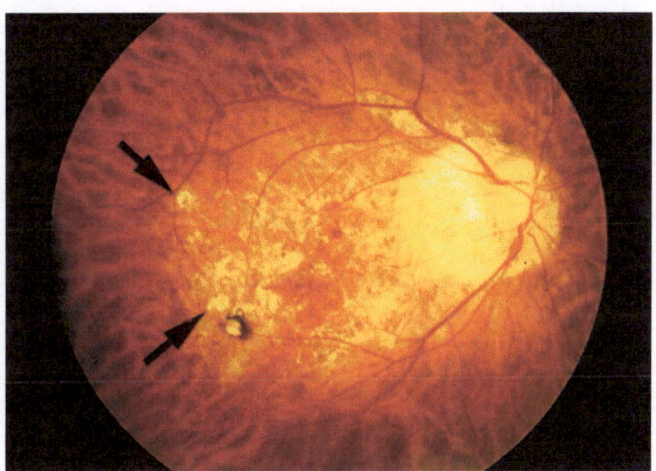

Fig. 27B. One year later (September 1991), two other spotty lesions of patchy atrophy are clearly visible (*arrows*)

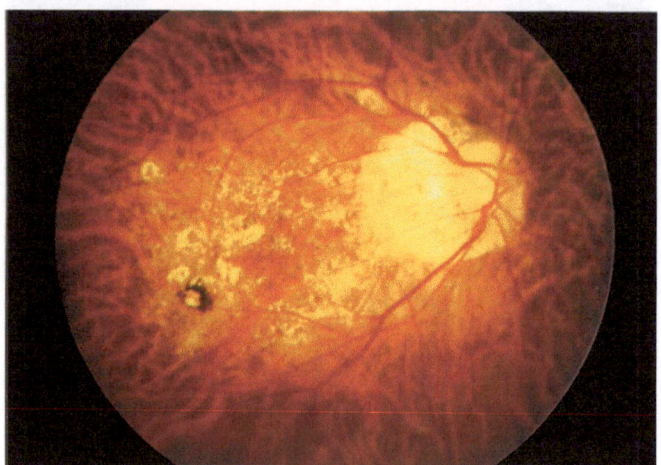

Fig. 27C. Two years after the initial examination (April 1992), the margins of patchy lesions temporal to the macula have become sharp

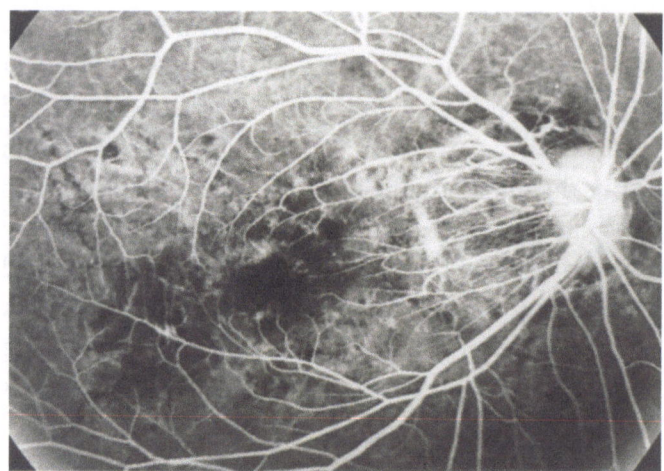

Fig. 27E. Fluorescein fundus angiogram 1 year after the initial examination (August 1991). At 33 sec after dye injection, all spotty lesions of patchy atrophy are hypofluorescent in the early phase. A wide choroidal filling delay is observed around the patchy atrophy. Diffuse atrophy shows irregular hyperfluorescence around the macula

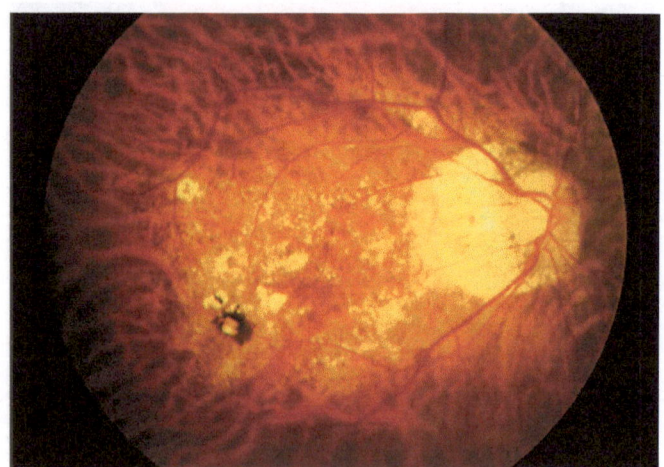

Fig. 27D. Three years after the initial examination (April 1993), all spotty lesions of patchy atrophy have slightly enlarged

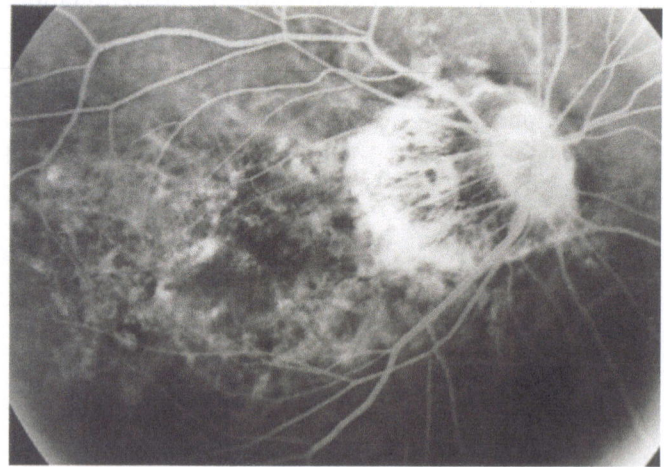

Fig. 27F. Fluorescein fundus angiogram 1 year after the initial examination (August 1991). At 8 min after dye injection, spotty lesions of patchy atrophy show tissue staining in the late phase

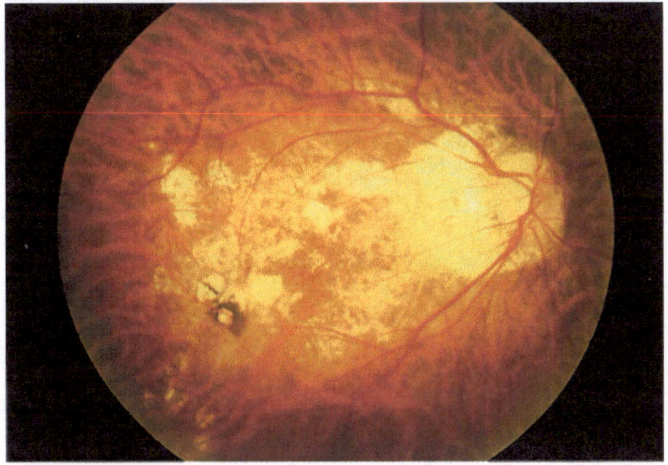

Fig. 27G. Right fundus 4 years after the initial examination (April 1993) shows all the rapidly enlarged spotty lesions of patchy atrophy of the previous year. New spotty lesions of patchy atrophy have appeared temporal to the peripapillary crescent, superior to the macula, and inferotemporal to the original lesions

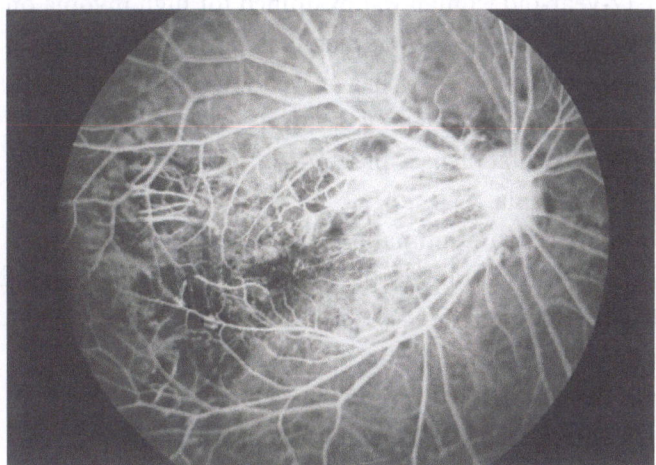

Fig. 27I. Fluorescein fundus angiogram 6 years after the initial examination (June 1993). At 21 sec after dye injection, patchy lesions show hypofluorescence in the early phase of the angiogram. A wide hypofluorescence is seen around the patchy lesion inferotemporal to the macula. Large choroidal vessels are seen within the patchy atrophy

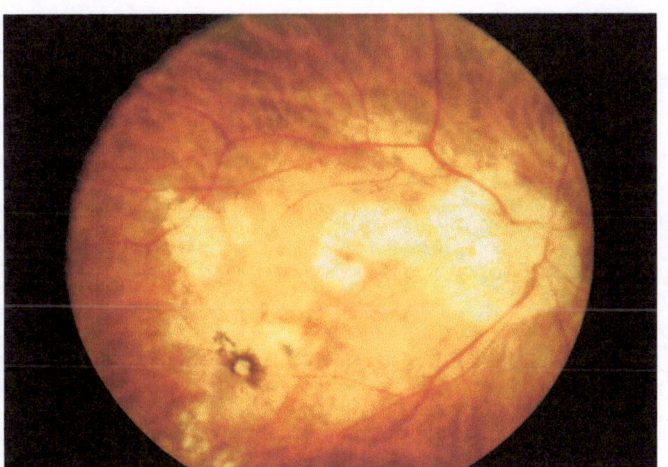

Fig. 27H. Right fundus 6 years after the initial examination (June 1993). All patchy lesions have further enlarged and coalesced. Visual acuity is 0.1, and the refractive error is −16.00 D

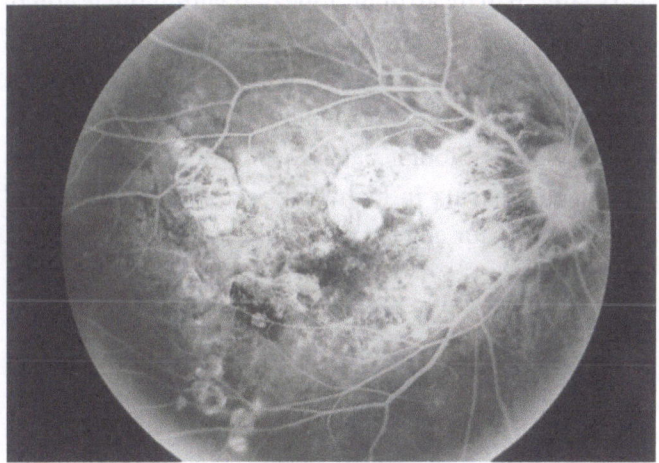

Fig. 27J. Fluorescein fundus angiogram 6 years after the initial examination (June 1993). At 7 min after dye injection, patchy lesions are hyperfluorescent because of tissue staining in the late phase

Case 28

A 17-year-old woman was examined for high myopia on October 23, 1981. She was diagnosed as having myopia at age 3 years, when she began wearing glasses. Her prescription was changed every few years, and she started wearing contact lenses in 1977. No family members had severe myopia.

In the initial examination, the patient's best corrected visual acuity was 0.3 in the right eye and 1.0 in the left. The refractive error was −18.75 D sphere in the right eye and −9.75 D sphere in the left, and the axial length measurements were 30.6 mm in the right eye and 26.7 mm in the left. Intraocular pressures and anterior segments were normal in both eyes. We describe the long-term fundus changes in her right eye.

Summary

This young woman was followed up for 14 years, since 1981. During the first several years of follow-up, only diffuse atrophy was seen inferior to the optic disc. Eight years later, patchy atrophy appeared within the lesion of diffuse atrophy. Patchy atrophy gradually enlarged and finally coalesced with the peripapillary crescent. As the patchy atrophy enlarged, shallow posterior staphyloma was formed. Although patchy atrophy usually appears around the macula in highly myopic eyes, it developed along the inferior edge of the staphyloma in this patient.

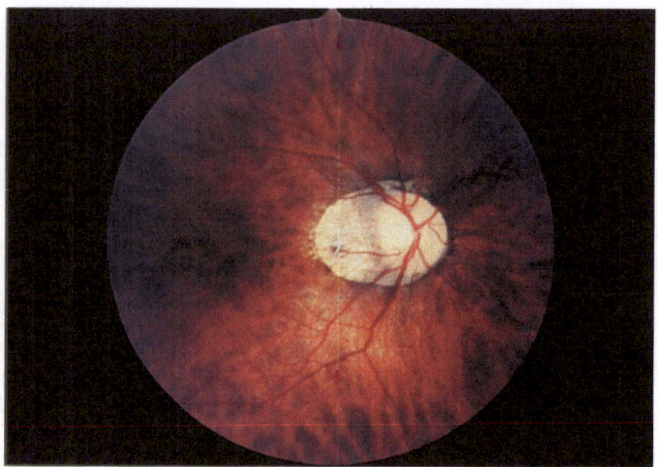

Fig. 28A. Right fundus at the initial examination (October 1981) shows spotty or linear lesions of diffuse atrophy inferior to the optic disc. The optic disc tilts temporally. Temporal peripapillary crescent is seen. No posterior staphyloma is present

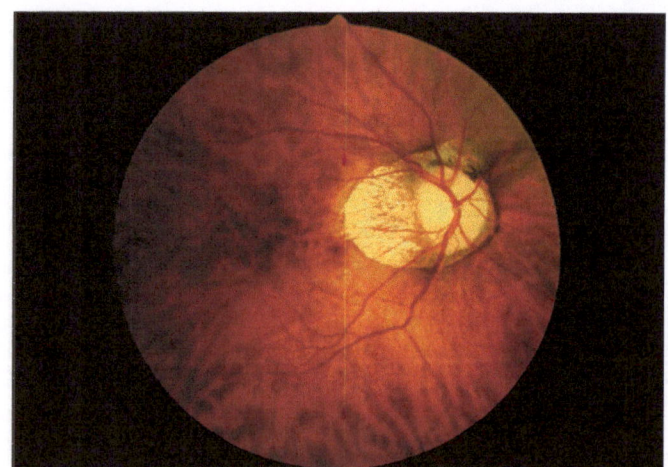

Fig. 28B. Five years after the initial examination (June 1986), spotty and linear lesions of diffuse atrophy have slightly enlarged inferior to the optic disc. Visual acuity is 0.3, and the refractive error is −19.50 D

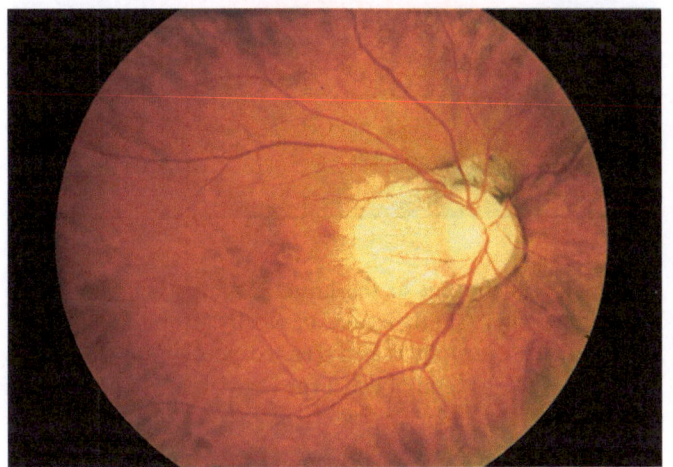

Fig. 28C. Six years after the initial examination (June 1987), spotty and linear lesions of diffuse atrophy have enlarged around the optic disc

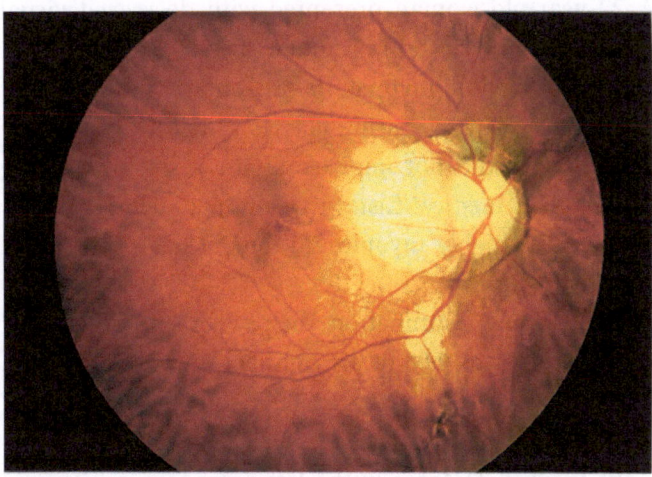

Fig. 28E. Nine years after the initial examination (November 1990), a spotty lesion of patchy atrophy and diffuse atrophy have enlarged. Posterior staphyloma has formed

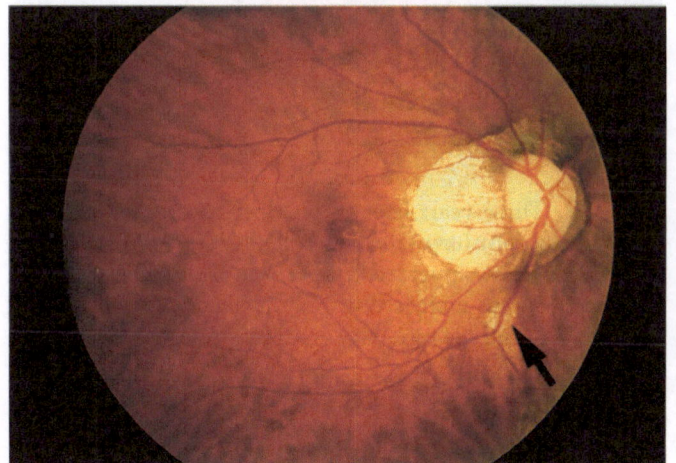

Fig. 28D. Eight years after the initial examination (June 1989), a spotty lesion of patchy atrophy has appeared within the lesion of diffuse atrophy (*arrow*)

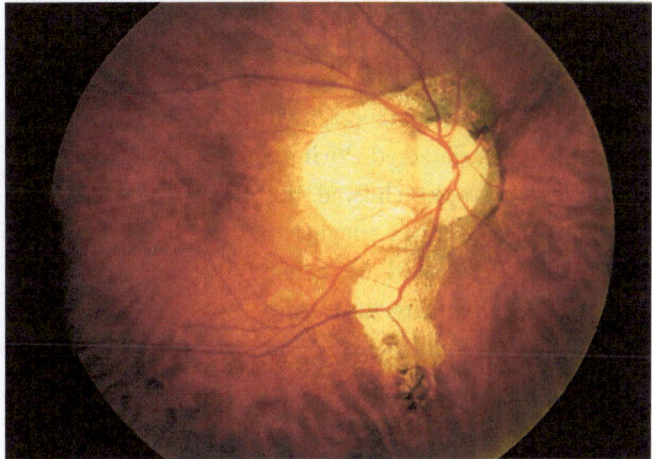

Fig. 28F. Twelve years after the initial examination (July 1993), patchy atrophy has enlarged and is continuous with the peripapillary crescent. Visual acuity is 0.3, and the refractive error is −24.00 D

Case 29

A 22-year-old-woman presented with decreased visual acuity in both eyes on December 15, 1978. She was diagnosed as having myopia before entering elementary school. She began wearing glasses at age 10 years. Her visual acuity did not improve as the result of wearing glasses. Her medical history was noncontributory. Her mother was highly myopic. All four of her siblings had myopia.

In the initial examination, the patient's best corrected visual acuity was 0.08 in the right eye and 0.4 in the left. The refractive error was −21.00 D sphere in both eyes, and the axial length measurements were 31.2 mm in the right eye and 31.4 mm in the left. Intraocular pressures and anterior segments were normal in both eyes. We describe the long-term fundus changes in the left eye.

Summary

This woman was followed up for 17 years, since 1978. During the follow-up period, spotty lesions of patchy atrophy enlarged and coalesced. Nine years after the initial examination, patchy atrophy covered a large area of the posterior fundus. Diffuse atrophy also enlarged with the enlarged patchy atrophy. Although no axial length elongation was detected during this period, a series of fundus photographs showed the dislocation of retinal vessels. These findings suggest that the enlargement of patchy atrophy could be caused by the continuous expansion of the posterior fundus.

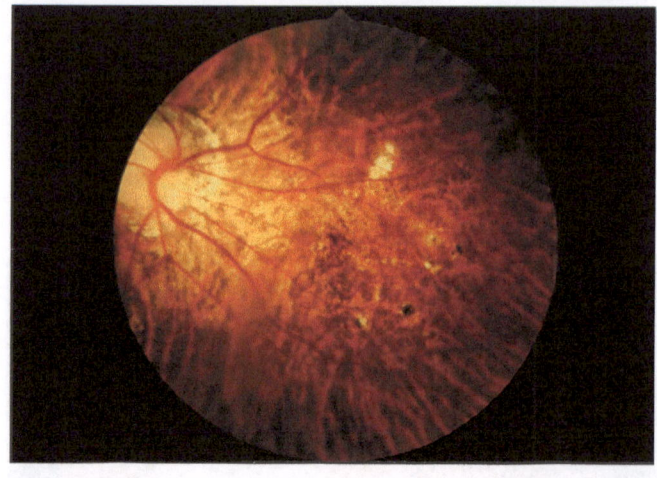

Fig. 29A. Left fundus at the initial examination (December 1978) shows small spotty lesions of patchy atrophy around the macula. Diffuse atrophy is also seen temporal to the optic disc. The optic disc tilts temporally. Type II posterior staphyloma is present

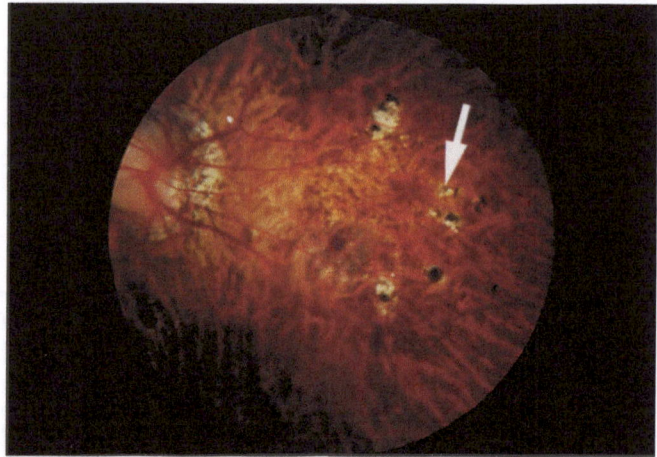

Fig. 29B. Three years later (September 1982), spotty lesions of patchy atrophy have enlarged. A new spotty lesion of patchy atrophy has also appeared temporal to the macula (*arrow*). Pigmentation has increased within the patchy atrophy. Visual acuity is 0.4, and the refractive error is −21.00 D

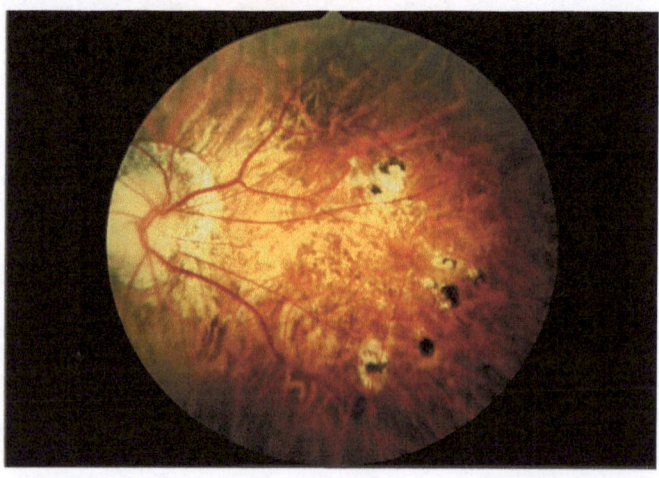

Fig. 29C. Six years after the initial examination (December 1984), patchy atrophy and diffuse atrophy have continued to enlarge

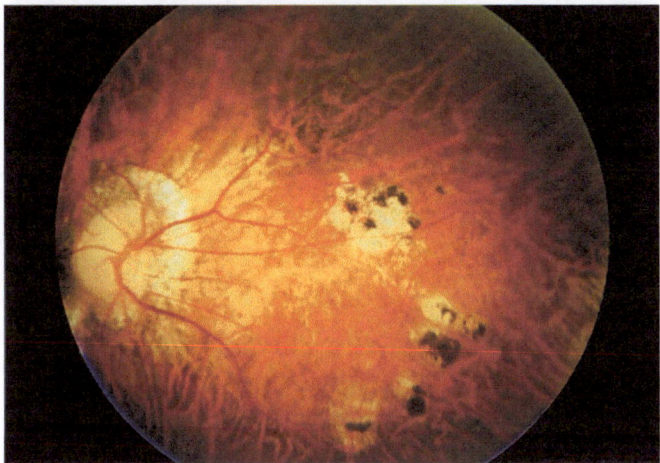

Fig. 29D. Eleven years after the initial examination (September 1989), patchy lesions have further enlarged and coalesced. Spotty lesions of diffuse atrophy have progressed into an enlarged lesion of diffuse atrophy

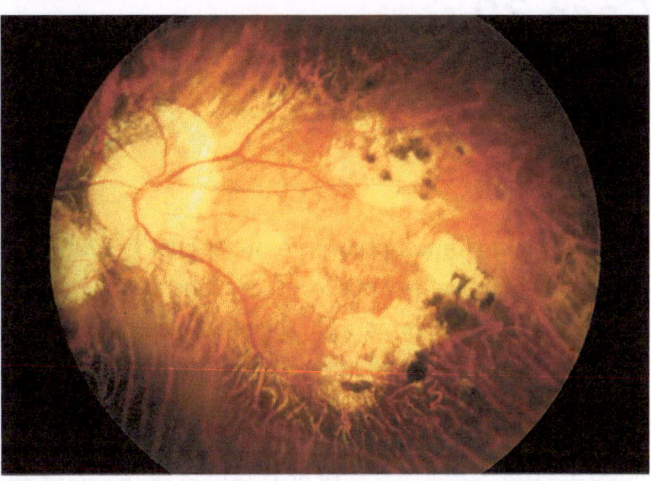

Fig. 29F. Fifteen years after the initial examination (October 1993), the patchy lesions have coalesced and have formed two large lesions of patchy atrophy temporal to the macula. Diffuse atrophy and peripapillary crescent have also enlarged. Visual acuity is 0.2, and the refractive error is $-21.00\,\mathrm{D}$

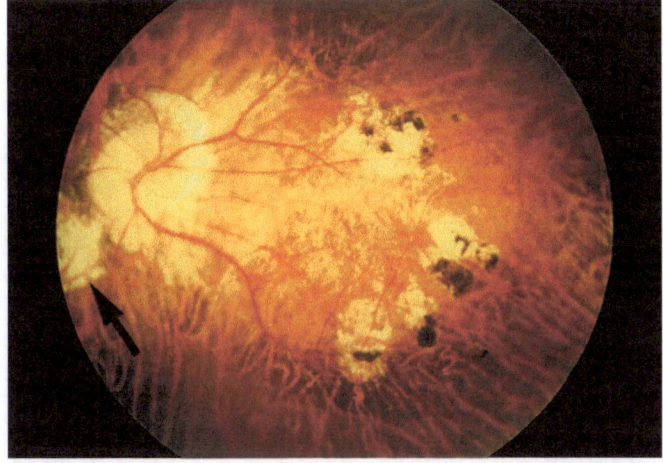

Fig. 29E. Twelve years after the initial examination (March 1991), patchy lesions have enlarged and coalesced still further. Another area of patchy atrophy is seen nasal to the optic disc (*arrow*)

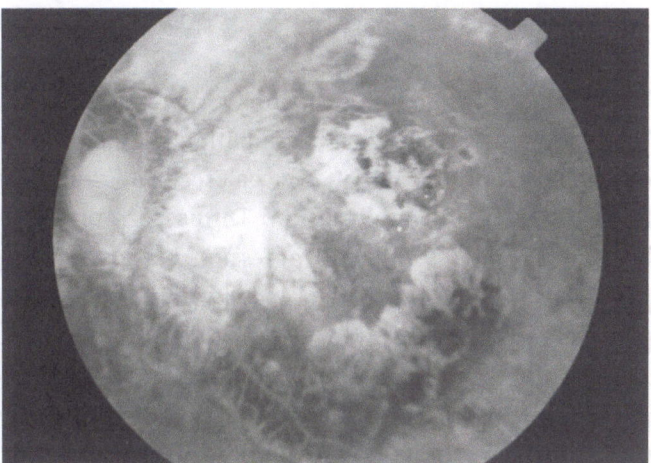

Fig. 29G. Fluorescein fundus angiogram 17 years after the initial examination (April 1996). At 8 min after dye injection, large patchy atrophy is continuous with peripapillary crescent inferior to the macula. Patchy atrophy has enlarged along the inferior edge of the posterior staphyloma. The macular lesion is surrounded by the enlarged patchy atrophy

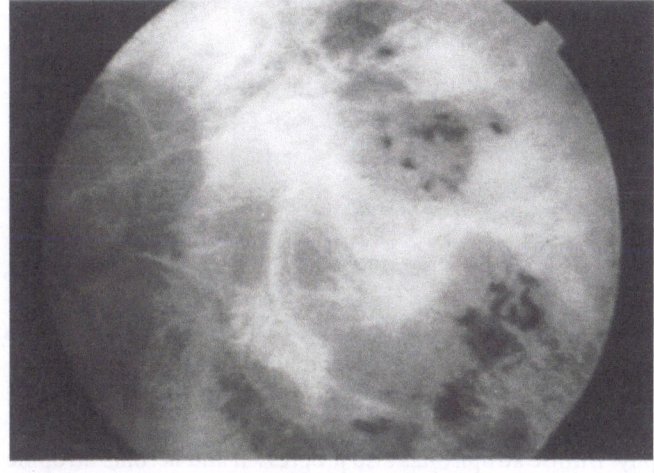

Fig. 29H. Indocyanine green angiogram 17 years after the initial examination (April 1996). The late phase of the angiogram shows a large area of hypofluorescence corresponding to the patchy atrophy

Case 30

A 69-year-old woman presented on August 1, 1986, with decreased visual acuity in the left eye. She was diagnosed with myopia as an infant. She began wearing glasses at age 13 years. All three of her children are highly myopic.

In the initial examination, the patient's best corrected visual acuity was 0.3 in the right eye and 0.04 in the left. The refractive error was −18.00 D sphere in the right eye and −20.00 D sphere in the left, and the axial length measurements were 31.1 mm in both eyes. Intraocular pressures and anterior segments were normal in both eyes. Nuclear cataract was observed bilaterally. We describe the long-term fundus changes of both eyes.

Summary

This woman was followed up for 9 years, since 1986. Three years after the initial examination, patchy lesions of patchy atrophy in her left eye coalesced and gradually formed a large atrophic lesion. Diffuse atrophy also became atrophic with the progression of surrounding patchy atrophy. In this patient, patchy and diffuse atrophy were already observed at the initial examination. Although there were no obvious ophthalmoscopic findings suggesting choroidal neovascularization, it is likely that myopic choroidal neovascularization existed before her initial visit to our high myopia clinic. Patchy atrophy sometimes progresses rapidly in the area of previous bleeding or retinal edema caused by choroidal neovascularization.

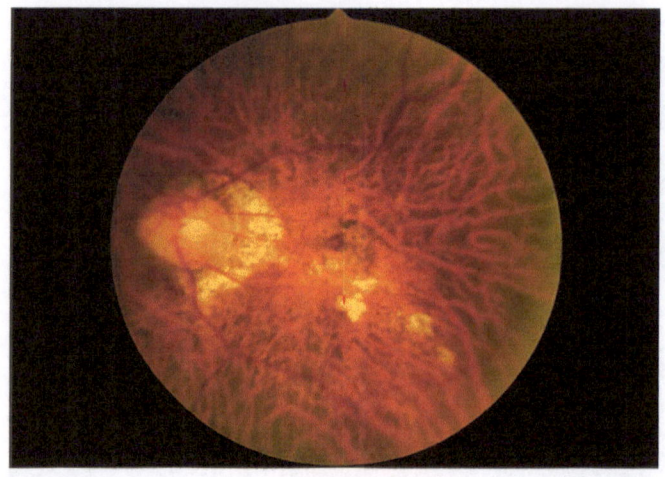

Fig. 30A. Left fundus at the initial examination (August 1986) shows four spotty lesions of patchy atrophy inferior to the macula. Spotty or linear lesions of diffuse atrophy are also seen in the macula. The optic disc tilts temporally. A temporal peripapillary crescent is seen. Type I posterior staphyloma is present. No choroidal neovascular membrane is observed ophthalmoscopically

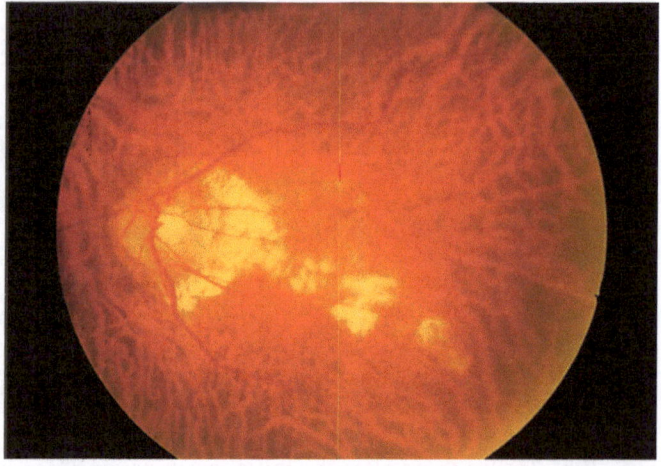

Fig. 30B. Three years later (January 1989), the spotty lesions of patchy atrophy inferior to the macula have enlarged. Spotty or linear lesions of diffuse atrophy have increased. Visual acuity is 0.04, even though the macular lesion is not involved with the patchy atrophy

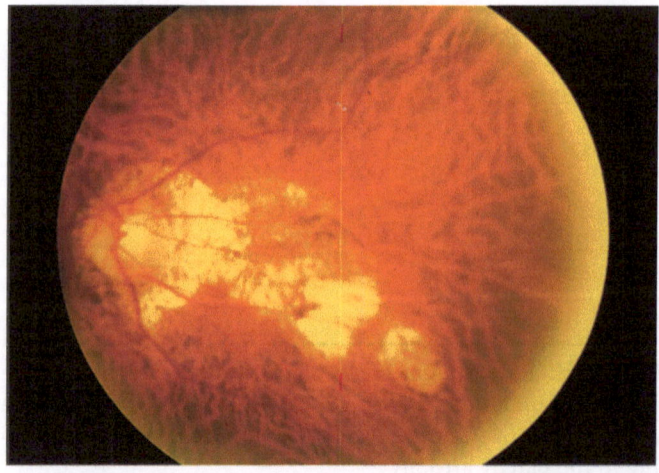

Fig. 30C. Five years after the initial examination (June 1991), the spotty lesions of patchy atrophy have further enlarged, coalesced, and progressed into patchy lesions of patchy atrophy. Diffuse atrophy has also progressed and become atrophic

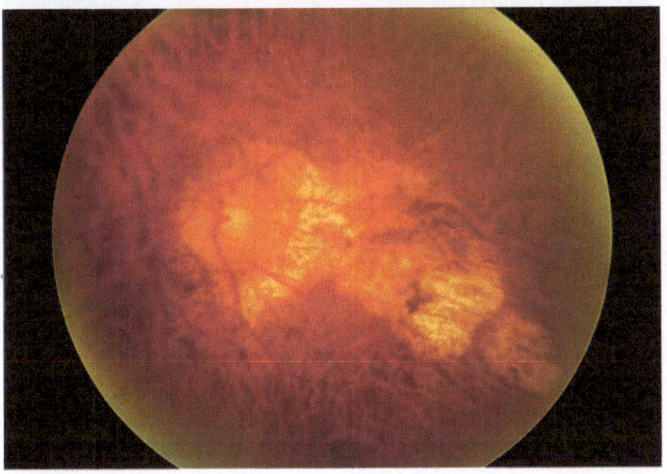

Fig. 30D. Six years after the initial examination (October 1992), the patchy lesions of patchy atrophy have coalesced and formed a large patchy lesion. Diffuse atrophy in the macula also has become atrophic. The margin of diffuse atrophy is blurring. Visual acuity is 0.05, and the refractive error is −21.00 D

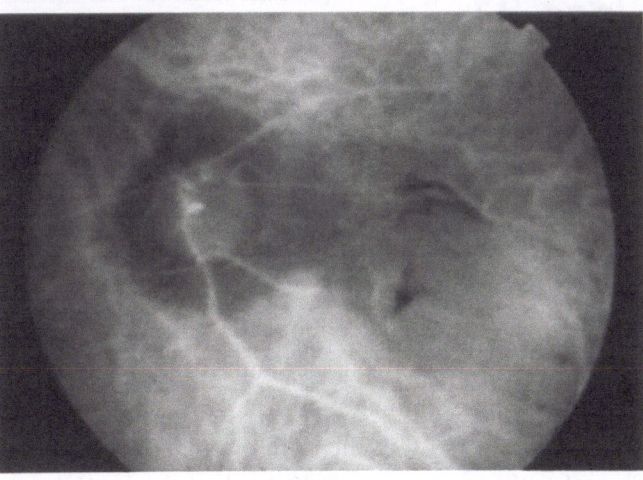

Fig. 30F. Indocyanine green fundus angiogram 10 years after the initial examination (February 1996) shows a large hypofluorescent area in the macula corresponding to the hyperfluorescent area seen by fluorescein angiography

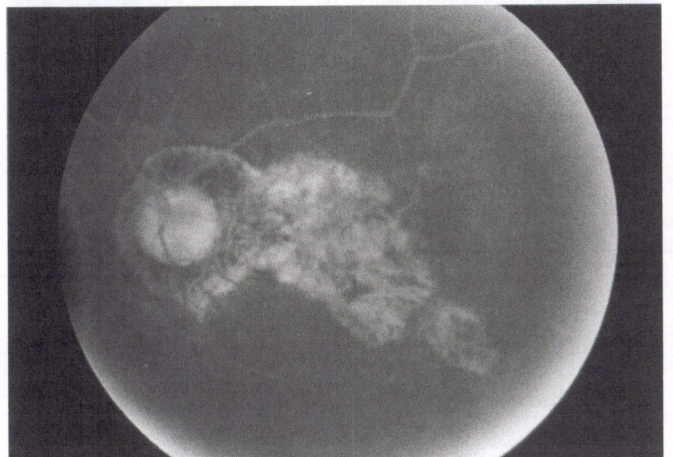

Fig. 30E. Fluorescein fundus angiogram 5 years after the initial examination (June 1991). At 8 min after dye injection, patchy atrophy and diffuse atrophy are detected as one large hyperfluorescent area caused by tissue staining

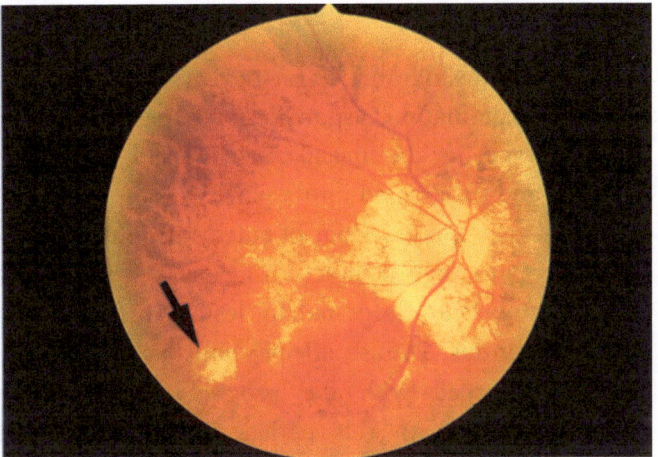

Fig. 30G. Right fundus at the initial examination (August 1986). The poorly defined patchy lesion of patchy atrophy is seen inferior to the macula (*arrow*). A temporal peripapillary crescent is seen. Type I posterior staphyloma is present

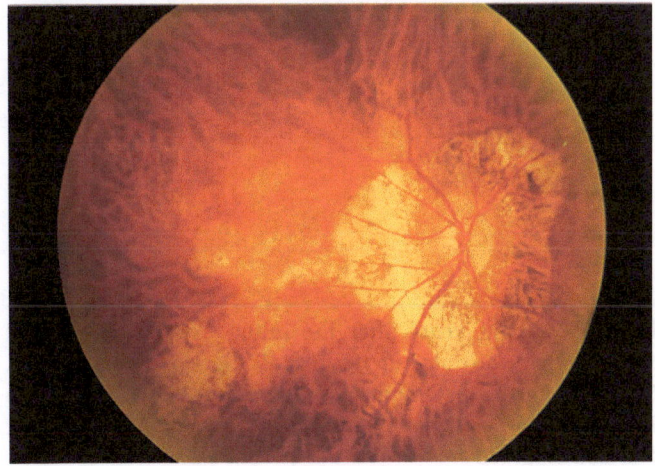

Fig. 30H. Right fundus 6 years after the initial examination (October 1992). The patchy lesion of patchy atrophy has enlarged. Visual acuity is 0.2, and the refractive error is −24.00 D

Case 31

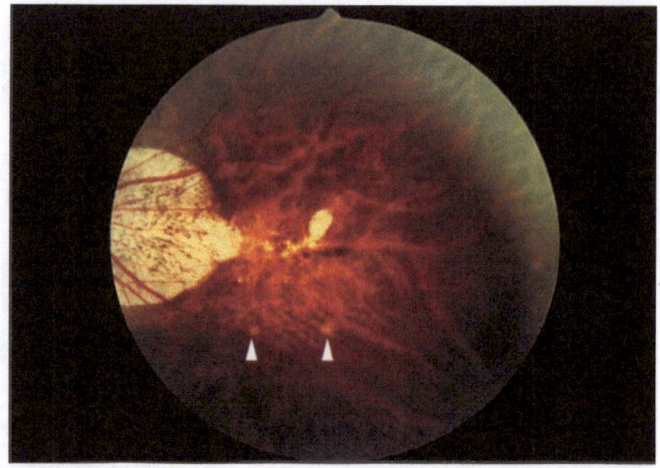

Fig. 31A. Left fundus at the initial examination (August 1981) shows a spotty lesion of patchy atrophy in the macula. Two other spotty lesions of patchy atrophy are visible inferior to the macula (*arrowheads*). A temporal peripapillary crescent is seen. Posterior staphyloma is present

A 55-year-old woman presented with myodesopsia in both eyes on August 28, 1981. She had noticed myodesopsia in the left eye about 10 years ago, and in the right eye about 1 year ago. Her aunt is highly myopic.

In the initial examination, the patient's best corrected visual acuity was 1.0 in the right eye and 0.1 in the left. The refractive error was −2.25 D sphere in the right eye and −12.00 D sphere in the left, and the axial length measurements were 24.2 mm in the right eye and 28.3 mm in the left. Intraocular pressures and anterior segments were normal in both eyes. We describe the long-term fundus changes in her left eye.

Summary

This woman was followed up for 14 years, since 1981. At the initial examination, a spotty lesion of patchy atrophy was observed in the macula. This lesion gradually enlarged and progressed into a patchy lesion of patchy atrophy. Other spotty lesions of patchy atrophy also appeared and gradually coalesced. Thirteen years after the initial examination, large patchy lesions occupied the posterior fundus. Diffuse atrophy and a peripapillary crescent enlarged with the progression of patchy atrophy. As seen in this patient, spotty lesions of patchy atrophy may enlarge rapidly and form large chorioretinal atrophy in the posterior fundus in highly myopic eyes.

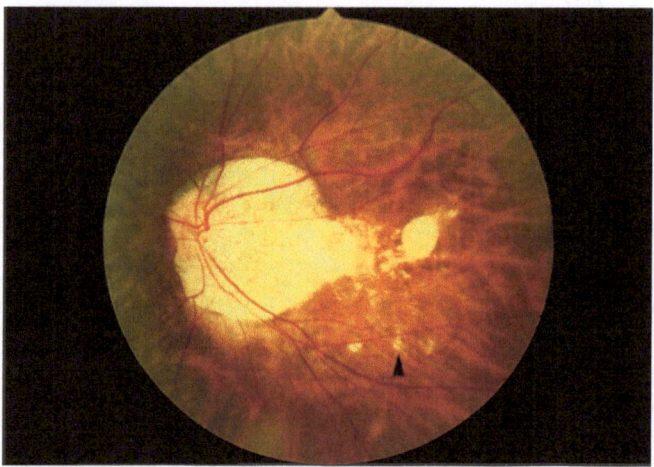

Fig. 31B. Four years later (May 1985), patchy atrophy in the macula has enlarged. A new spotty lesion of patchy atrophy appears inferior to the macula (*arrowhead*). Spotty or linear lesions of diffuse atrophy are observed around the peripapillary crescent. Visual acuity is 0.08, and the refractive error is −13.00 D

Fig. 31C. Eight years after the initial examination (April 1989), patchy atrophy in the macula has enlarged further. Spotty lesions of patchy atrophy inferior to the macula have increased. Diffuse atrophy around the peripapillary crescent has also enlarged

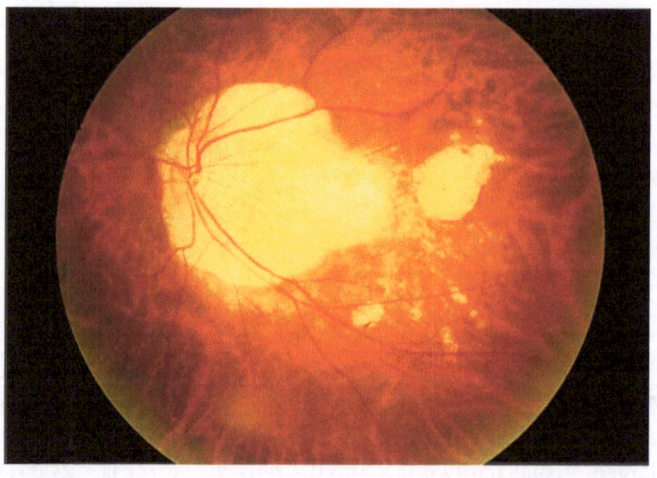

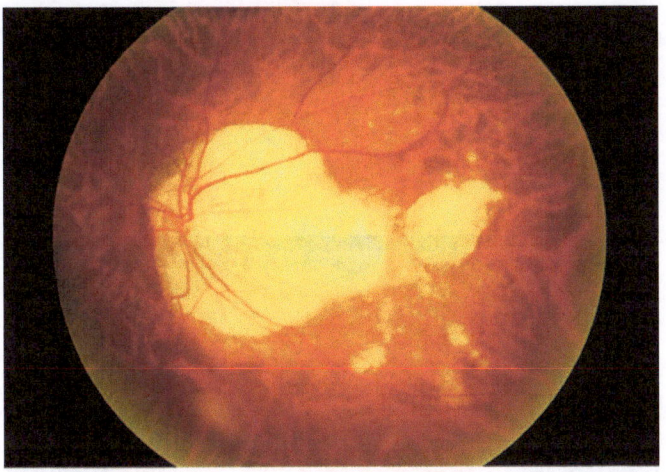

Fig. 31D. Nine years after the initial examination (March 1990), spotty lesions of patchy atrophy inferior to the macula have enlarged further

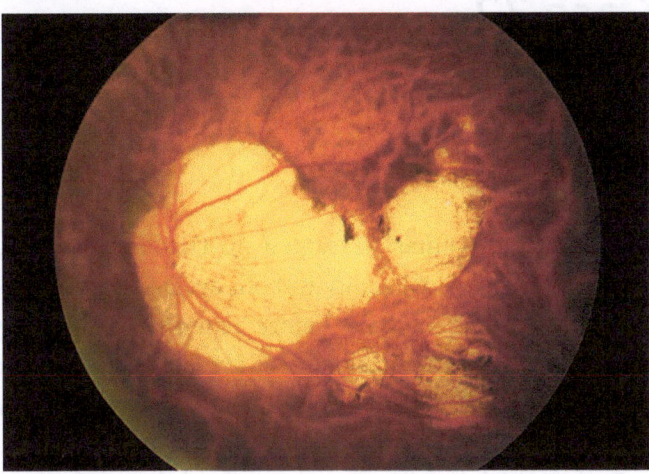

Fig. 31F. Thirteen years after the initial examination (June 1994), patchy atrophy in the posterior fundus has enlarged and coalesced

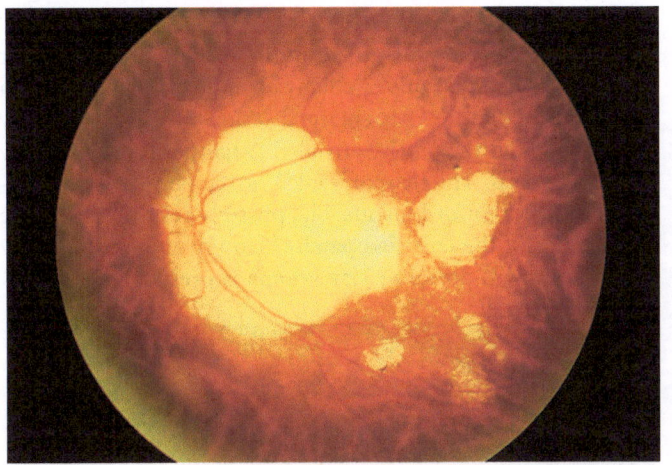

Fig. 31E. Ten years after the initial examination (April 1991), spotty lesions of patchy atrophy inferior to the macula have continued to enlarge. Patchy atrophy in the macula and peripapillary crescent has also enlarged. Visual acuity is 0.04, and the refractive error is −13.75 D

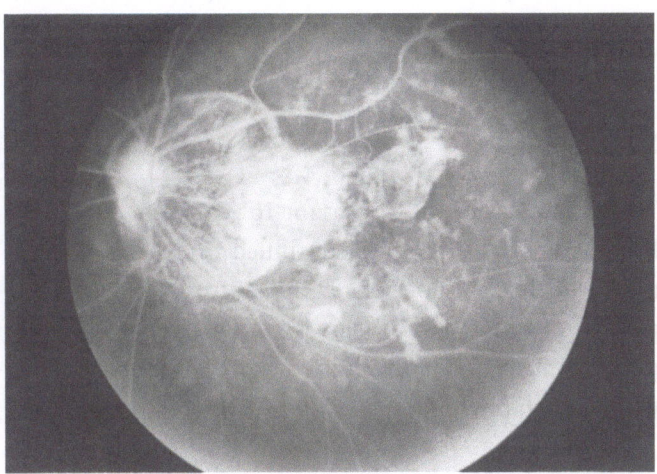

Fig. 31G. Fluorescein fundus angiogram 8 years after the initial examination (April 1989). At 4 min after dye injection, patchy atrophy shows hyperfluorescence. The center of the patchy atrophy in the macula remains hypofluorescent

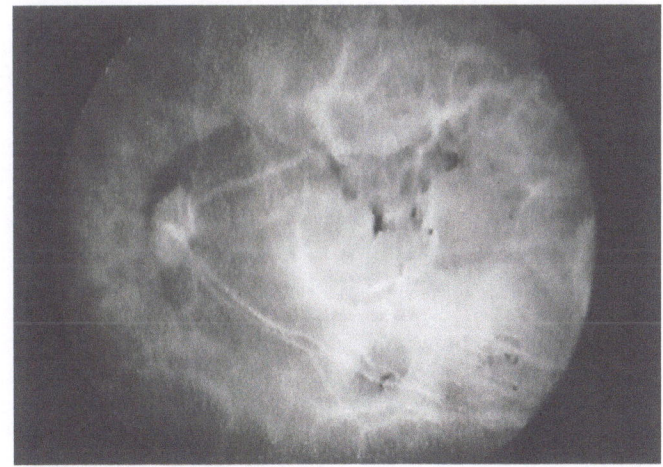

Fig. 31H. Indocyanine green fundus angiogram 12 years after the initial examination (September 1993). Patchy atrophy is hypofluorescent in the late phase

Case 32

A 54-year-old woman presented on October 19, 1979, with decreased visual acuity in both eyes. She was diagnosed as having myopia before entering elementary school. She began wearing glasses for distance vision at age 14 years. Her vision had gradually decreased in both eyes since 1971. One of her five siblings is highly myopic.

In the initial examination, the patient's best corrected visual acuity was 0.3 in both eyes. The refractive error was −30.00 D sphere in the right eye and −24.00 D sphere in the left, and the axial length measurements were 31.7 mm in the right eye and 30.4 mm in the left. Intraocular pressures and anterior segments were normal in both eyes. Mild cataractous changes were noted. We describe the long-term fundus changes in both eyes.

Summary

This woman was followed up for 16 years, since 1979. All lesions of patchy atrophy continued to enlarge and coalesce during this period. Diffuse atrophy around the patchy atrophy also progressed. The progression of patchy and diffuse atrophy was noted only within the posterior staphyloma.

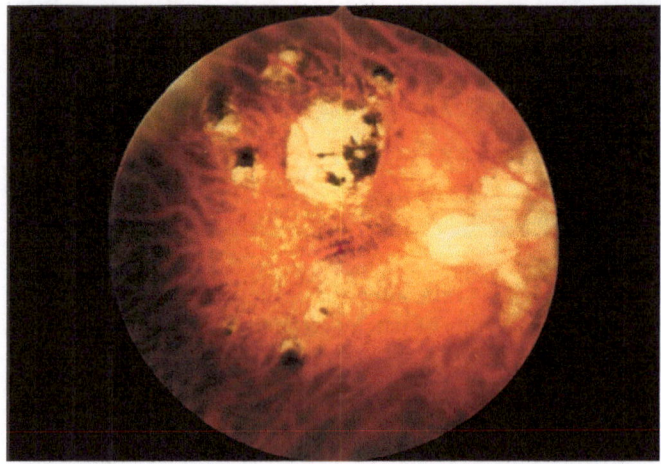

Fig. 32A. Right fundus at the initial examination (October 1979) shows eight lesions of patchy atrophy of various sizes in the posterior fundus. An enlarged lesion of diffuse atrophy appears around the patchy atrophy. A temporal peripapillary crescent is seen. The temporal edge of the peripapillary crescent protrudes toward the macula, possibly resulting from the coalescence of the enlarged patchy atrophy and peripapillary crescent. Type II posterior staphyloma is present

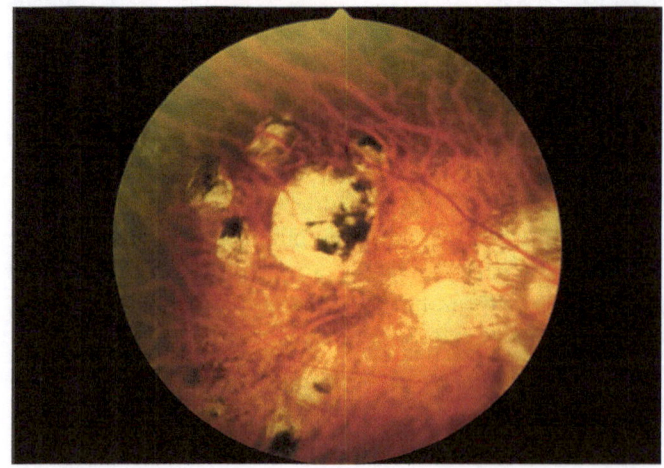

Fig. 32B. Five years later (October 1984), all lesions of patchy atrophy have enlarged. Visual acuity is 0.3, and the refractive error is −26.00 D

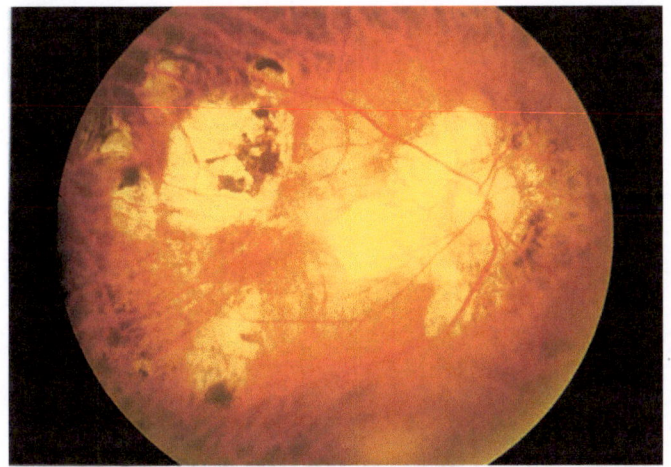

Fig. 32C. Twelve years after the initial examination (October 1991), all lesions of patchy atrophy have enlarged further and are coalescing. Diffuse atrophy has also enlarged and covers the entire posterior fundus

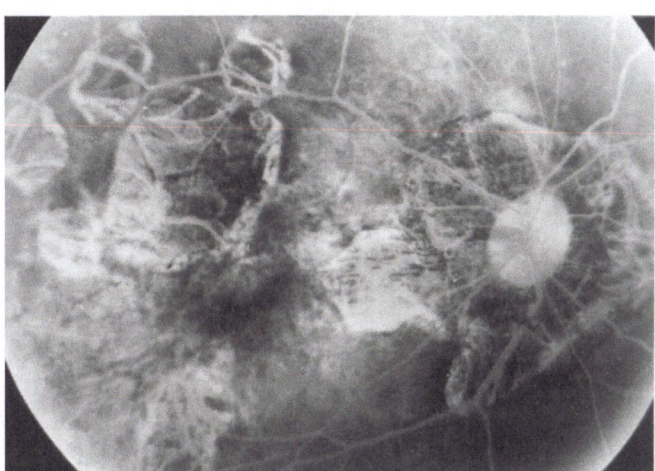

Fig. 32E. Fluorescein fundus angiogram 12 years after the initial examination (October 1991). Six minutes after dye injection, patchy atrophy shows late hyperfluorescence, particularly at the margins. Large-sized choroidal vessels are visible within the lesion of patchy atrophy

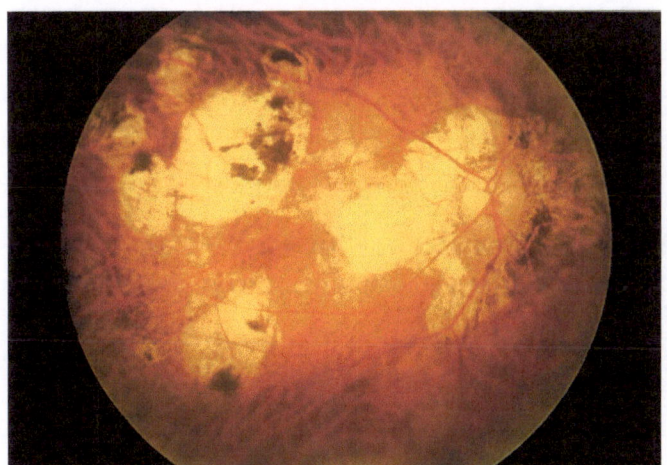

Fig. 32D. Fifteen years after the initial examination (August 1994), all lesions of patchy atrophy have enlarged further and have coalesced. The fovea is not involved with the patchy atrophy

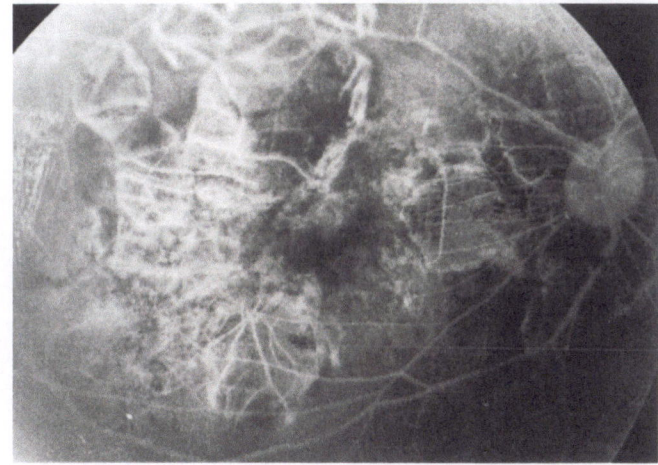

Fig. 32F. Fluorescein fundus angiogram 15 years after the initial examination (May 1994). At 1 min after dye injection, all lesions of patchy atrophy show a choroidal filling defect. The area of patchy atrophy has enlarged in the past 3 years

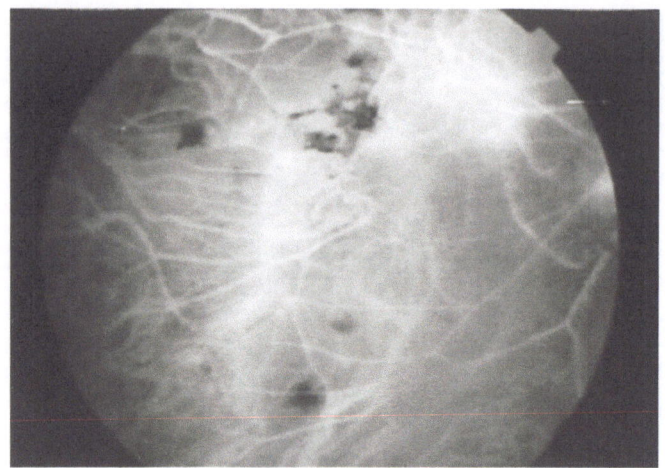

Fig. 32G. Indocyanine green fundus angiogram 15 years after the initial examination (May 1994). Patchy atrophy is relatively hypofluorescent because of a choroidal filling defect. Pigmentation within the lesion of patchy atrophy shows blocked fluorescence

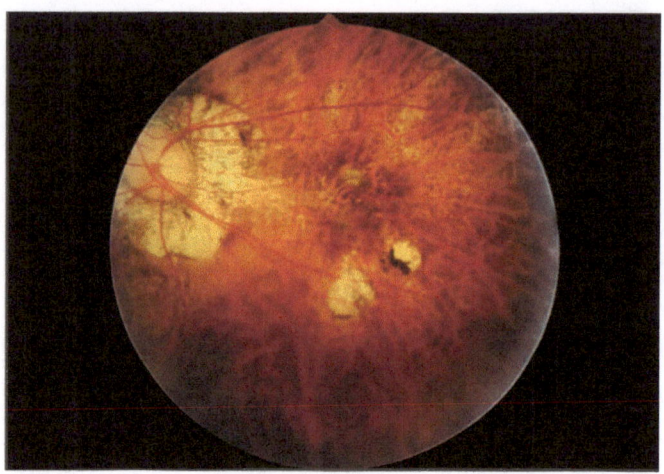

Fig. 32I. Five years later (October 1984), the lesions of patchy atrophy and diffuse atrophy have enlarged. Visual acuity is 0.3, and the refractive error is −24.00 D

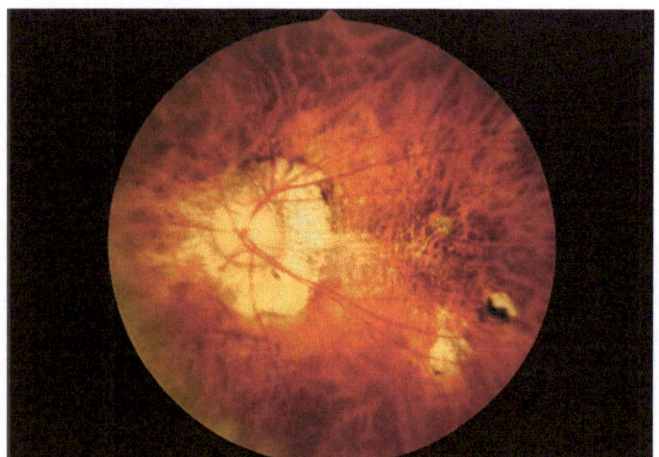

Fig. 32H. Left fundus at the initial examination (October 1979) shows two lesions of patchy atrophy inferior to the macula. Pigmentation is seen within the lesions. Myopic choroidal neovascular membrane is observed in the macula. A wide annular crescent is seen around the optic disc. Type II posterior staphyloma is present

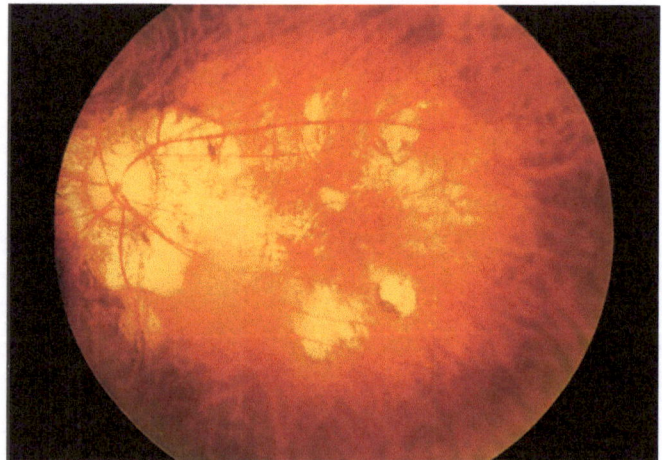

Fig. 32J. Twelve years after the initial examination (October 1991), the lesions of patchy atrophy have enlarged further. Another lesion of patchy atrophy is newly formed inferior to the peripapillary crescent. Diffuse atrophy has progressed and covers the entire posterior fundus

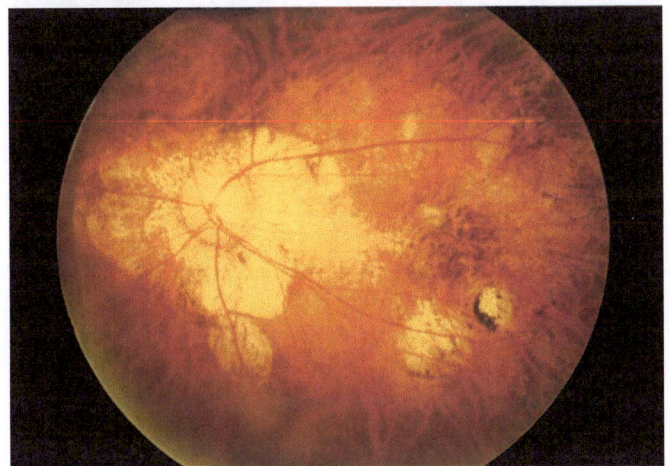

Fig. 32K. Fifteen years after the initial examination (October 1994), newly formed patchy atrophy inferior to the peripapillary crescent has enlarged and is moving closer to the peripapillary crescent. The lesions of patchy atrophy inferior to the macula have also enlarged

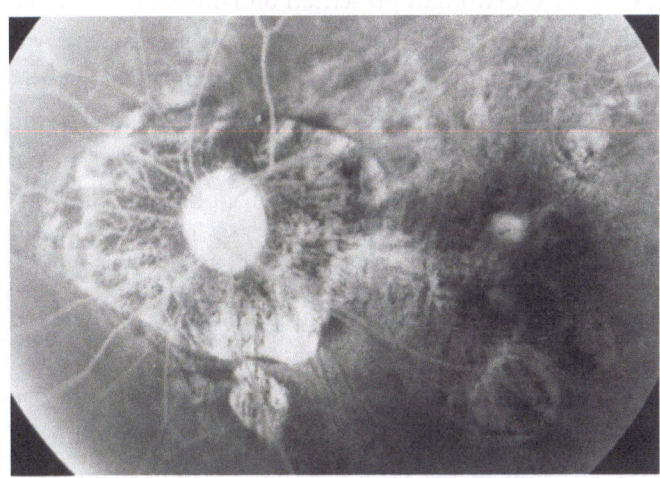

Fig. 32M. Fluorescein fundus angiogram 12 years after the initial examination (October 1991). At 8 min after dye injection, all lesions of patchy atrophy appear hyperfluorescent in the late phase. No dye leakage is seen from the choroidal neovascular membrane in the macula

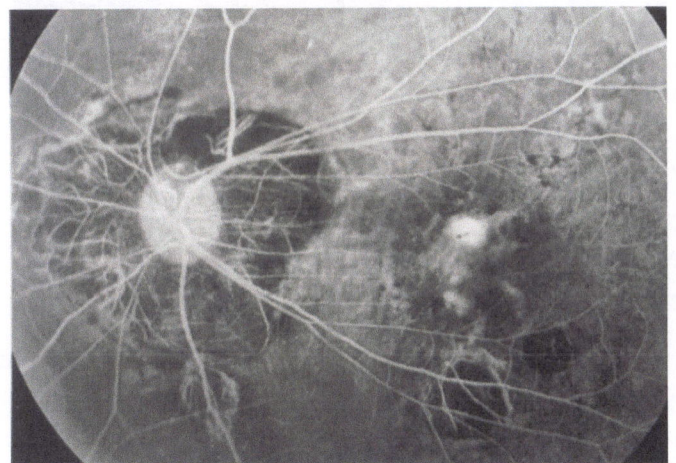

Fig. 32L. Fluorescein fundus angiogram 12 years after the initial examination (October 1991). At 38 sec after dye injection, all lesions of patchy atrophy are hypofluorescent because of a choroidal filling defect in the early phase. Choroidal neovascular membrane in the macula is hyperfluorescent

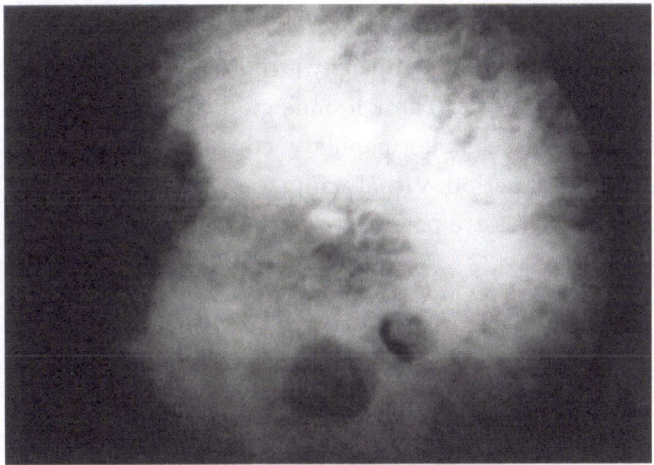

Fig. 32N. Indocyanine green fundus angiogram taken 15 years after the initial examination (May 1994). The lesions of patchy atrophy inferior to the macula are hypofluorescent in the late phase. Choroidal neovascular membrane appears slightly hyperfluorescent

Case 33

A 44-year-old-woman presented on November 13, 1981, with decreased visual acuity in both her eyes. She was diagnosed with myopia as an infant. Her visual acuity did not improve with wearing glasses. She began wearing contact lenses at age 13 years. The best corrected visual acuity at that time was about 0.4 in both eyes. She suffered from hepatitis at the age of 23. No family members had severe myopia.

In the initial examination, the patient's best corrected visual acuity was 0.4 in the right eye and 0.5 in the left. The refractive error was $-9.00\,D$ sphere in the right eye and $-12.00\,D$ in the left. The axial length measurements were 28.8 mm in the right eye and 29.8 mm in the left. Intraocular pressures and anterior segments were normal, other than slight bilateral keratoconus. We describe the long-term fundus changes in her right eye.

Summary

This woman was followed up for 14 years, since 1981. Until 1987, her right fundus showed diffuse atrophy only. No patchy atrophy was observed at that time. In 1990, many spotty lesions of patchy atrophy appeared temporal to the macula. These lesions gradually enlarged and finally coalesced. Peripapillary crescent also enlarged during that period. Visual acuity was maintained in spite of the progressive patchy atrophy.

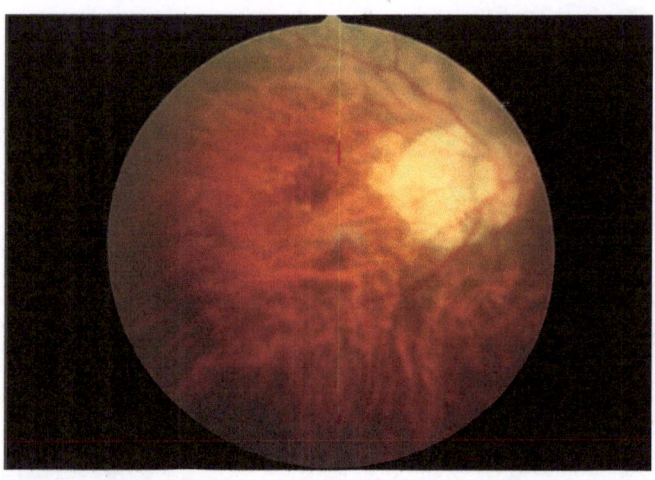

Fig. 33A. Right fundus at the initial examination (November 1981) shows spotty or linear lesions of diffuse atrophy in the macula. Patchy atrophy is not seen. The optic disc tilts temporally. Temporal peripapillary crescent is seen. Type I posterior staphyloma is present

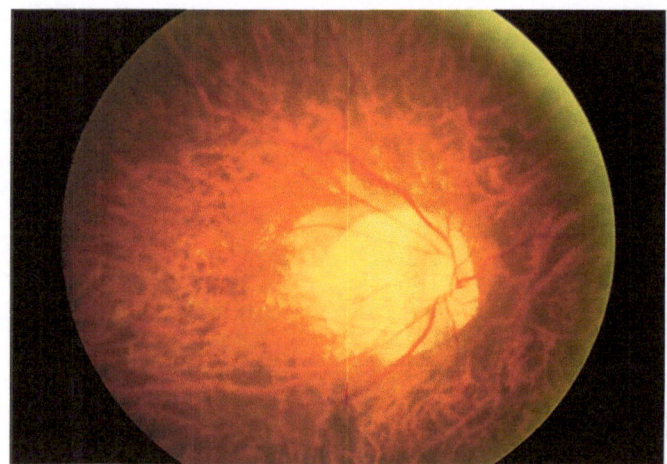

Fig. 33B. Six years after the initial examination (October 1987), spotty and linear lesions of diffuse atrophy have increased in the macula. The best corrected visual acuity is 0.4

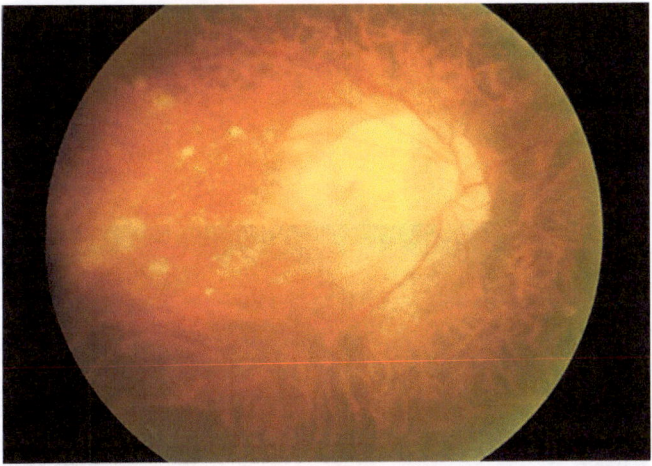

Fig. 33C. Ten years after the initial examination (October 1991), many spotty lesions of patchy atrophy have appeared around the macula. Diffuse atrophy has also enlarged. The best corrected visual acuity is 0.4

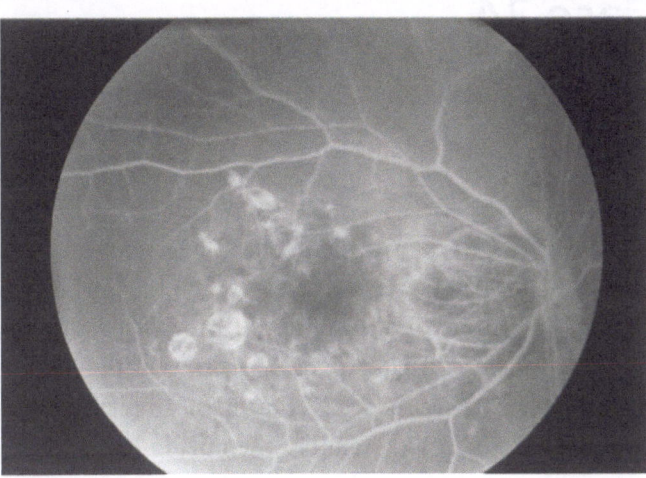

Fig. 33F. Fluorescein fundus angiogram 10 years after the initial examination (October 1991). At 2 min after dye injection, many spotty lesions of patchy atrophy show hyperfluorescence. The center of the lesions remains hypofluorescent

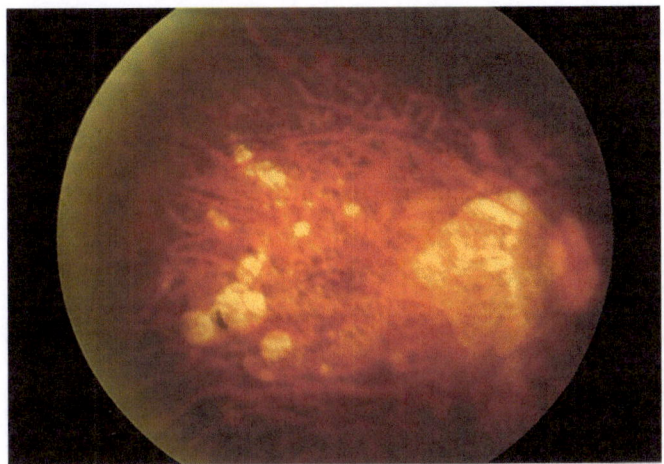

Fig. 33D. Eleven years after the initial examination (October 1992), spotty lesions of patchy atrophy have enlarged and coalesced

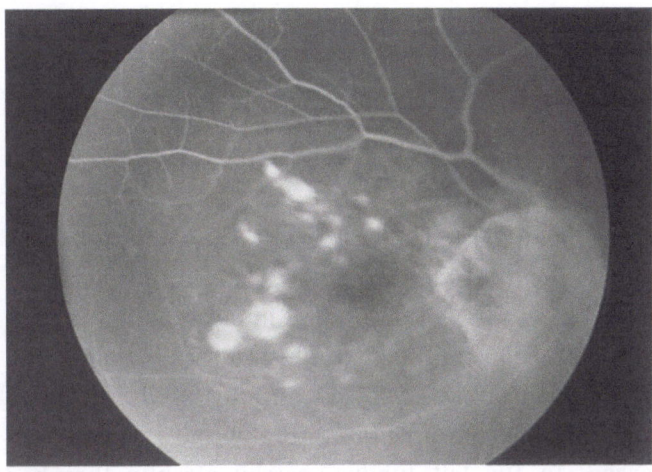

Fig. 33G. Fluorescein fundus angiogram 10 years after the initial examination (October 1991). At 7 min after dye injection, all spotty lesions of patchy atrophy are hyperfluorescent

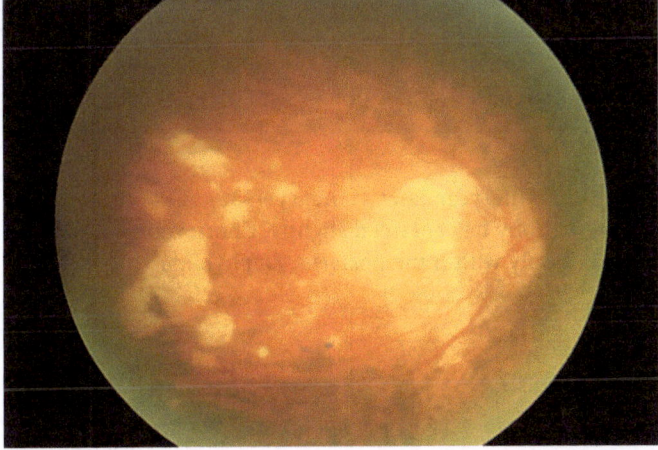

Fig. 33E. Thirteen years after the initial examination (October 1994), the patchy lesions have enlarged and coalesced into several large lesions. Diffuse atrophy and peripapillary crescent have also increased

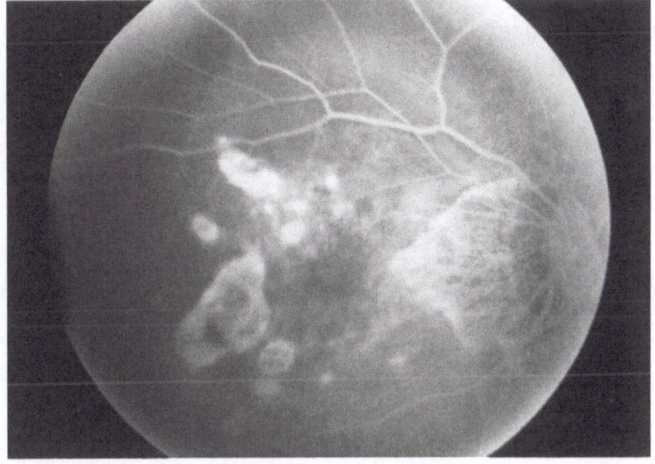

Fig. 33H. Fluorescein fundus angiogram 13 years after the initial examination (June 1994). At 7 min after dye injection, enlarged spotty lesions are hyperfluorescent. The foveal lesion is not involved in the enlargement of patchy atrophy

Case 34

A 47-year-old-woman presented with decreased visual acuity in both her eyes on January 24, 1985. She was diagnosed with myopia as an infant. Her vision did not improve much with glasses. She began wearing contact lenses about 15 years ago. Her medical history was noncontributory. No family members had severe myopia.

In the initial examination, the patient's best corrected visual acuity was 0.1 in the right eye and 0.2 in the left. The refractive error was -18.00 D sphere in the right eye and -22.00 D in the left. The axial length measurements were 29.8 mm in the right eye and 30.7 mm in the left. Intraocular pressures and anterior segments were normal in both eyes. We describe the long-term fundus changes of both eyes.

Summary

This woman was followed up for 10 years, since 1985. The progression of patchy atrophy was observed in both her eyes during this period. At the initial examination, an enlarged lesion of diffuse atrophy was seen in both fundi. In the right fundus, patchy atrophy newly appeared within the lesion of diffuse atrophy and gradually enlarged. In the left fundus, patchy atrophy that had already existed at the initial examination gradually enlarged. These areas coalesced with one another and finally occupied a large part of both posterior fundi. Patchy atrophy seen within lesions of diffuse atrophy in eyes with deep staphyloma tends to progress rapidly, as seen in this patient.

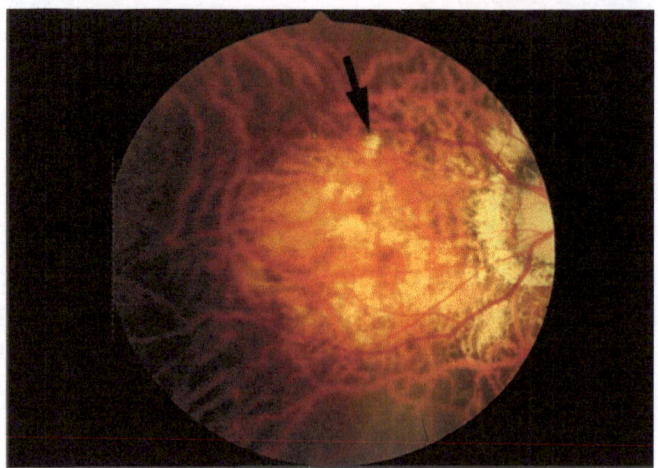

Fig. 34A. Right fundus at the initial examination (January 1985) shows a small spotty lesion of patchy atrophy superior to the macula (*arrow*). An enlarged lesion of diffuse atrophy is visible in the posterior fundus. The optic disc tilts temporally. A temporal peripapillary crescent is seen. Type II posterior staphyloma is present

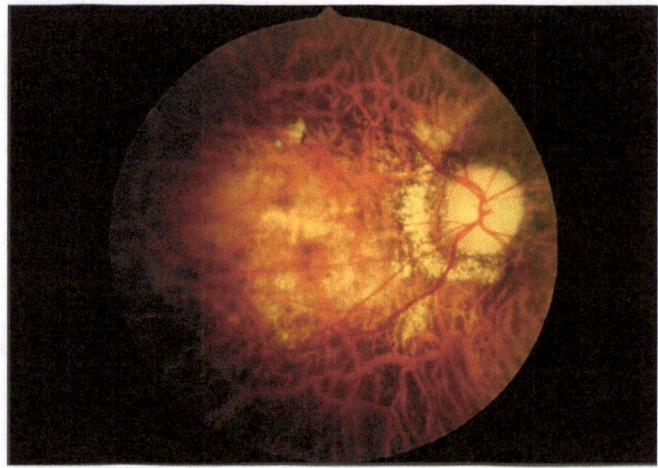

Fig. 34B. One year later (January 1986), a spotty lesion of patchy atrophy has enlarged slightly. Chorioretinal atrophy is observed only within the posterior staphyloma

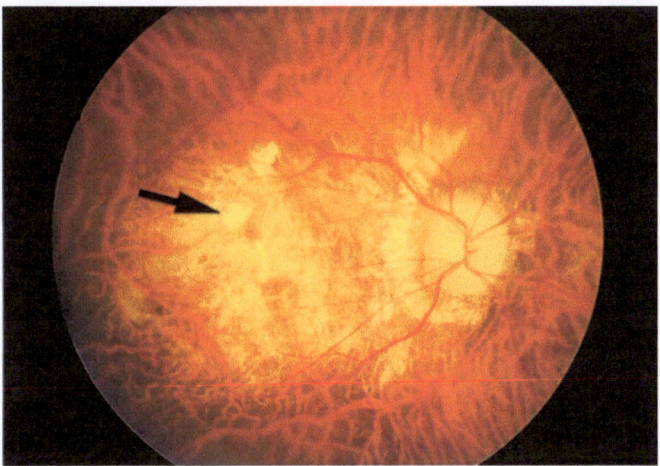

Fig. 34C. Three years after the initial examination (April 1988), a new spotty lesion of patchy atrophy has appeared temporal to the macula (*arrow*). An enlarged lesion of diffuse atrophy covers the entire posterior fundus

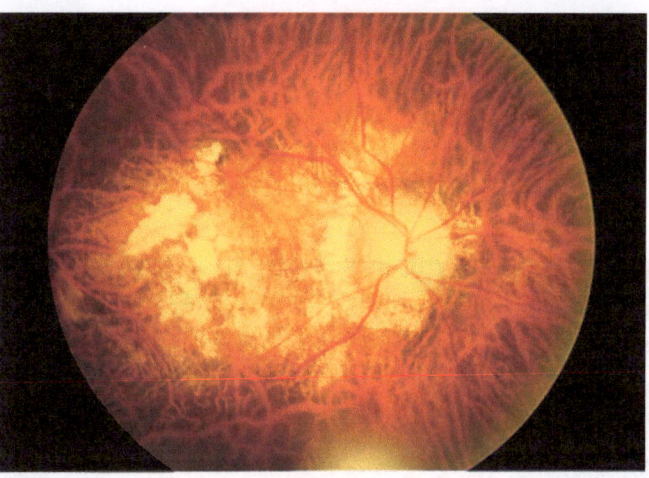

Fig. 34E. Five years after the initial examination (January 1990), spotty lesions of patchy atrophy have enlarged further and progressed into patchy lesions. The edges of the patchy lesions are irregular. The shapes of the patchy lesions are not rounded, which are different from typical patchy lesions

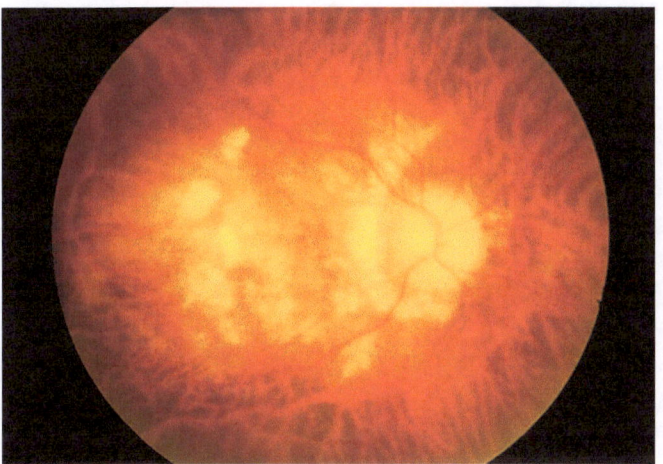

Fig. 34D. Four years after the initial examination (January 1989), spotty lesions of patchy atrophy have enlarged

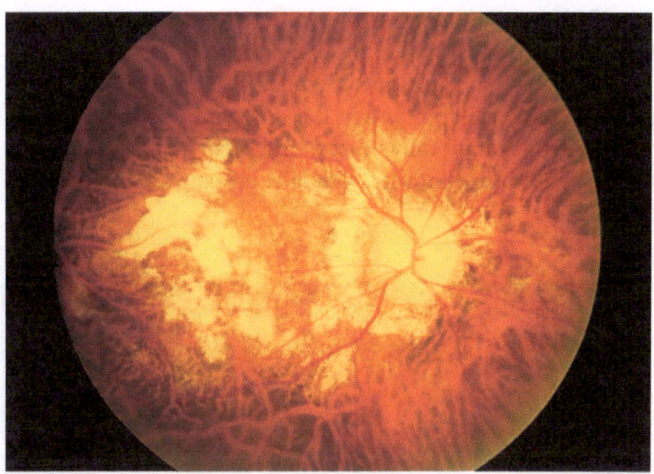

Fig. 34F. Seven years after the initial examination (January 1992), patchy lesions have further enlarged and coalesced

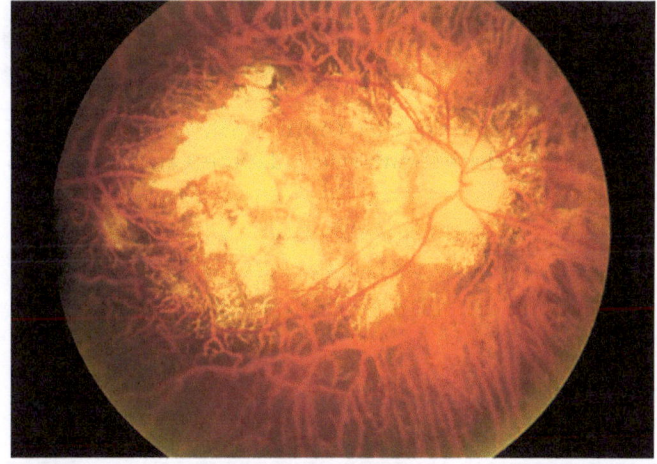

Fig. 34G. Eight years after the initial examination (July 1993), patchy lesions have increased and enlarged. Visual acuity is 0.1, and the refractive error is −18.00 D

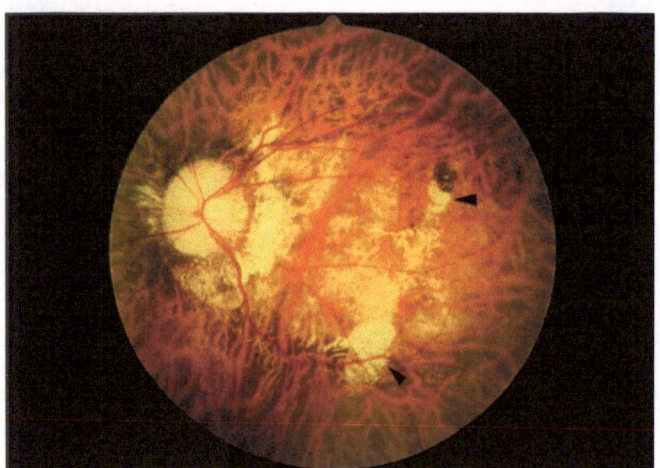

Fig. 34H. Left fundus at the initial examination (January 1985) shows two spotty lesions of patchy atrophy superior and inferior to the macula (*arrowheads*). An enlarged lesion of diffuse atrophy is seen within the posterior staphyloma. The optic disc tilts temporally. A temporal peripapillary crescent is seen. Type II posterior staphyloma is present

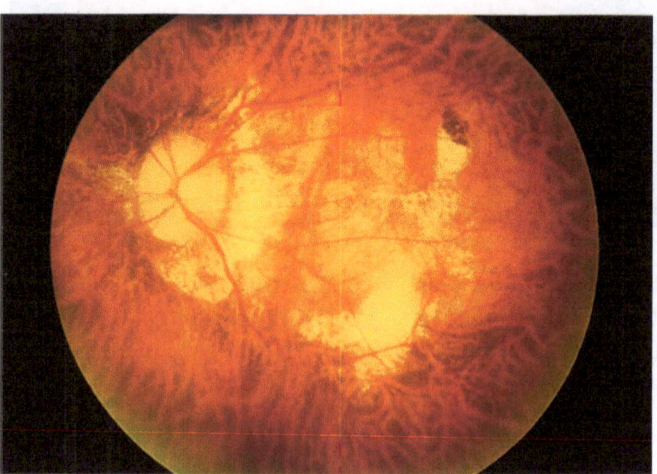

Fig. 34J. Five years after the initial examination (July 1990), spotty lesions of patchy atrophy have enlarged

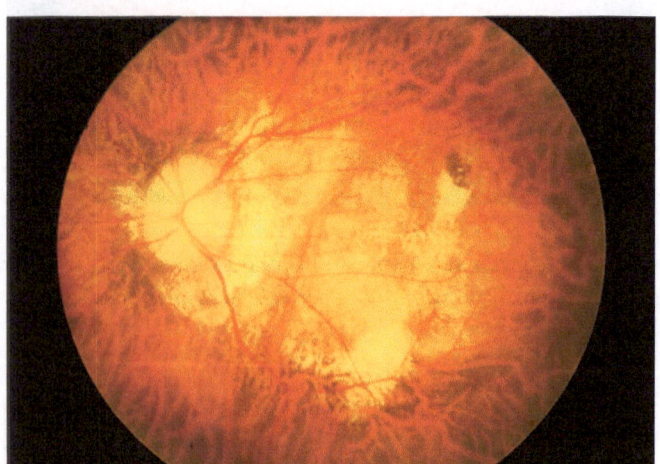

Fig. 34I. Three years later (April 1988), spotty lesions of patchy atrophy have slightly enlarged. Diffuse atrophy has also enlarged

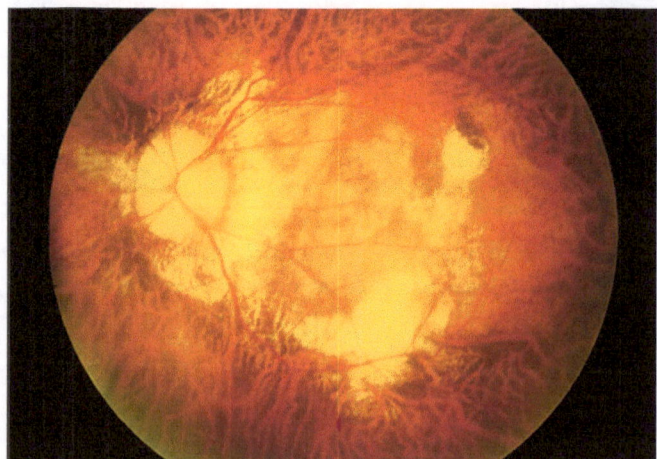

Fig. 34K. Eight years after the initial examination (July 1993), the patchy atrophy inferior to the macula has increased alongside the inferior edge of the staphyloma. Another area of patchy atrophy superior to the macula has enlarged toward the macula

Case 35

A 23-year-old man was examined for bilateral high myopia on July 17, 1973. His vision began to decrease when he was in the upper grades of elementary school, and he began wearing glasses for distance vision when he was in junior high school. His medical history was noncontributory. No family members had severe myopia.

In the initial examination, the patient's best corrected visual acuity was 1.2 in both eyes. The refractive error was −13.00 D sphere in both eyes, and the axial length measurements were 30.0 mm in the right eye and 30.1 mm in the left. Intraocular pressures and anterior segments were normal in both eyes. We describe the long-term fundus changes in his right eye.

Summary

This man was followed up for 23 years, since 1973. A large patchy lesion was already observed inferotemporal to the macula at the initial examination. This lesion did not enlarge rapidly during the entire follow-up period. However, spotty lesions of patchy atrophy appeared around the original patchy atrophy, enlarged rapidly, and coalesced with the original one 7–12 years after the initial examination. Visual acuity was well maintained because the macula was not involved with the progression of patchy atrophy. Posterior staphyloma was visible ophthalmoscopically 10 years after the initial examination. The patient's myopia rapidly progressed by 9.0 D for 23 years, since age 23.

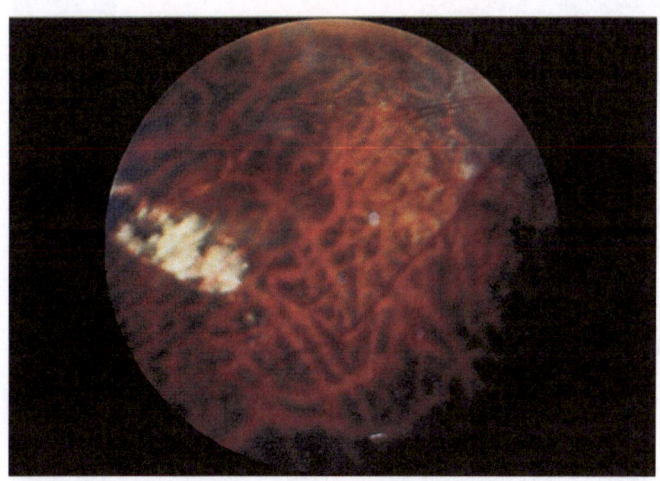

Fig. 35A. Right fundus at the initial examination (July 1973) shows an oval patchy atrophy inferotemporal to the macula. No posterior staphyloma is present

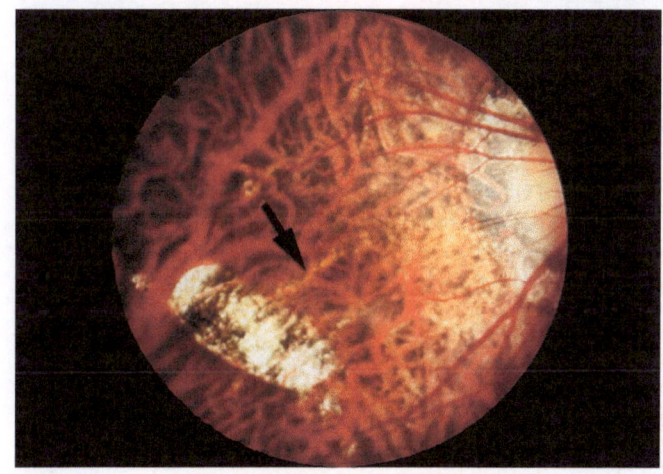

Fig. 35B. Three years later (July 1976), several spotty lesions of patchy atrophy have appeared around the patchy lesion. A lacquer crack lesion is seen across the macula (*arrow*). Spotty or linear lesions of diffuse atrophy are observed temporal to the optic disc. Visual acuity is 1.0, the refractive error is −17.00 D

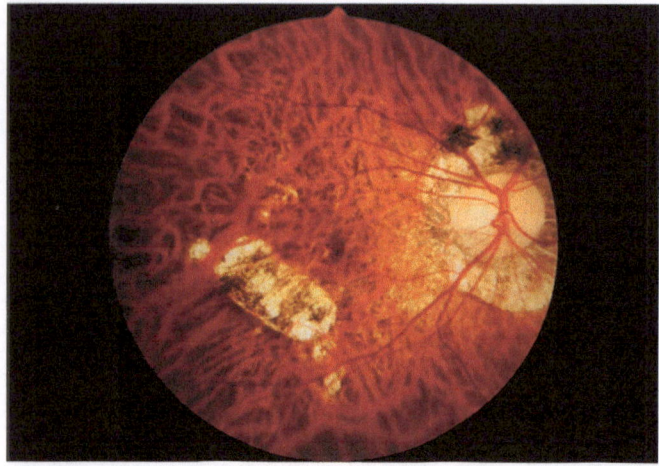

Fig. 35C. Seven years after the initial examination (August 1980), spotty lesions around the original patchy atrophy have enlarged. Their margins have become clear

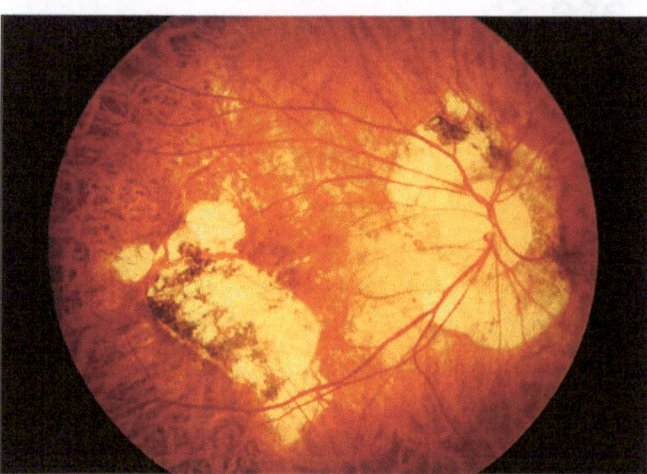

Fig. 35F. Seventeen years after the initial examination (December 1990), the size of the patchy lesions is almost the same. The peripapillary crescent has slightly enlarged

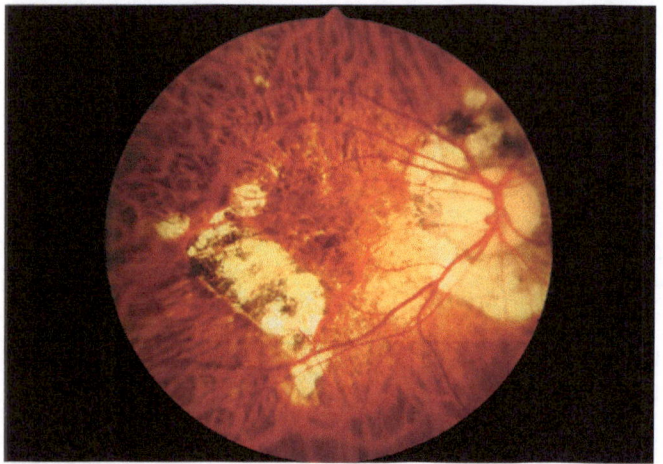

Fig. 35D. Twelve years after the initial examination (March 1985), the spotty lesions of patchy atrophy have continued to enlarge and coalesce with the original patchy atrophy, forming one large patchy lesion temporal to the macula

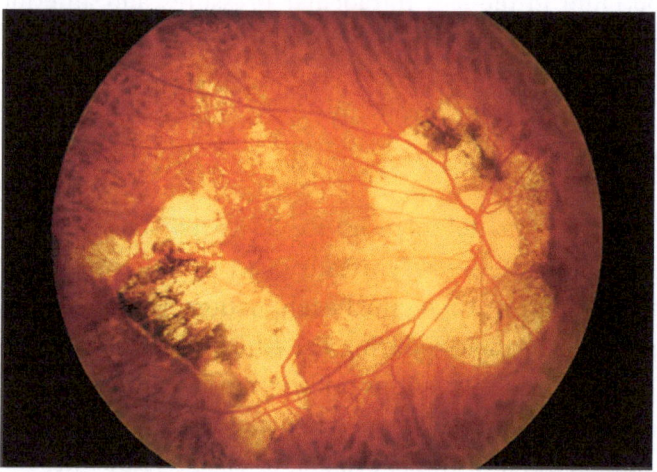

Fig. 35G. Twenty-one years after the initial examination (August 1994), the patchy lesion has further enlarged toward the macula. An enlarged lesion of diffuse atrophy covers the entire posterior fundus. Visual acuity is 0.8, and the refractive error is −22.00 D

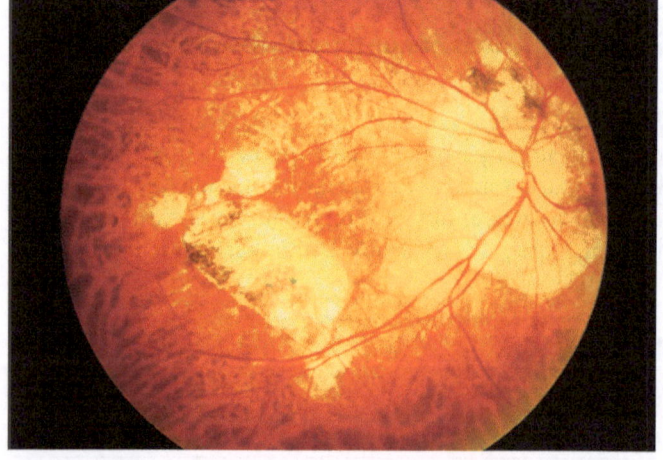

Fig. 35E. Fourteen years after the initial examination (July 1987), the large patchy lesion has enlarged toward the macula. Spotty or linear lesions of diffuse atrophy have progressed into an enlarged lesion of diffuse atrophy in the posterior fundus. Type I posterior staphyloma is present

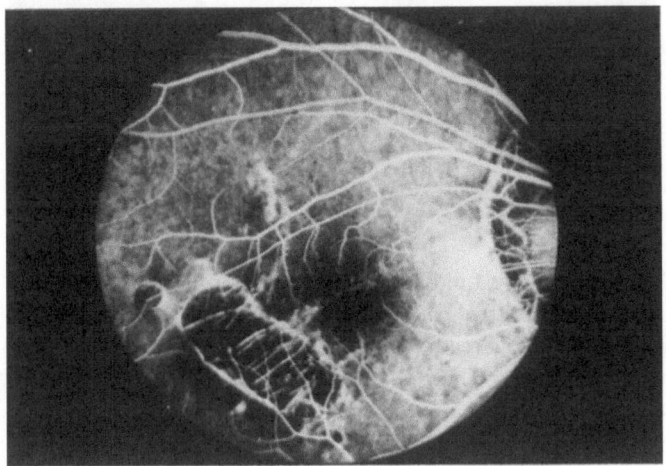

Fig. 35H. Fluorescein fundus angiogram 4 years after the initial examination (August 1977). All lesions of patchy atrophy show choroidal filling defect in the early phase. Lacquer crack lesions show linear hyperfluorescence in the macula

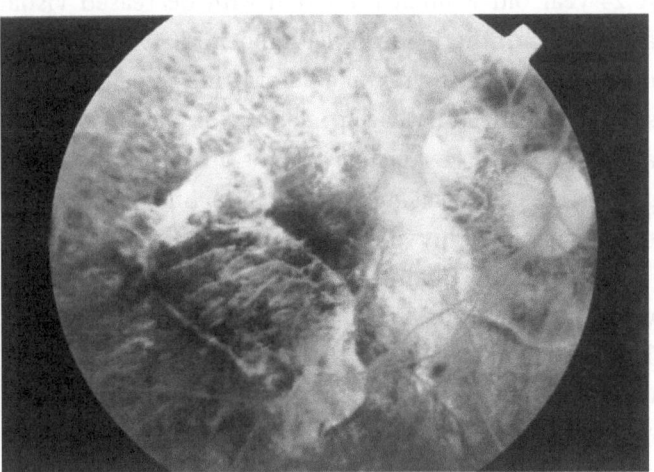

Fig. 35J. Fluorescein fundus angiogram 23 years after the initial examination (January 1996). At 4 min after dye injection, patchy atrophy has slightly enlarged, and is hyperfluorescent, especially in the superior and inferior parts

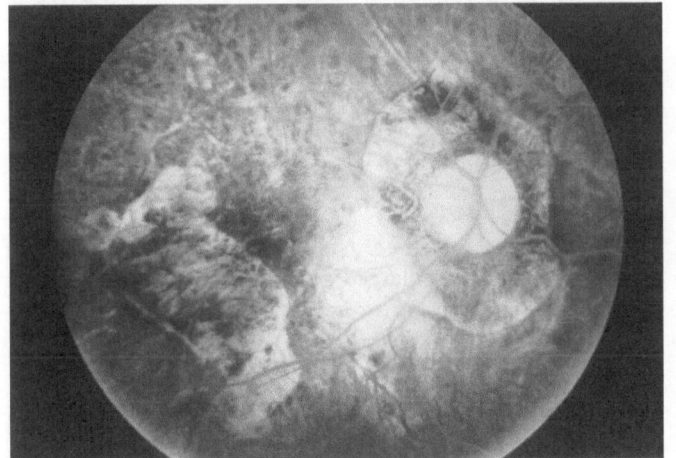

Fig. 35I. Fluorescein fundus angiogram 19 years after the initial examination (August 1992). At 6 min after dye injection, patchy atrophy shows hyperfluorescence because of tissue staining, especially at the edge of the lesion. An enlarged lesion of diffuse atrophy shows irregular staining along the choroidal vessels

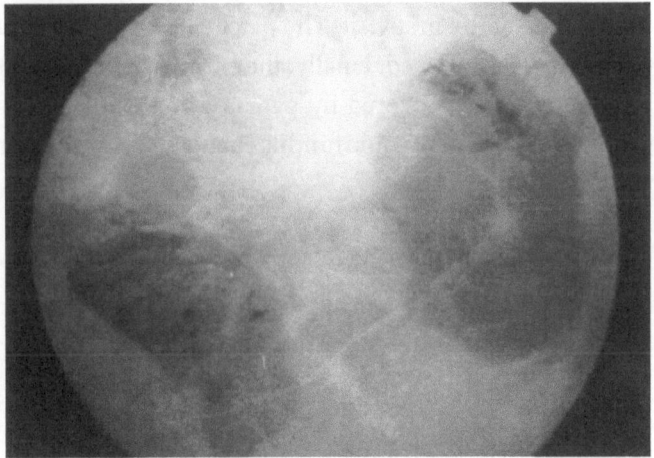

Fig. 35K. Indocyanine green fundus angiogram 23 years after the initial examination (January 1996). In the late phase, the patchy atrophy and the peripapillary crescent are hypofluorescent. The superior and inferior edges of the patchy atrophy are less hypofluorescent than the central part of the lesion

Case 36

A 24-year-old woman presented with decreased visual acuity in both her eyes on December 15, 1978. She was diagnosed as having myopia before entering elementary school. She began wearing glasses for distance vision at age 14 years. Her vision did not improve much with glasses. Her medical history was noncontributory. Her mother is highly myopic.

In the initial examination, the patient's best corrected visual acuity was 0.08 in the right eye and 0.3 in the left. The refractive error was −21.00 D sphere in both eyes, the axial length measurements were 30.9 mm in the right eye and 30.5 mm in the left. Intraocular pressures and anterior segments were normal in both eyes. We decribe the long-term fundus changes in her right eye.

Summary

This woman was followed up for 17 years, since 1978. Patchy lesions of patchy atrophy were already observed at the initial examination. Patchy atrophy including the macula led to decreased visual acuity in the right eye also by the time of the first visit. The patchy lesions gradually enlarged and coalesced. Finally, the entire macular lesion became atrophic, covered by patchy atrophy. The progressive pattern of myopic fundus changes in this patient was from P_2 to MA.

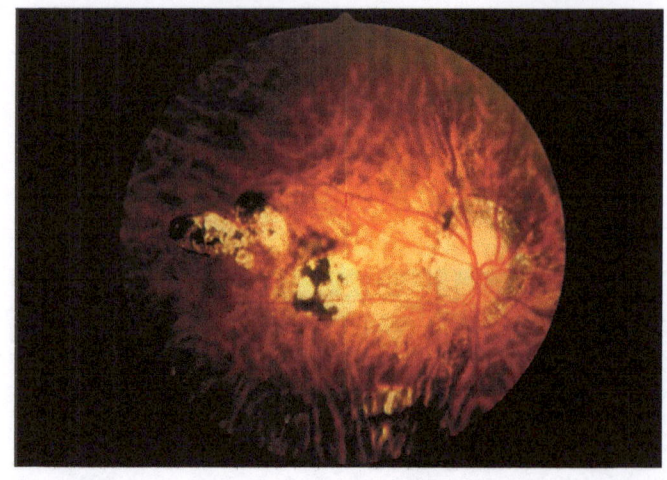

Fig. 36A. Right fundus at the initial examination (December 1978) shows three patchy lesions of patchy atrophy in the macula. An enlarged lesion of diffuse atrophy is observed around the patchy atrophy. The optic disc tilts temporally. A narrow annular crescent is seen around the optic disc. Type II posterior staphyloma is present

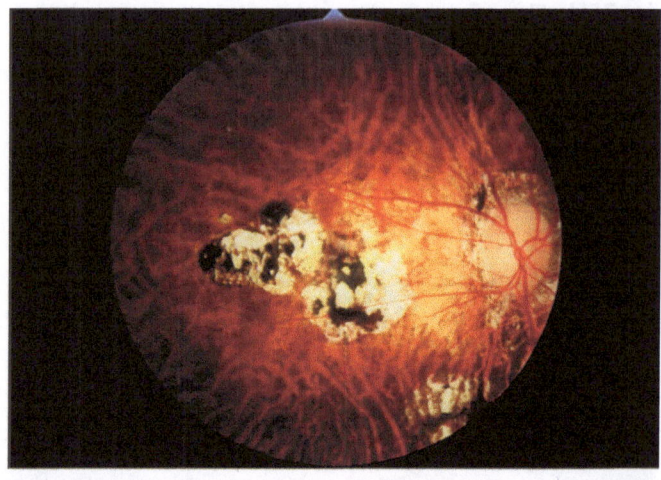

Fig. 36B. Three years later (July 1982), the patchy lesions of patchy atrophy have enlarged and coalesced. Visual acuity is 0.04, and the refractive error is −20.00 D

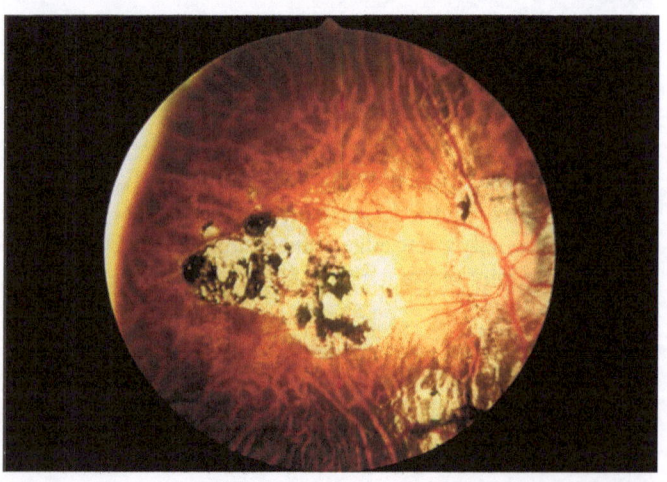

Fig. 36C. Seven years after the initial examination (December 1985), the patchy lesions of patchy atrophy have coalesced and formed one large atrophic lesion in the macula

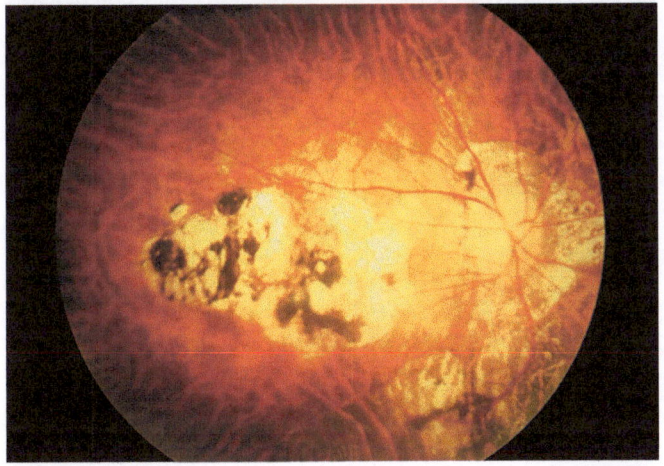

Fig. 36D. Ten years after the initial examination (December 1988), the patchy lesions of patchy atrophy have enlarged and covered the macular lesion. The patchy lesion alongside the inferior edge of the staphyloma has also enlarged and coalesced with the peripapillary crescent inferior to the optic disc. Visual acuity is 0.05, and the refractive error is −22.00 D

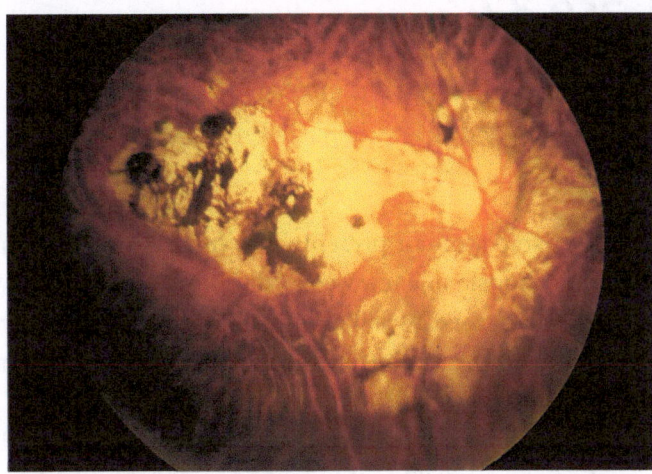

Fig. 36F. Fifteen years after the initial examination (October 1993), the patchy lesions of patchy atrophy in the macula have enlarged. Visual acuity is 0.03, and the refractive error is −23.00 D

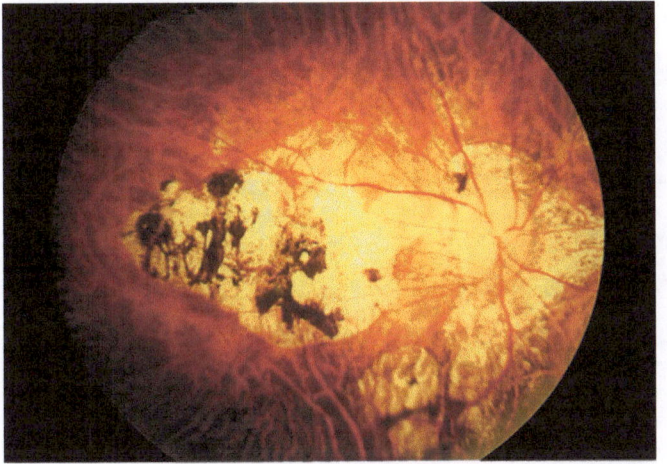

Fig. 36E. Twelve years after the initial examination (March 1991), the patchy lesions of patchy atrophy in the macula have further enlarged and coalesced with the peripapillary crescent. The peripapillary crescent has also enlarged in all directions

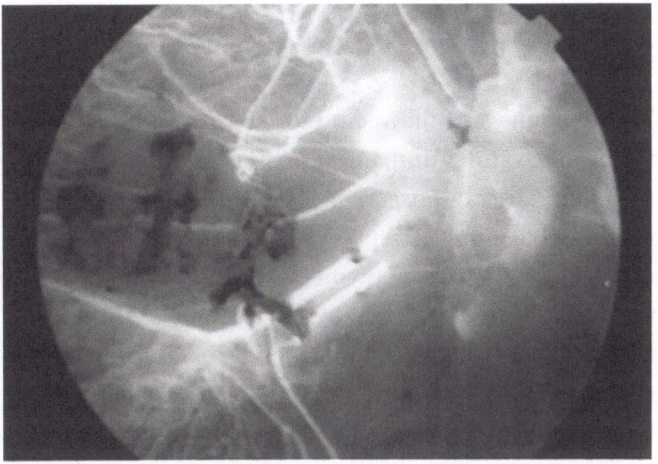

Fig. 36G. Indocyanine green fundus angiogram 17 years after the initial examination (April 1996). In the early phase of the angiogram, retrobulbar arteries are visible through the atrophic choroid in the macula. These arteries are pulsatile on a videoscreen. Large choroidal vessels are not observed in the macula

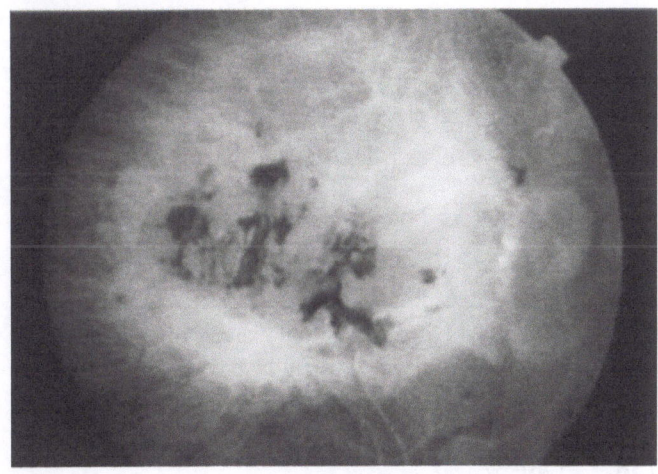

Fig. 36H. Indocyanine green fundus angiogram 17 years after the initial examination (April 1996). Patchy atrophy shows hypofluorescence in the late phase. Pigmentation within the patchy atrophy shows blocked fluorescence

Case 37

A 36-year-old woman presented on May 11, 1979, with metamorphopsia of a few weeks' duration in her left eye. She was diagnosed as having myopia as an infant. Her medical history was noncontributory. Her father and an aunt are highly myopic.

At the initial examination, the patient's best corrected visual acuity was 0.07 in the right eye and 0.7 in the left. The refractive error was −22.00 D sphere in the right eye and −19.00 D sphere in the left, and the axial length measurements were 31.8 mm in the right eye and 30.7 mm in the left. Intraocular pressures and anterior segments were normal. We show the long-term fundus changes in her left eye.

Summary

This woman was followed up for 16 years, since 1979. At the initial examination, the patchy lesions of patchy atrophy were already observed, somewhat distant from the macular bleeding. After the macular bleeding was absorbed, a fibrovascular membrane was found. The patchy lesions of patchy atrophy seen at the initial examination gradually enlarged and coalesced with the choroidal neovascular membrane. They finally formed a large atrophic lesion in the macula.

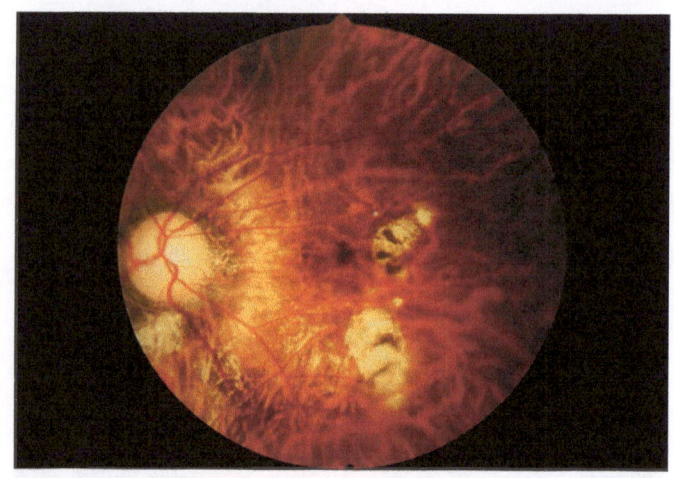

Fig. 37A. Left fundus at the initial examination (May 1979) shows macular bleeding and two patchy lesions of patchy atrophy superior and inferior to the macula. Spotty or linear lesions of diffuse atrophy are visible temporal to the optic disc. A narrow peripapillary crescent is seen. Type III posterior staphyloma is present

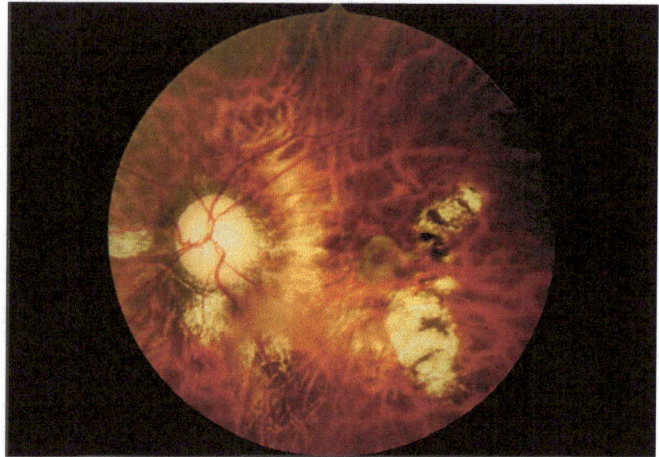

Fig. 37B. Four years later (September 1983), two patchy lesions of patchy atrophy have enlarged. A choroidal neovascular membrane is observed in the macula after the absorption of the bleeding. Visual acuity has decreased to 0.04

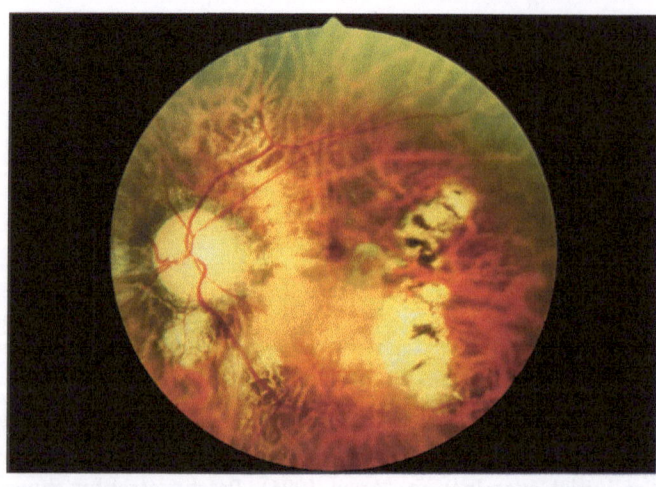

Fig. 37C. Six years after the initial examination (September 1985), patchy lesions of patchy atrophy have slightly enlarged. Choroidal neovascular membrane in the macula is unchanged

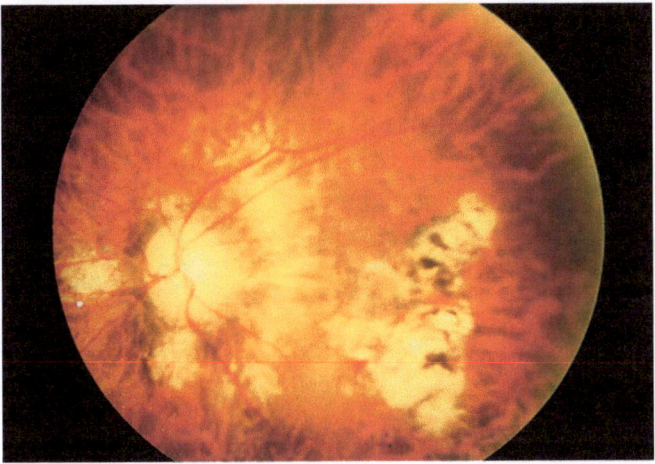

Fig. 37D. Ten years after the initial examination (September 1989), the patchy lesions of patchy atrophy have coalesced with the choroidal neovascular membrane and formed one large atrophic area in the macula. An enlarged area of diffuse atrophy is seen temporal to the optic disc. Visual acuity is 0.1, and the refractive error is −21.00 D

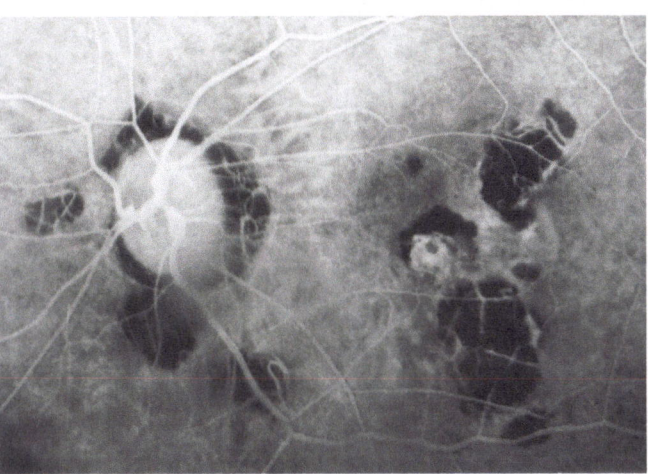

Fig. 37F. Fluorescein fundus angiogram 2 years after the initial examination (May 1981). At 64 sec after dye injection, two patchy lesions of patchy atrophy show choroidal filling defect in the early phase. The choroidal neovascular membrane is hyperfluorescent and surrounded by a blocked fluorescence produced by the bleeding

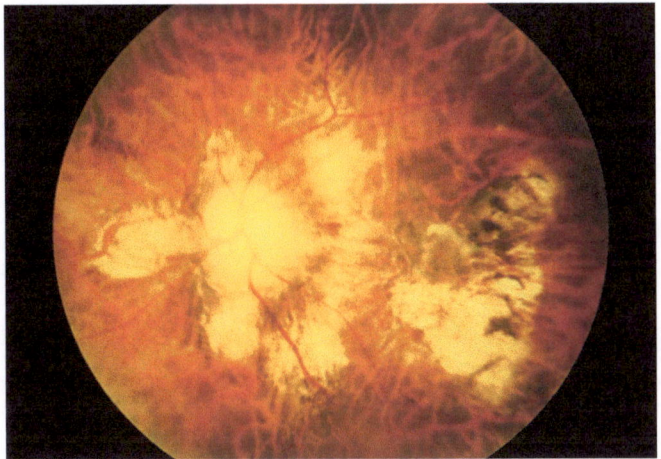

Fig. 37E. Fifteen years after the initial examination (October 1994), the large macular atrophy including the choroidal neovascular membrane has slightly enlarged

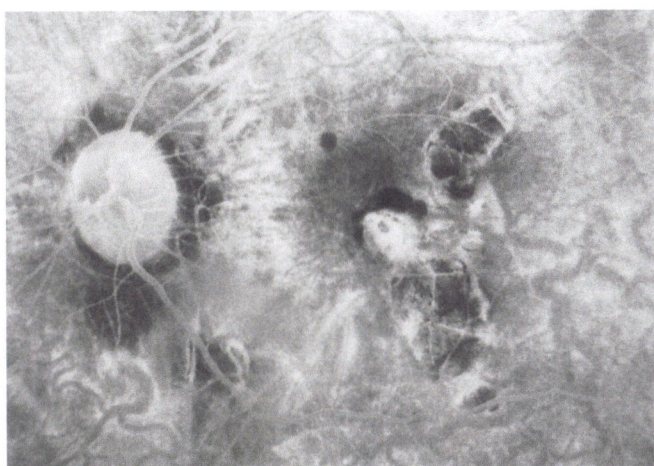

Fig. 37G. Fluorescein fundus angiogram 2 years after the initial examination (May 1981). At 5 min after dye injection, the edges of the patchy lesions of patchy atrophy are hyperfluorescent in the late phase. The choroidal neovascular membrane shows slight dye leakage

Fig. 37H. Fluorescein fundus angiogram 15 years after the initial examination (October 1994). At 43 sec after dye injection, the choroidal filling defect corresponding to the patchy lesions of patchy atrophy has enlarged

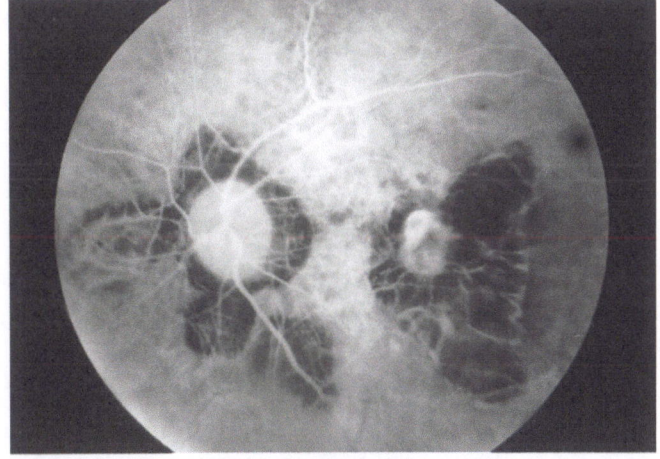

Myopic Choroidal Neovascularization (Fuchs' Spot)

Myopic choroidal neovascular membrane shows less activity, as compared with other neovascular maculopathies. The activity of a choroidal neovascular membrane is usually low in highly myopic eyes. Bleeding is absorbed quickly, and the neovascular membrane spontaneously shrinks and regresses without the episode of rebleeding in many cases. However, atrophic lesions gradually form around regressed neovascular membranes in highly myopic eyes and lead to further decrease of visual acuity. The development of chorioretinal atrophy around the neovascular membrane is influenced by many factors, including axial length, posterior staphyloma, choroidal circulation in the posterior fundus, or surrounding diffuse atrophy.

Ophthalmoscopic and angiographic findings of the atrophic lesion around regressed neovascular membrane are very similar to those of patchy atrophy. After the choroidal neovascular membrane completely regresses, it is difficult to differentiate chorioretinal atrophy with regressed neovascular membrane from patchy atrophy without choroidal neovascularization ophthalmoscopically. However, in the early developmental period of chorioretinal atrophy, fluorescein angiography shows hyperfluorescence as the result of a window defect. This finding demonstrates that the retinal pigment epithelial atrophy first appears in the chorioretinal atrophy developing around the choroidal neovascularization.

Myopic choroidal neovascularization and the subsequent formation of chorioretinal atrophy cause severe visual decrease in highly myopic eyes. Long-term follow-up is necessary for the later development of chorioretinal atrophy around the regressed choroidal neovascular membrane in highly myopic eyes.

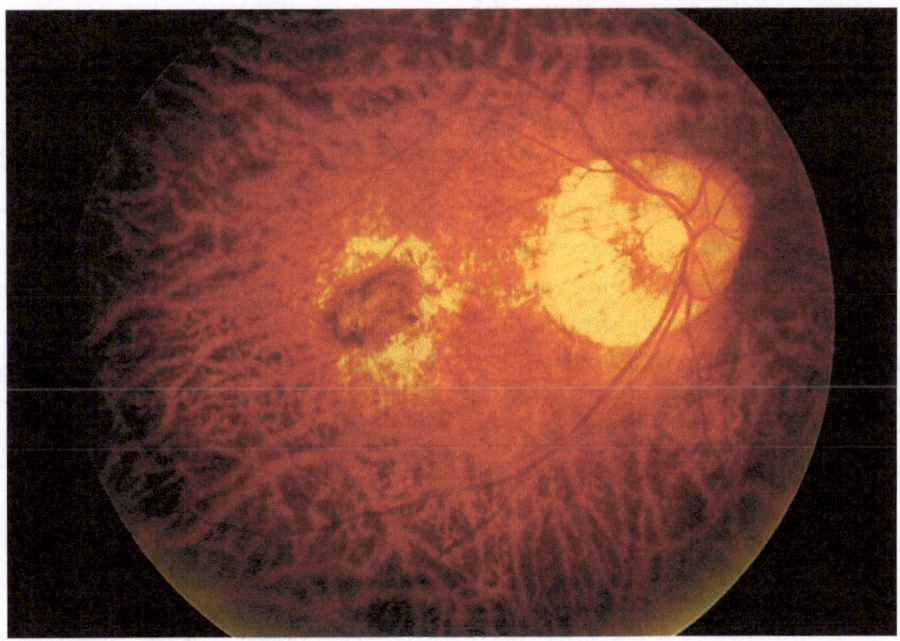

Fig. 45B. *(see page 182)*

Cases 38–52

Abbreviations *T*: Tessellated fundus; *D*: Diffuse chorioretinal atrophy; *Lc*: Lacquer crack lesion; *P*: Patchy atrophy; *NS*: Simple macular hemorrhage; *HN*: Neovascular macular hemorrhage; *MA*: Chorioretinal atrophy of the macula. For details, refer to Table 3.1 and Fig. 7.1.

Case 38

A 14-year-old girl presented on April 20, 1977, with visual decrease in the right eye. She noticed meta-morphopsia in the right eye in February 1977, visited a general practitioner, and was referred to our high myopia clinic for macular bleeding in the left eye. Her medical history was noncontributory. Her father and one of her four siblings are myopic.

In the initial examination, the patient's best corrected visual acuity was 0.3 in the right eye and 0.7 in the left. The refractive error was −17.0 D sphere in both eyes. The axial length measurements were 28.6 mm in the right eye and 28.0 mm in the left. Intraocular pressures were normal in both eyes. We describe the long-term fundus changes in her right eye.

Summary

This young woman was followed up for 9 years, since the age of 14. She is the youngest patient among those with Fuchs' spot in our high myopia clinic. At the initial examination, macular bleeding was already absorbed. A pigmented Fuchs' spot was seen in the macular lesion of her right fundus. The activity of choroidal neovascular membrane was not very high. Fluorescein angiography at the initial examination showed only slight dye leakage in the late phase. After rebleeding in 1979, the choroidal neovascular membrane regressed and shrank into yellowish-white fibrous tissue with no other episodes of rebleeding. Chorioretinal atrophy was finally formed around the Fuchs' spot. The developmental pattern of chorioretinal atrophy around Fuchs' spot in this patient was typical.

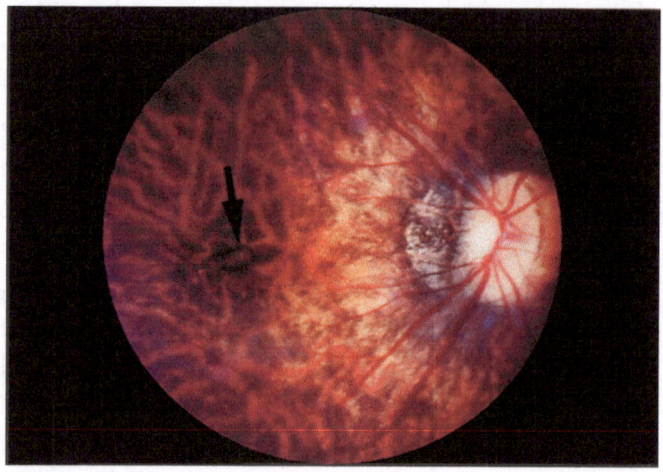

Fig. 38A. Right fundus at the initial examination (April 1977) shows a pigmented Fuchs' spot in the macula (*arrow*). Macular bleeding is already absorbed. Spotty and linear lesions of diffuse atrophy are observed temporal to the optic disc

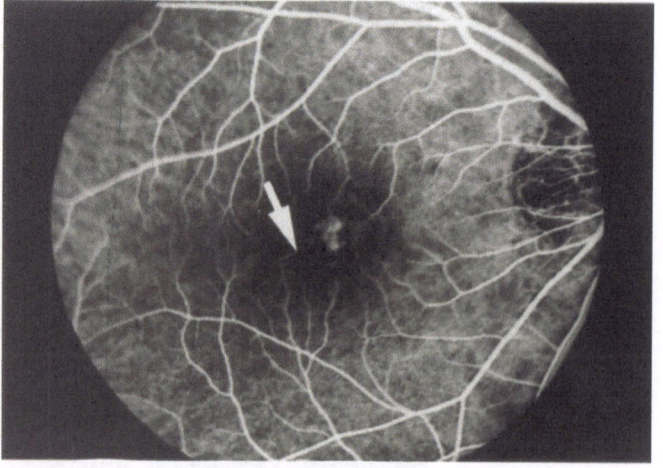

Fig. 38B. Fluorescein fundus angiogram at the initial examination (April 1977). At 1 min after dye injection, the choroidal neovascular membrane is hyperfluorescent. Linear hyperfluorescence similar to lacquer crack lesions is seen across the neovascular membrane (*arrow*)

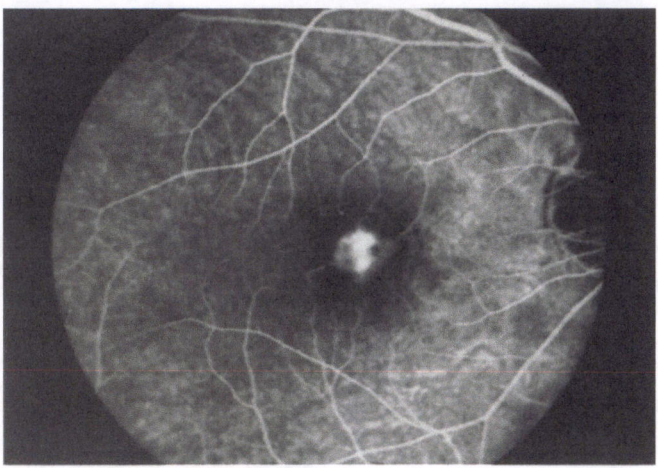

Fig. 38C. Fluorescein fundus angiogram at the initial examination (April 1977). At 8 min after dye injection, the choroidal neovascular membrane shows slight dye leakage in the late phase

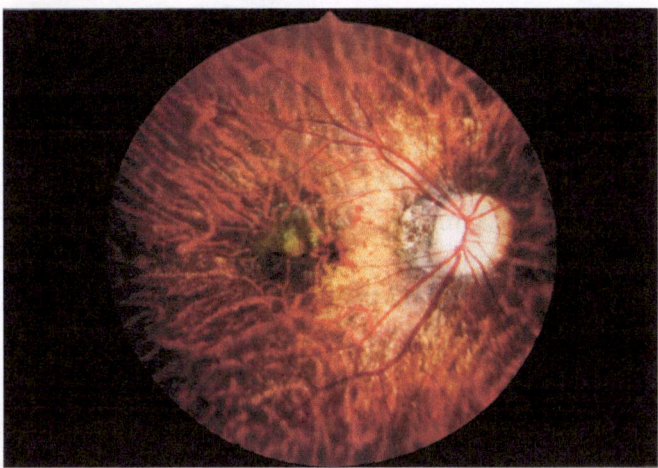

Fig. 38D. Two years after the initial examination (February 1979), rebleeding has occurred nasal to the Fuchs' spot. The Fuchs' spot has enlarged. Visual acuity is 0.5, and the refractive error is −14.75 D

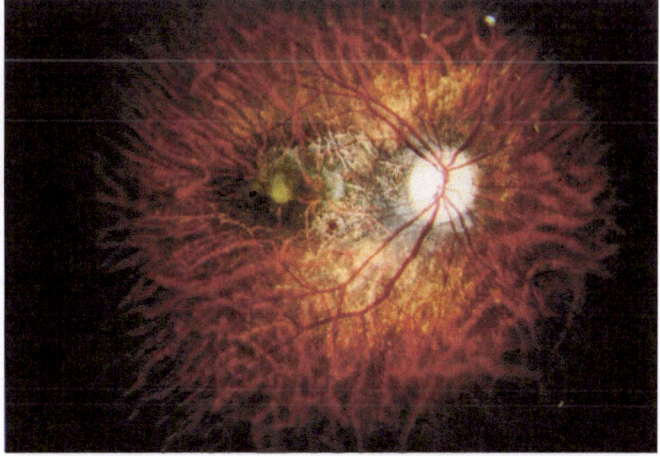

Fig. 38E. Five years after the initial examination (October 1982), the choroidal neovascular membrane has shrunk and regressed into a yellowish-white fibrovascular tissue. Rebleeding did not occur after 1979. Chorioretinal atrophy with pigmentation appears around the Fuchs' spot. Another fibrous tissue is seen nasal to the Fuchs' spot. Visual acuity is 0.3, and the refractive error is −16.5 D

Case 39

A 45-year-old woman presented on November 4, 1988, with decreased visual acuity in her left eye. She was diagnosed as having myopia as an elementary school student. She began wearing glasses for distance vision in junior high school. She reported a central scotoma in her left eye in April 1988. She visited a general practitioner and underwent fluorescein fundus angiography, which showed macular bleeding in the left eye. She was referred to our high myopia clinic for further examination of the macular bleeding in the left eye. No family members had severe myopia.

In the initial examination, the patient's best corrected visual acuity was 0.3 in the right eye and 0.3 in the left. The refractive error was −16.00 D sphere in the right eye and −15.50 D sphere in the left. Axial length measurements were 28.3 mm in the right eye and 28.1 mm in the left. Intraocular pressures and anterior segments were normal in both eyes. We show the long-term fundus changes in her left eye.

Summary

This woman was followed up for 6 years, since 1988. She visited our high myopia clinic because of a central scotoma in the left eye caused by macular bleeding with choroidal neovascular membrane. Choroidal neovascular membrane in the left eye was not very active. It transformed into the regressive stage without producing extensive bleeding or hard exudates. A small chorioretinal atrophy has formed around the regressed choroidal neovascular membrane after the regression of choroidal neovascularization.

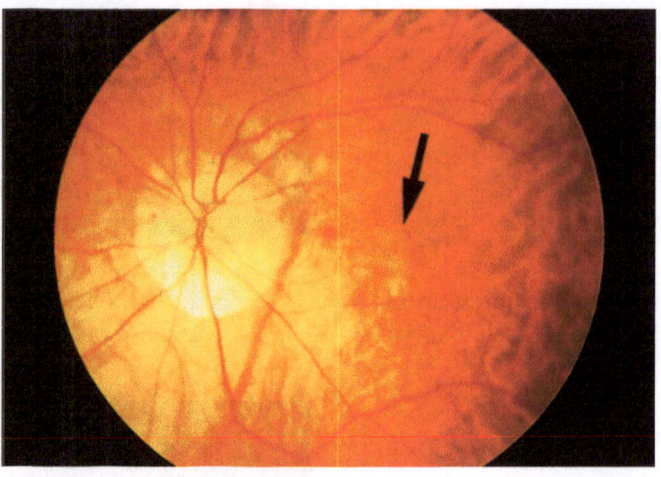

Fig. 39A. Left fundus at the initial examination (November 1988) shows a choroidal neovascular membrane with bleeding in the macula (*arrow*). Diffuse atrophy is prominent inferior to the optic disc. The optic disc tilts inferotemporally. Annular peripapillary crescent is seen. No posterior staphyloma is present

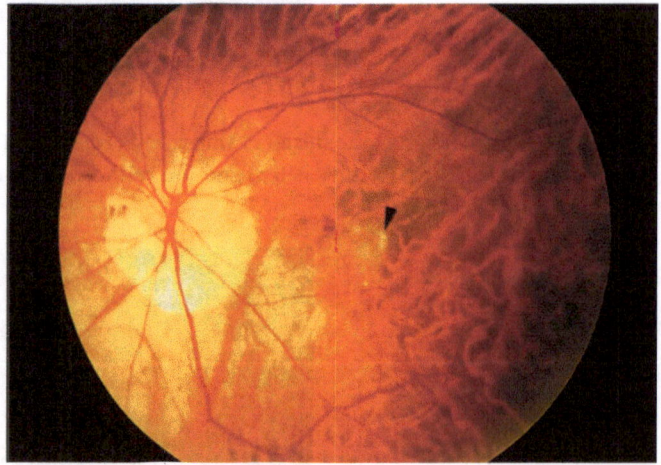

Fig. 39B. Two years later (January 1990), the bleeding is completely absorbed. A small chorioretinal atrophy has appeared superior to the choroidal neovascular membrane (*arrowhead*). Visual acuity is 0.2, and the refractive error is −15.50 D

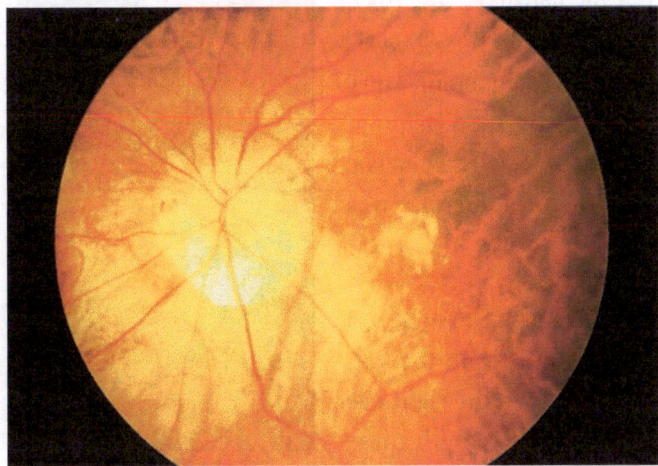

Fig. 39C. Three years after the initial examination (January 1991), chorioretinal atrophy superior to the choroidal neovascular membrane has enlarged. Visual acuity is 0.1, and the refractive error is −15.50 D

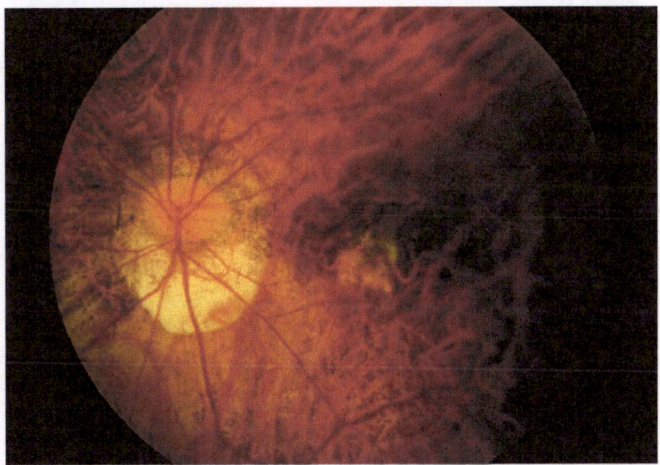

Fig. 39D. Six years after the initial examination (March 1994), chorioretinal atrophy around the choroidal neovascular membrane has enlarged further, and its margins are becoming clear. Visual acuity is 0.04, and the refractive error is −15.50 D

Case 40

A 24-year-old woman presented on February 26, 1982, with a gradual loss of visual acuity in both eyes. She was diagnosed with myopia when she was in elementary school. She began wearing glasses for distance vision at age 11 years. Her myopia progressed, especially when she was in junior high school. Her medical history was noncontributory. Her father and one of her uncles are highly myopic.

In the initial examination, the patient's best corrected visual acuity was 0.8 in the right eye and 1.2 in the left. The refractive error was −14.00 D sphere in the right eye and −12.50 D sphere in the left. The axial length measurements were 27.7 mm in the right eye and 27.7 mm in the left. We describe the long-term fundus changes in her left eye.

Summary

This highly myopic patient developed choroidal neovascularization, which caused a severe decrease in vision in her left eye. Choroidal neovascularization sometimes occurs in young, highly myopic eyes with slight tessellated fundus changes, as seen in this patient. Choroidal neovascular membrane gradually enlarged even after the laser photocoagulation was performed. Annular chorioretinal atrophy was later formed around the regressed neovascular membrane.

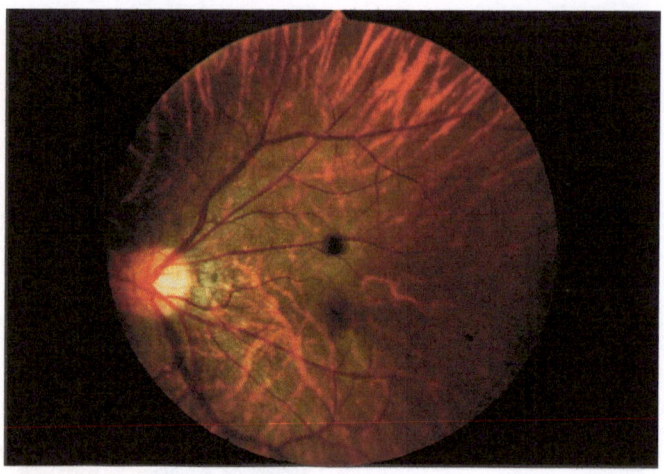

Fig. 40A. Left fundus at the initial examination (February 1982) shows a tessellated fundus. The optic disc tilts temporally. A narrow papillary crescent is seen temporal to the optic disc. No posterior staphyloma is present

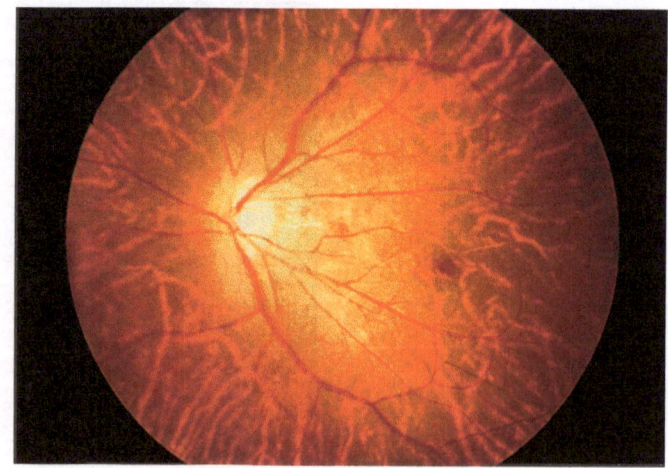

Fig. 40B. Seven years later (May 1989), spotty and linear lesions of diffuse atrophy are observed temporal to the optic disc. Visual acuity is 1.2, and the refractive error is −13.00 D

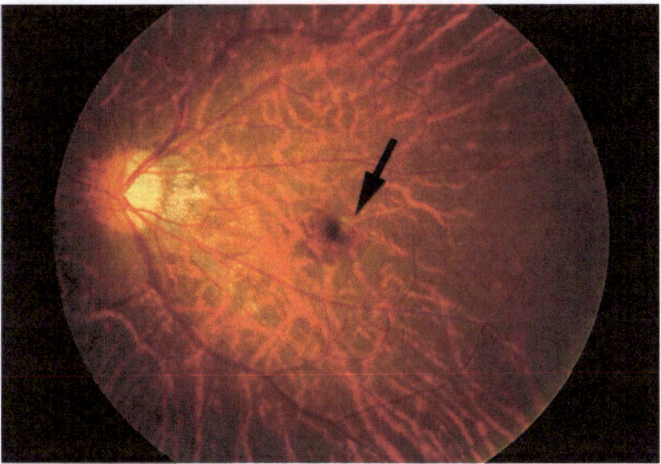

Fig. 40C. Eight years after the initial examination (May 1990), macular bleeding has occurred. Choroidal neovascular membrane is observed within the bleeding (*arrow*). Visual acuity has dropped to 0.06

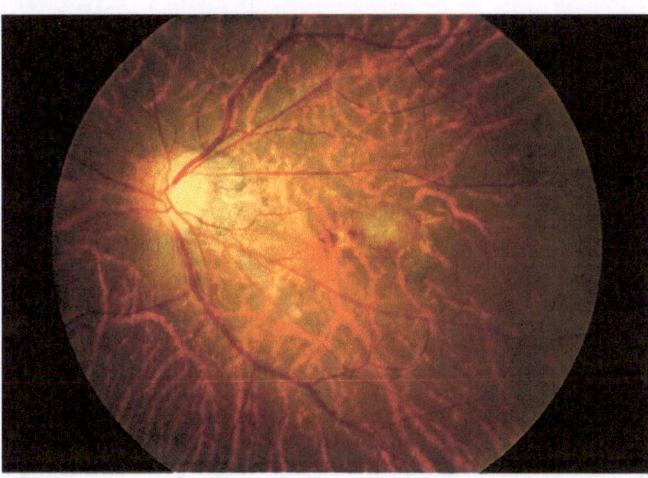

Fig. 40E. Ten years after the initial examination (May 1992), the choroidal neovascular membrane has enlarged. Macular bleeding is still observed around the membrane. Visual acuity has improved to 0.3

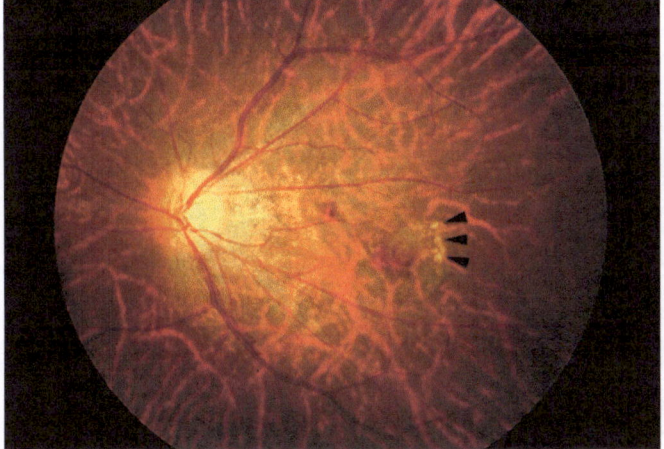

Fig. 40D. Eight years after the initial examination (July 1990), we performed laser photocoagulation on her choroidal neovascular membrane using the following laser conditions (krypton red, duration time, 0.1 sec; spot size, 200 μm; power, 0.11 watts; number of burns, 5). Laser scars are seen temporal to the neovascular membrane (*arrowheads*)

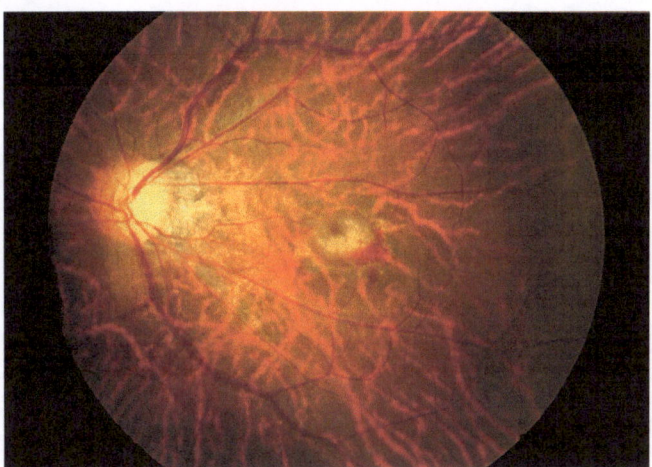

Fig. 40F. Eleven years after the initial examination (May 1993), macular bleeding still remains around the choroidal neovascular membrane. Visual acuity is 0.2, and the refractive error is −14.00 D

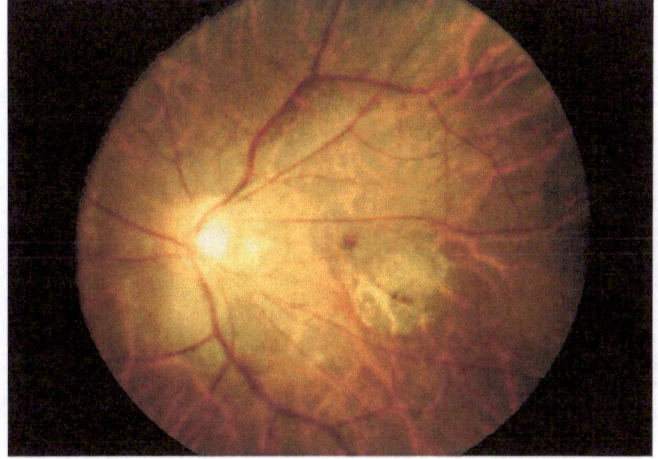

Fig. 40G. Fourteen years after the initial examination (October 1996), chorioretinal atrophy has developed around the neovascular membrane. Sclerotic choroidal vessels are visible within the lesion of the chorioretinal atrophy. Visual acuity is 0.03, and the refractive error is −14.00 D

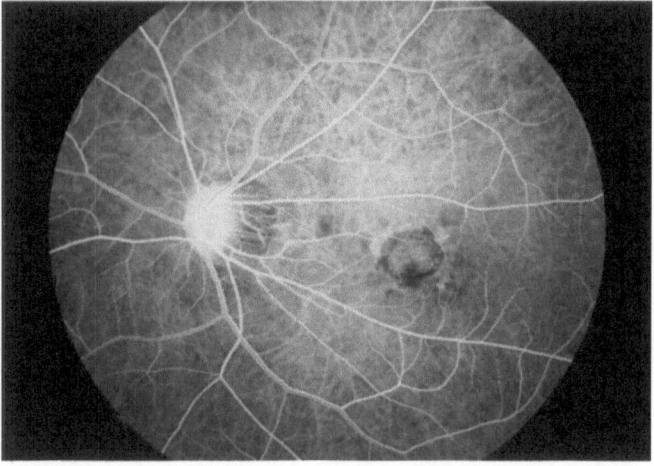

Fig. 40H. Fluorescein angiogram 9 years after the initial examination (January 1991). At 12 sec after dye injection, the choroidal neovascular membrane shows slight hyperfluorescence. Hyperfluorescence from a window defect is visible around the choroidal neovascular membrane

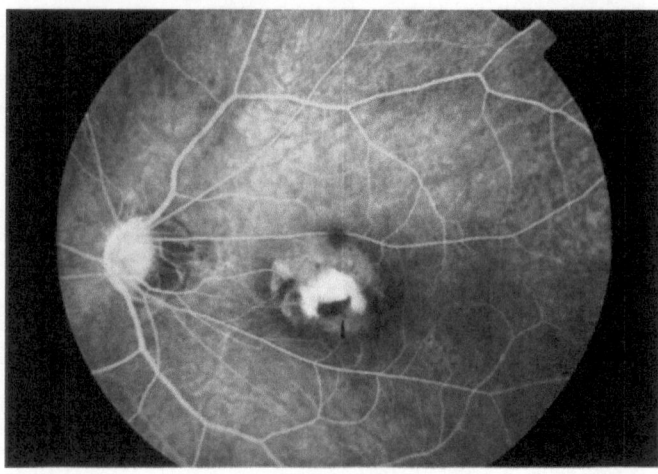

Fig. 40K. Fluorescein angiogram 12 years after the initial examination (September 1994). At 8 min after dye injection, choroidal neovascular membrane shows tissue staining. No dye leakage is obvious

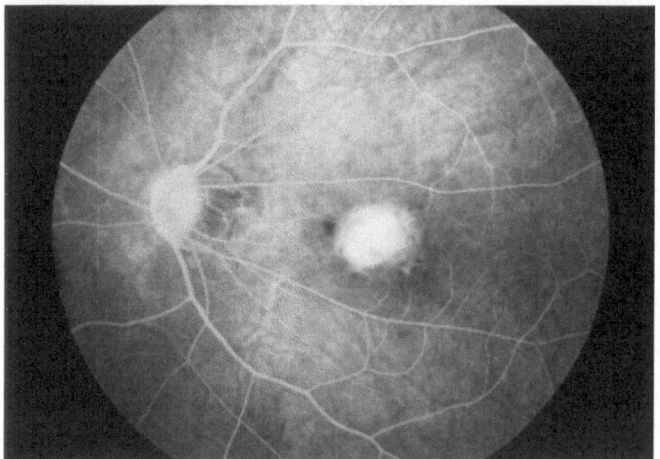

Fig. 40I. Fluorescein angiogram 9 years after the initial examination (January 1991). At 10 min after dye injection, dye leakage from the choroidal neovascular membrane is obvious

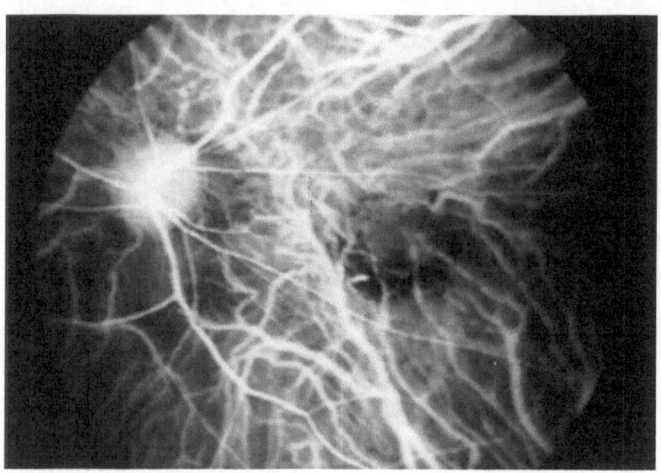

Fig. 40L. Indocyanine green fundus angiogram 14 years after the initial examination (April 1996). The choroidal neovascular membrane shows slight hyperfluorescence surrounded by a large hypofluorescence of the chorioretinal atrophy

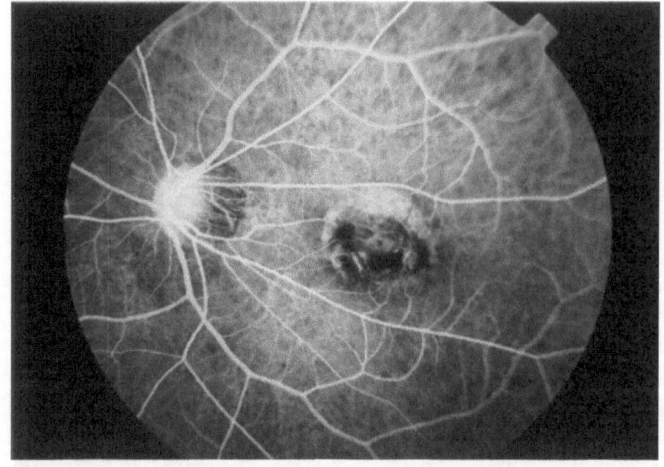

Fig. 40J. Fluorescein angiogram 12 years after the initial examination (September 1994). At 29 sec after dye injection, the choroidal neovascular membrane still appears hyperfluorescent. The window defect around the neovascular membrane has enlarged

Case 41

A 46-year-old woman presented on June 14, 1988, with decreased visual acuity in her right eye. She was diagnosed with myopia when she was in elementary school. She began wearing glasses for distance vision at age 10 years. She noticed a visual decrease in her right eye 4 months before the initial examination. Her medical history was noncontributory. No family members had severe myopia.

In the initial examination, the patient's best corrected visual acuity was 0.5 in the right eye and 1.0 in the left eye. The refractive error was $-11.00\,D$ sphere in the right eye and $-11.00\,D$ in the left, and the axial length measurements were 26.7 mm in the right eye and 26.2 mm in the left. Intraocular pressures and anterior segments were normal in both eyes. We describe the long-term fundus changes in her right eye.

Summary

This woman presented with a visual decrease in her right eye. Macular bleeding was observed around the choroidal neovascular membrane. After the bleeding was absorbed, the neovascular membrane shrank and regressed. An annular atrophic lesion formed around the regressed choroidal neovascular membrane. The choroidal neovascular membrane in her right eye occurred within the lacquer crack lesions and linear lesions of diffuse atrophy. This finding suggests a close relationship between lacquer crack lesions (or diffuse atrophy) and choroidal neovascularization. The progressive pattern of myopic fundus changes in this patient was from D_1 to NH_1 to HN_2 and to MA.

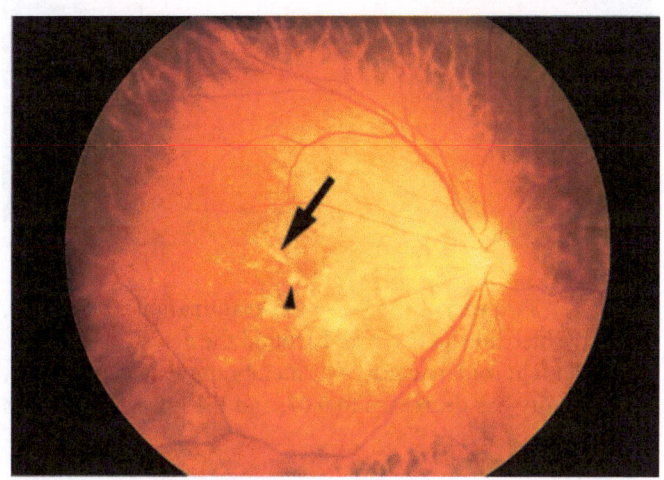

Fig. 41A. Right fundus at the initial examination (June 1988) shows lacquer crack lesions (*arrow*) and linear lesions of diffuse atrophy in the macula. A small choroidal neovascular membrane is observed in the fovea (*arrowhead*). An enlarged lesion of diffuse atrophy appears temporal to the optic disc. The optic disc tilts temporally. Type I posterior staphyloma is present

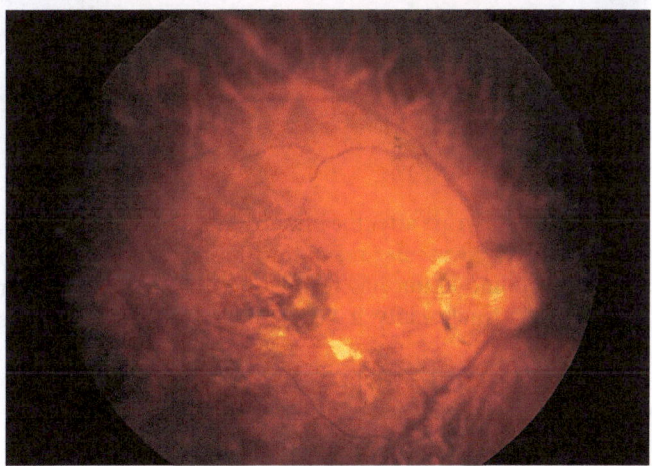

Fig. 41B. One year later (October 1989), a small bleeding is seen around the neovascular membrane. The choroidal neovascular membrane is surrounded by pigmentation. Patchy atrophy has enlarged inferior to the macula. In the right eye, visual acuity is 0.3, and the refractive error is $-11.00\,D$

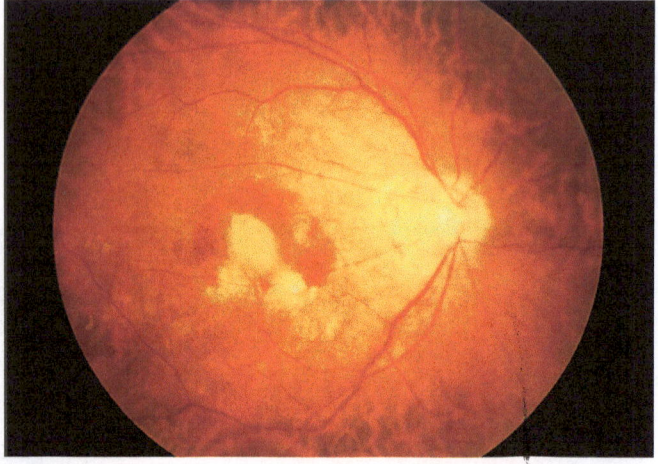

Fig. 41C. Two years after the initial examination (June 1990), extensive bleeding has occurred around the neovascular membrane. The choroidal neovascular membrane also has enlarged. Visual acuity has decreased to 0.07, and the refractive error is −11.00 D

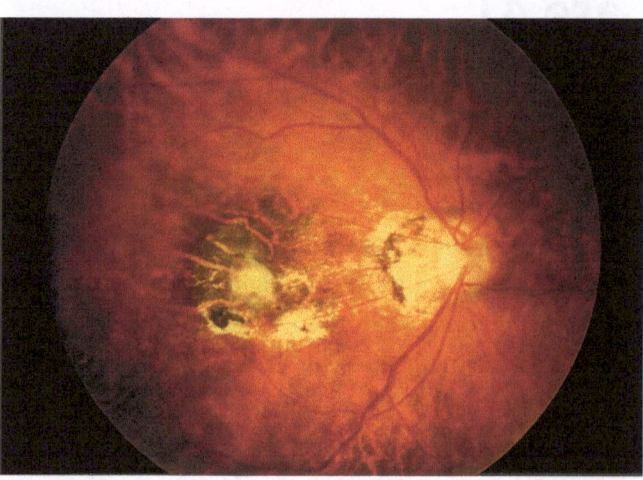

Fig. 41F. Five years after the initial examination (May 1993), the choroidal neovascular membrane has shrunk further. Pigmentation has increased within the atrophic lesion around the neovascular membrane

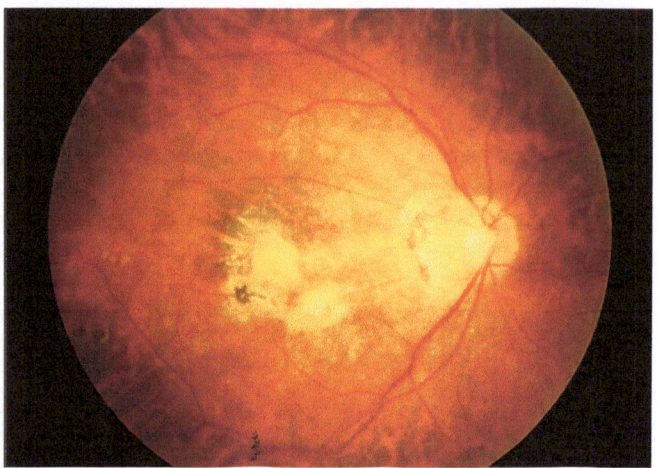

Fig. 41D. Four years after the initial examination (June 1992), the choroidal neovascular membrane has slightly shrunk. An annular atrophic lesion has formed around the neovascular membrane. Visual acuity is 0.1, and the refractive error is −11.00 D

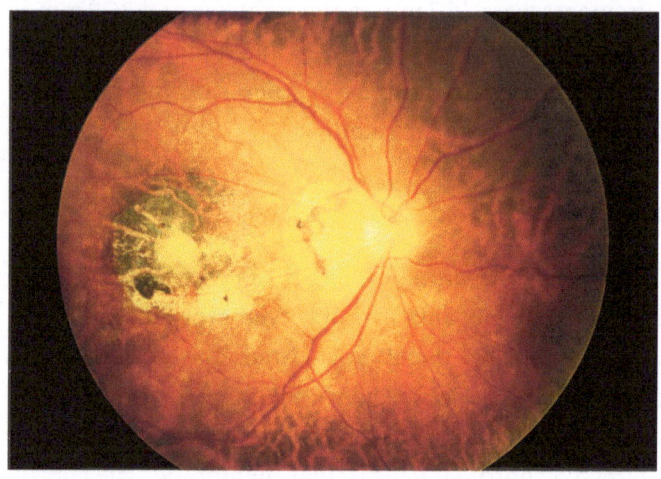

Fig. 41G. Six years after the initial examination (June 1994), the atrophic lesion around the neovascular membrane has enlarged toward the peripapillary crescent. Visual acuity is 0.1, and the refractive error is −11.00 D

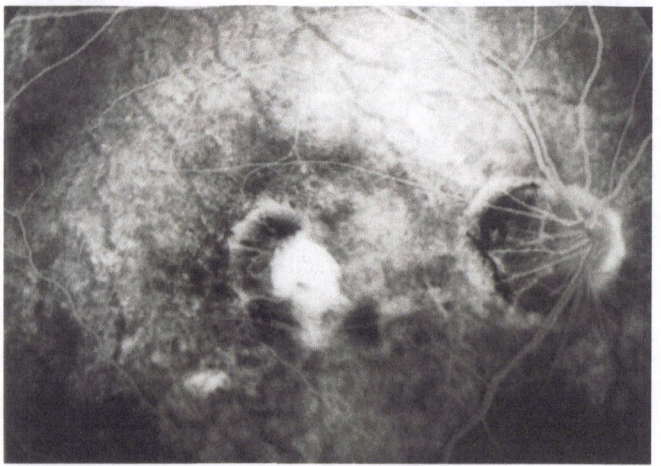

Fig. 41E. Fluorescein fundus angiogram 7 years after the initial examination (June 1992). At 3 min after dye injection, the choroidal neovascular membrane is hyperfluorescent. Slight dye leakage from the neovascular membrane is observed in the late phase. An atrophic lesion around the neovascular membrane shows hypofluorescence because of a choroidal filling defect

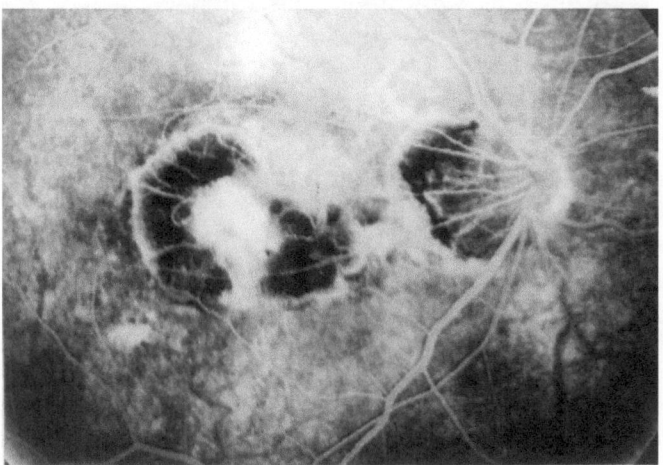

Fig. 41H. Fluorescein fundus angiogram 6 years after the initial examination (June 1994). At 2 min after dye injection, hypofluorescence corresponding to the atrophic lesion around the neovascular membrane has enlarged. The choroidal neovascular membrane is hyperfluorescent. Spotty hyperfluorescence is observed superotemporal to the choroidal neovascular membrane

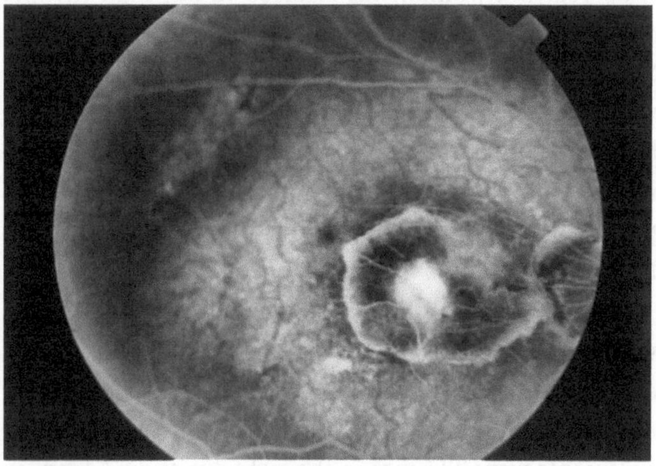

Fig. 41J. Fluorescein fundus angiogram 8 years after the initial examination (April 1996). At 6 min after dye injection, an annular atrophic lesion appears hyperfluorescent at the margin of the lesion. These angiographic findings are similar to those of patchy atrophy

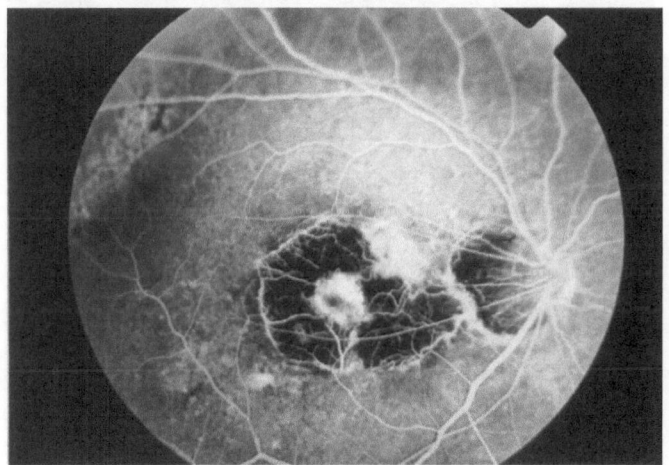

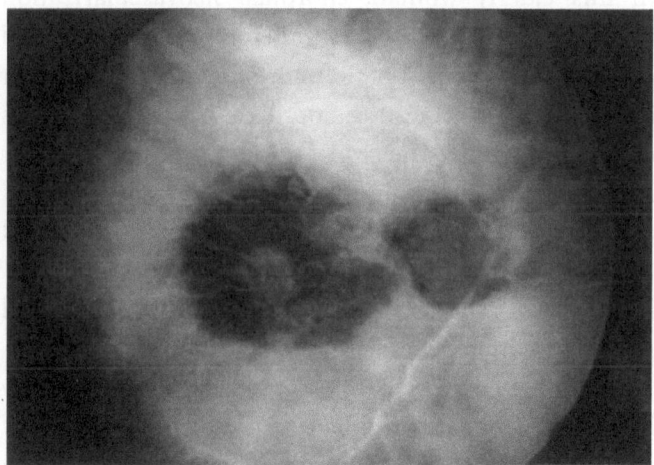

Fig. 41I. Fluorescein fundus angiogram 8 years after the initial examination (April 1996). At 33 sec after dye injection, hypofluorescence corresponding to the annular atrophy around the neovascular membrane has further enlarged and coalesced with the peripapillary crescent. Hyperfluorescence of choroidal neovascular membrane has slightly decreased

Fig. 41K. Indocyanine green fundus angiogram 8 years after the initial examination (April 1996). At 6 min after dye injection, the annular atrophy shows hypofluorescence. The choroidal neovascular membrane is slightly hyperfluorescent

Case 42

A 60-year-old woman was referred to our high myopia clinic on October 2, 1981, for myopic fundus changes. She was diagnosed as having bilateral myopia when she was in elementary school. She has not worn glasses because she has reported no difficulties. Fundus examinations have been performed annually by a general practitioner. Her medical history was noncontributory. No family members had severe myopia.

In the initial examination, the patient's best corrected visual acuity was 0.8 in the right eye and 0.8 in the left eye. The refractive error was −14.00 D sphere in the right eye and −13.00 D in the left, and the axial length measurements were 28.5 mm in the right eye and 27.4 mm in the left. Intraocular pressures and anterior segments were normal in both eyes. Mild cataractous changes were noted in the crystalline lens bilaterally. We describe the long-term fundus changes in both her right and left eyes.

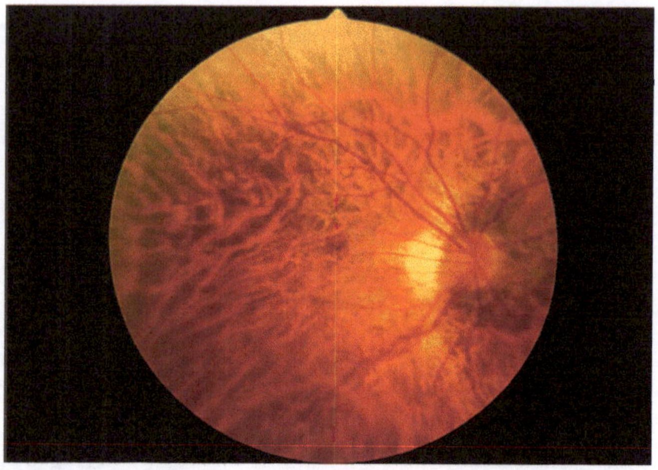

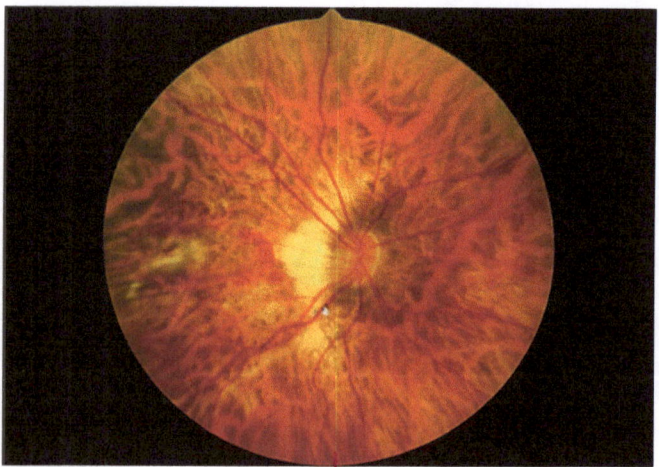

Fig. 42A. Right fundus at the initial examination (October 1981) shows slight diffuse atrophy around the optic disc. The optic disc tilts temporally. A temporal peripapillary crescent is seen. Posterior staphyloma is present around the optic disc. The red dot in the center is a photographic artifact

Summary

In this elderly woman, choroidal neovascularization occurred in both eyes. Before the choroidal neovascularization, both fundi showed only slight diffuse atrophy around the optic disc. Neither eye was extremely myopic. The size of the choroidal neovascular membrane in the right fundus was larger than that usually seen in a highly myopic fundus. Choroidal neovascularization in her right fundus was not accompanied by dense pigmentation and differed from a typical Fuchs' spot in appearance.

Choroidal neovascularization may occur in elderly highly myopic patients who are not extremely myopic and who show slight diffuse atrophy in the fundus. In these patients, age-related macular degeneration must be ruled out. This patient showed no obvious age-related fundus changes, such as senile drusen, before the onset of choroidal neovascularization. Moreover, the area of surrounding retinal edema and bleeding was small, as compared with typical age-related macular degeneration. These findings suggest that choroidal neovascularization in this woman is closely related to high myopia.

Fig. 42B. Three years later (October 1984), choroidal neovascularization with surrounding subretinal bleeding has occurred. Visual acuity has dropped to 0.03, and the refractive error is −13.00 D

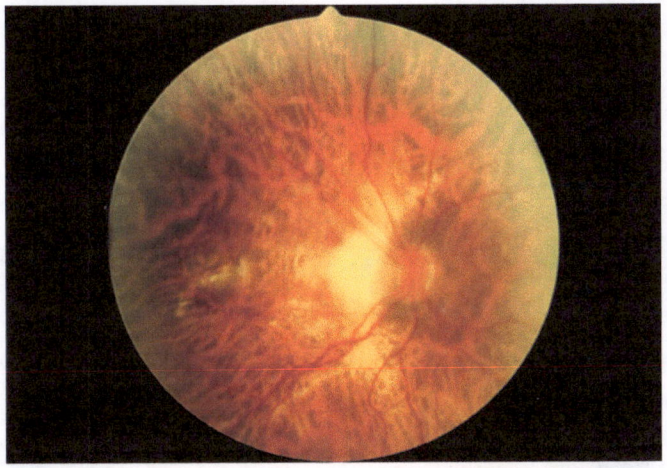

Fig. 42C. Four years after the initial examination (September 1985), subretinal bleeding has absorbed. Diffuse atrophy has gradually enlarged in the posterior fundus

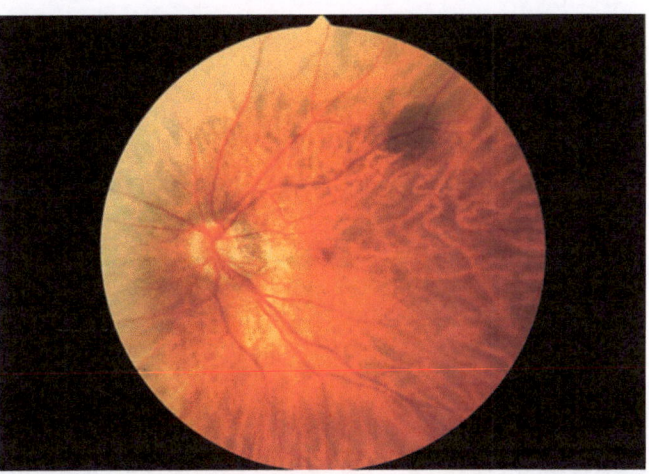

Fig. 42F. Left fundus at the initial examination (October 1981) shows a slight diffuse atrophy around the optic disc. The optic disc tilts temporally. A temporal peripapillary crescent is seen. No posterior staphyloma is present

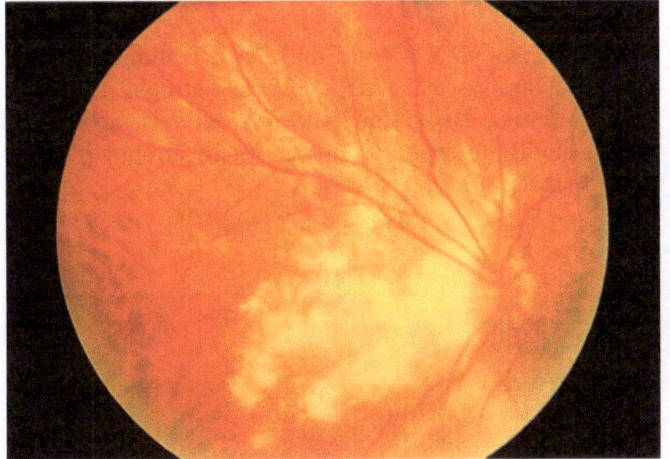

Fig. 42D. Seven years after the initial examination (July 1988), the macular lesion is occupied by irregularly shaped and yellowish-white atrophic lesions. Choroidal neovascularization has regressed and is less evident

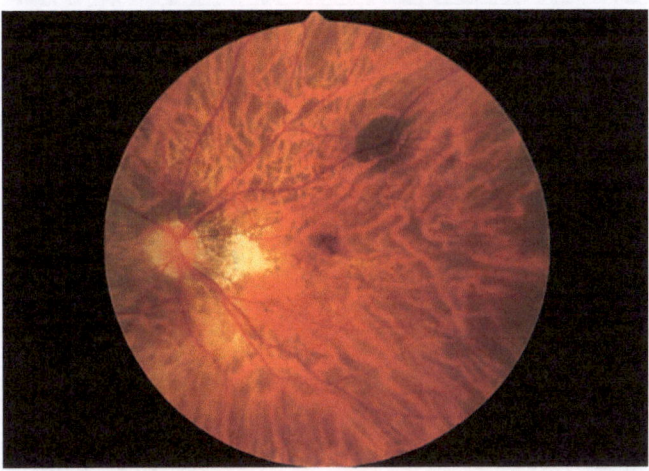

Fig. 42G. Three years later (October 1984), small choroidal neovascularization has appeared with surrounding retinal edema and bleeding. Visual acuity is 0.5, and the refractive error is −12.50 D

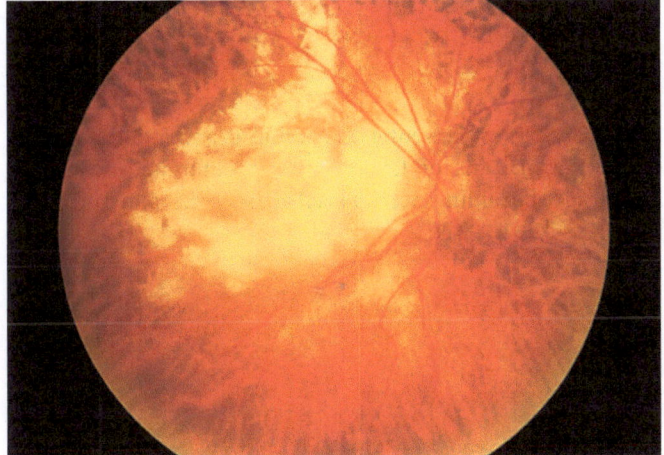

Fig. 42E. Nine years after the initial examination (October 1990), the margins of the atrophic lesion have become clear. The atrophic lesion has also enlarged. Diffuse atrophy has also increased. Visual acuity is 0.04, and the refractive error is −16.00 D

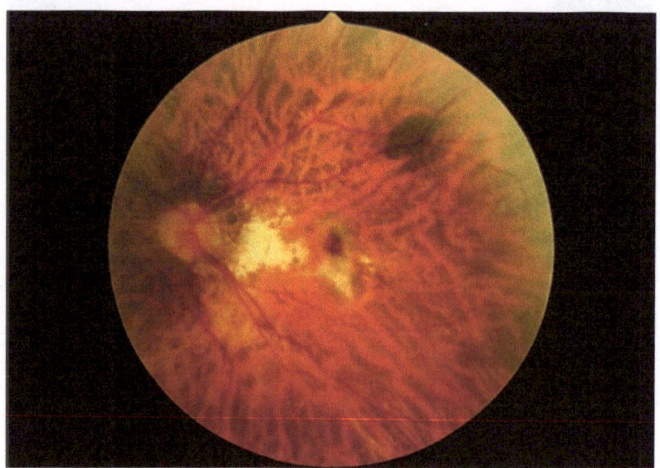

Fig. 42H. Four years after the initial examination (September 1985), a fibrovascular membrane of choroidal neovascularization has formed after the absorption of subretinal bleeding. Visual acuity is 0.1, and the refractive error is −12.50 D

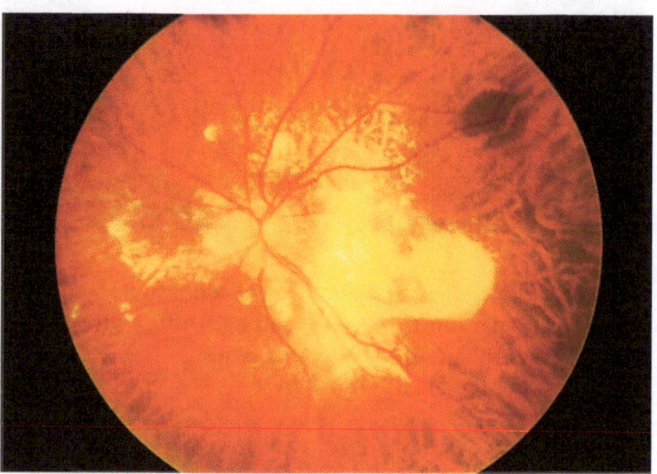

Fig. 42J. Eight years after the initial examination (July 1989), subretinal fibrovascular tissue and diffuse atrophy around the optic disc have enlarged simultaneously. Several small atrophic lesions similar to spotty lesions of patchy atrophy have appeared nasal to the optic disc

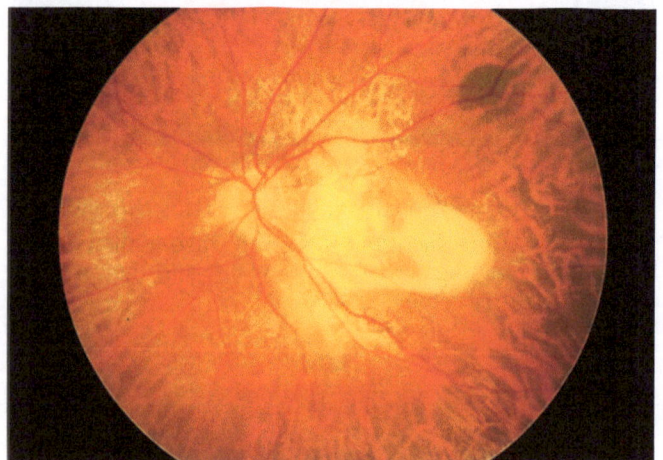

Fig. 42I. Six years after the initial examination (May 1987), the fibrovascular membrane has enlarged. Diffuse atrophy has also enlarged around the optic disc

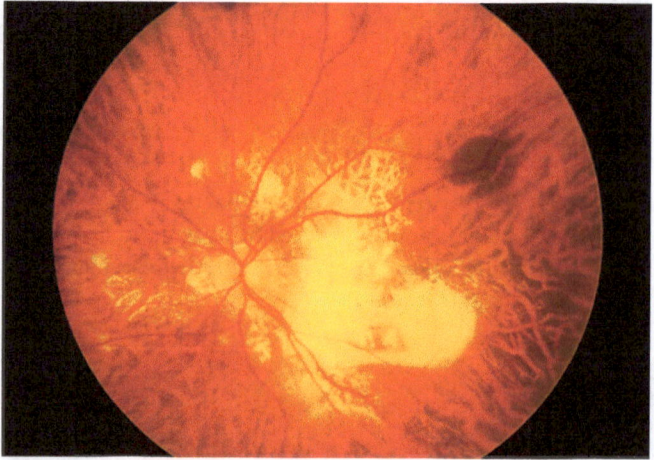

Fig. 42K. Nine years after the initial examination (October 1990), the margins of fibrovascular membrane and diffuse atrophy are becoming clear. Visual acuity is 0.1, and the refractive error is −12.00 D

Case 43

A 50-year-old woman presented with decreased visual acuity in her right eye on October 3, 1986. She was diagnosed with myopia when she was in elementary school. Her myopia progressed in the right eye after she entered high school. At that time, corrected visual acuity in the right eye was 0.8. She noticed blurred vision in the right eye 5 months before her initial examination in our high myopia clinic. One month later, she noticed a central scotoma in the right eye. Her medical history was noncontributory. No family members had severe myopia.

In the initial examination, the patient's best corrected visual acuity was 0.5 in the right eye and 1.2 in the left. The refractive error was −17.00 D sphere in the right eye and −4.00 D sphere in the left, and axial length measurements were 29.3 mm in the right eye and 24.3 mm in the left. Intraocular pressures and anterior segments were normal in both eyes. We describe the long-term fundus changes in her right eye.

Summary

This woman was followed up for 10 years, since 1986. She presented with decreased visual acuity caused by myopic choroidal neovascularization in the right eye. The activity of choroidal neovascular membrane was low. Subretinal bleeding was absorbed quickly. Visual acuity in the right eye was maintained for 5 years after the initial examination. Atrophic lesions, however, gradually formed around the regressed neovascular membranes and caused additional visual decrease in the right eye.

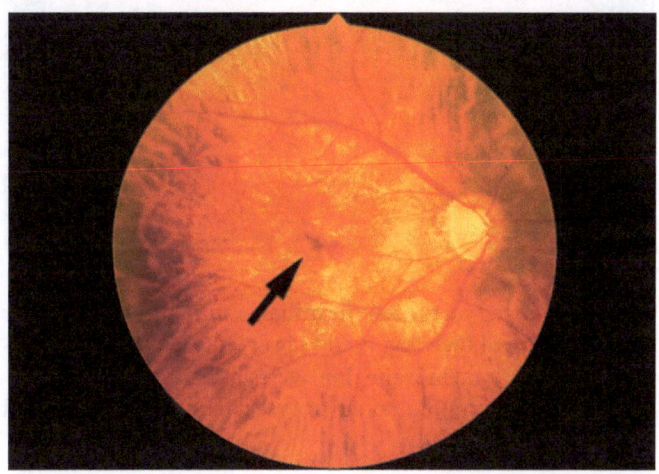

Fig. 43A. Right fundus at the initial examination (October 1986) shows subretinal bleeding and a pigmented fibrovascular membrane in the macula (*arrow*). Spotty or linear lesions of diffuse atrophy are seen in the posterior fundus. The optic disc tilts temporally. A narrow peripapillary crescent is observed. Type I posterior staphyloma is present

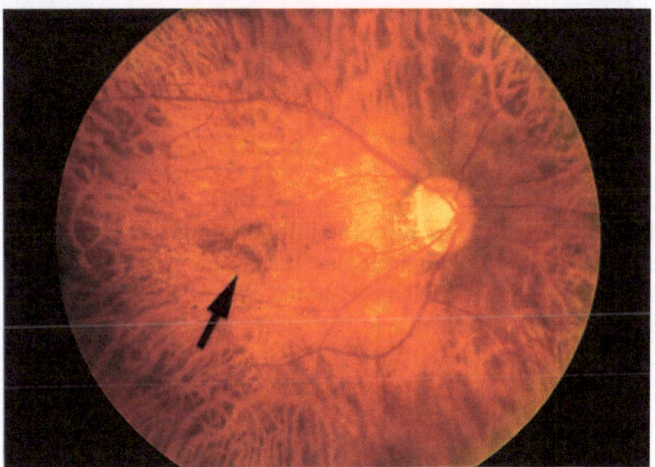

Fig. 43B. Two years later (December 1988), the choroidal neovascular membrane has slightly enlarged (*arrow*). Visual acuity is 0.5, and the refractive error is −17.00 D. The subretinal bleeding has almost absorbed

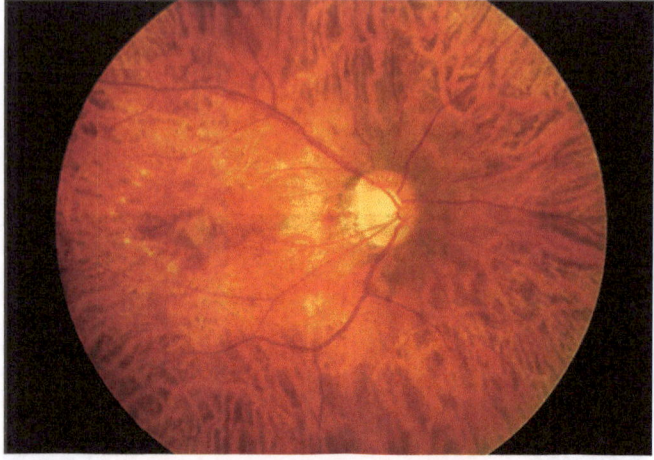

Fig. 43C. Three years after the initial examination (December 1989), subretinal bleeding is still observed around the choroidal neovascular membrane. Linear lesions of diffuse atrophy have increased temporal to the neovascular membrane. Visual acuity is 0.4

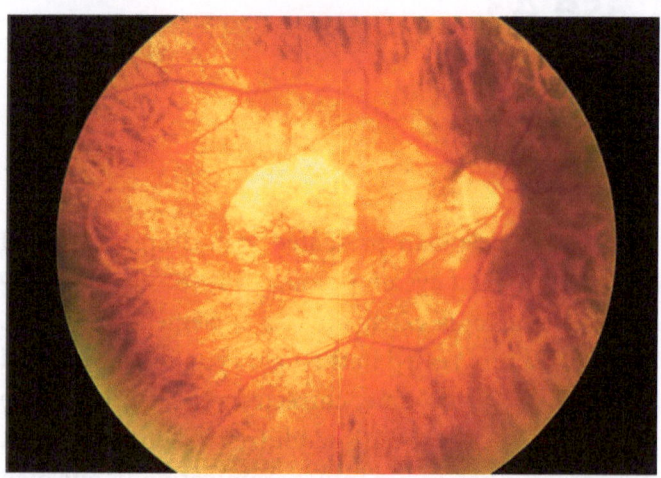

Fig. 43F. Seven years after the initial examination (December 1993), a semicircular atrophic lesion has developed superior to the regressed neovascular membrane. Visual acuity has further decreased to 0.1

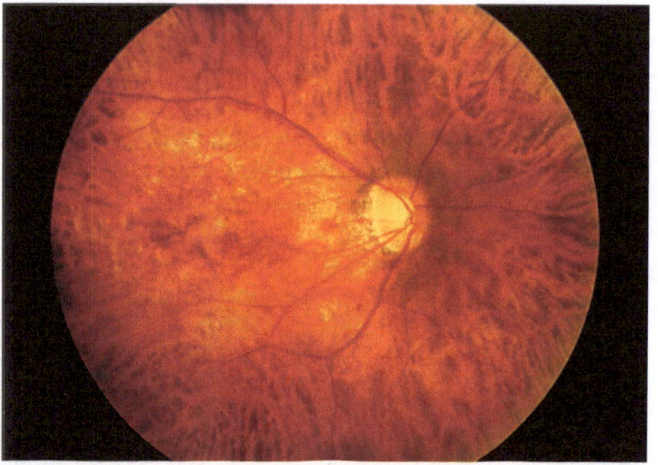

Fig. 43D. Five years after the initial examination (February 1991), the choroidal neovascular membrane is regressing. No retinal bleeding or edema is noted around the neovascular membrane. Visual acuity is 0.5

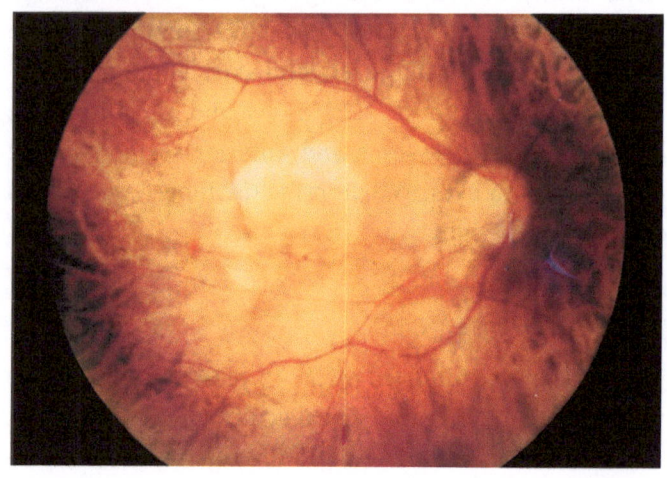

Fig. 43G. Nine years after the initial examination (January 1995), the atrophic lesion around the regressed neovascular membrane has enlarged. Visual acuity is 0.1, and the refractive error is −17.00 D

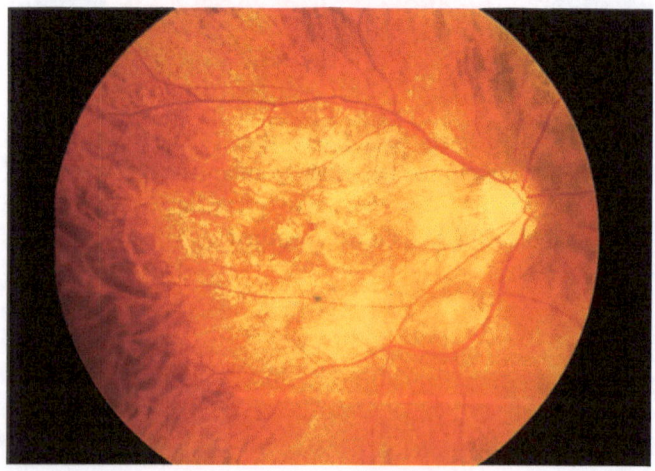

Fig. 43E. Five years after the initial examination (December 1991), the choroidal neovascular membrane is becoming unclear. Diffuse atrophy covers the entire posterior fundus. Visual acuity has decreased to 0.3

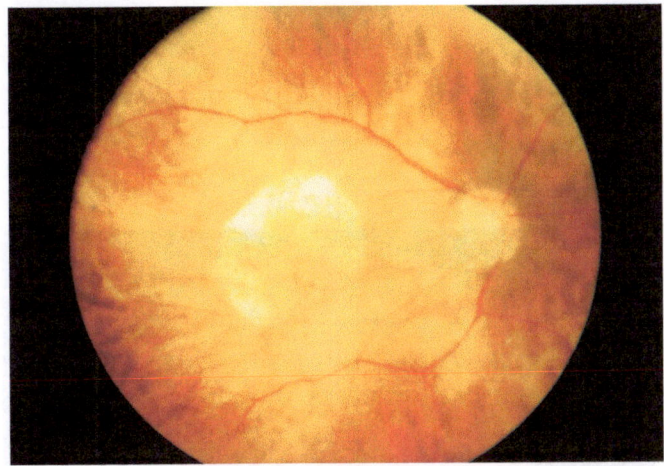

Fig. 43H. Ten years after the initial examination (April 1996), the atrophic lesion has further enlarged around the neovascular membrane, and its margins are clear. The original neovascular membrane is difficult to detect ophthalmoscopically. Visual acuity is 0.1, and the refractive error is −17.00 D

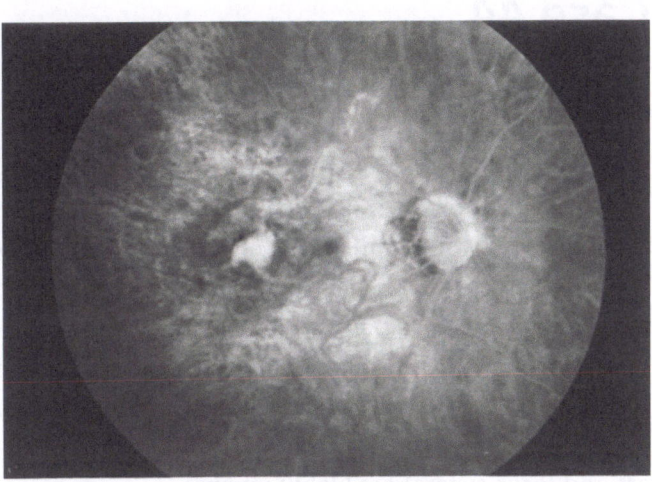

Fig. 43J. Fluorescein fundus angiogram 5 years after the initial examination (December 1991). At 6 min after dye injection, the choroidal neovascular membrane shows tissue staining. No dye leakage is obvious. The atrophic lesion around the neovascular membrane also is hyperfluorescent because of tissue staining in the late phase

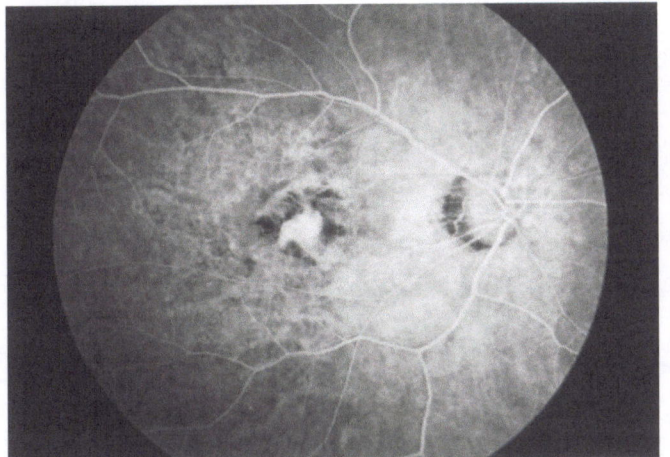

Fig. 43I. Fluorescein fundus angiogram 5 years after the initial examination (December 1991). At 37 sec after dye injection, the choroidal neovascular membrane shows hyperfluorescence. The atrophic lesion around the neovascular membrane shows hypofluorescence from a choroidal filling defect

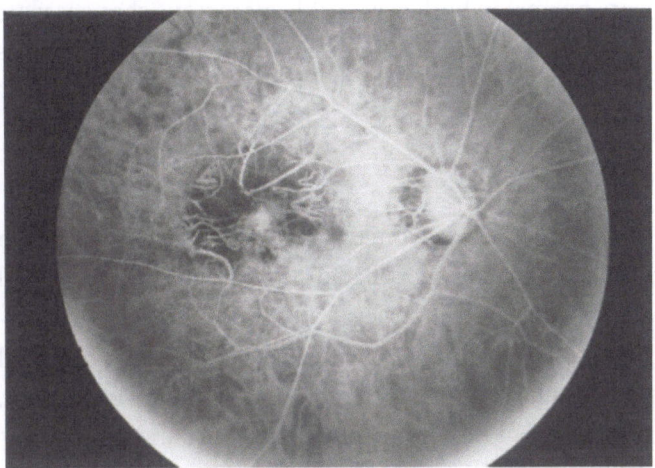

Fig. 43K. Fluorescein fundus angiogram 9 years after the initial examination (January 1995). At 41 sec after dye injection, the choroidal neovascular membrane is slightly hyperfluorescent. The atrophic lesion around the choroidal neovascular membrane shows a choroidal filling defect. Large choroidal vessels are visible within the atrophic lesion

Fig. 43L. Fluorescein fundus angiogram 9 years after the initial examination (January 1995). At 8 min after dye injection, the choroidal neovascular membrane shows slight hyperfluorescence. The atrophic lesion around the neovascular membrane is hyperfluorescent because of tissue staining in the late phase. The angiographic findings of the atrophic lesion are similar to those of typical patchy atrophy

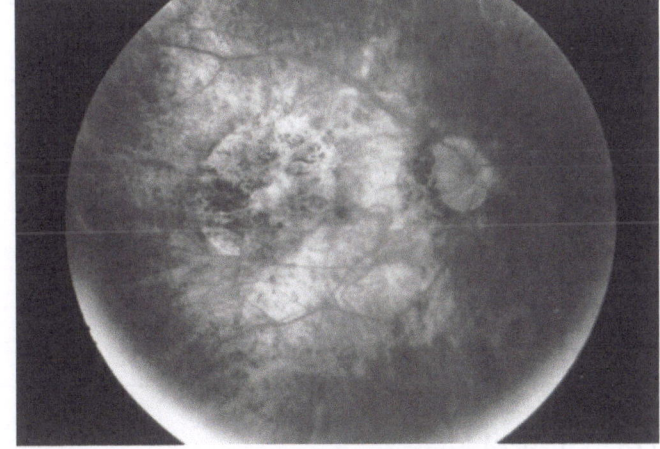

Case 44

A 56-year-old woman presented on November 11, 1983, with decreased vision in her right eye. She was diagnosed with myopia as an elementary school student. She began wearing glasses for distance vision in high school. Her medical history was noncontributory. Both of her parents are slightly myopic. Her five siblings (two brothers and three sisters) are highly myopic.

In the initial examination, the patient's best corrected visual acuity was 0.08 in the right eye and 0.9 in the left eye. The refractive error was $-16.5\,D$ sphere in the right eye and $-13.75\,D$ in the left, and the axial length measurements were 28.5 mm in the right eye and 27.1 mm in the left. Intraocular pressures and anterior segments were normal in both eyes. Mild cataractous changes were noted in her left eye. We describe the long-term fundus changes in her left eye.

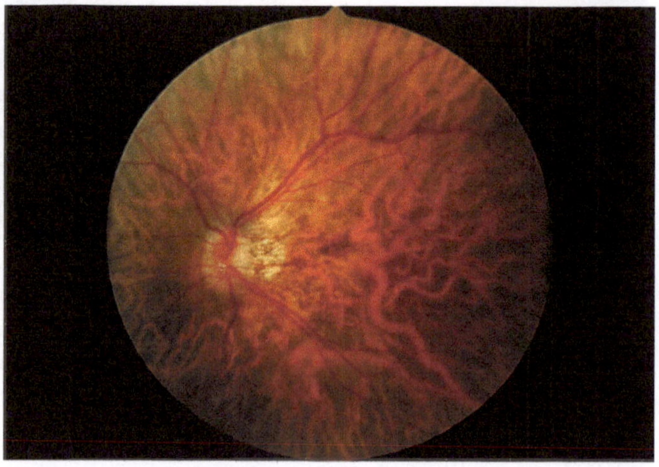

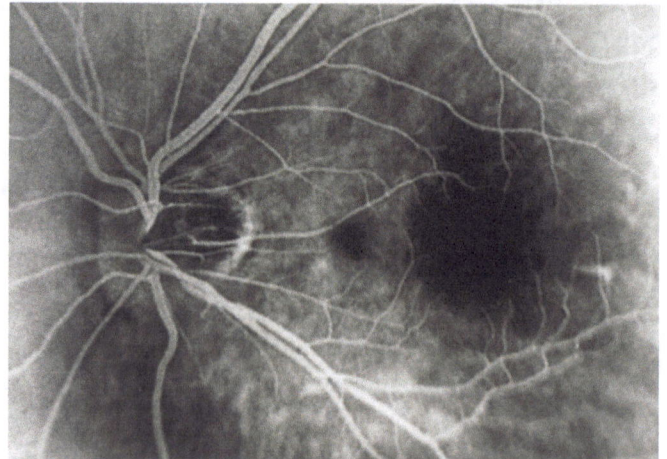

Fig. 44A. Left eye at the initial examination (November 1983) shows a tessellated fundus. The optic disc tilts temporally. Type I posterior staphyloma is present

Summary

In this elderly woman, choroidal vascularization occurred in her tessellated fundus. Her final visual acuity dropped to legal blindness. The progressive course in her left fundus after the choroidal neovascularization was typical of a myopic Fuchs' spot. An atrophic lesion gradually formed around the choroidal neovascularization, until the entire macula became atrophic. The progressive pattern of myopic fundus changes in this patient was from T to D_1 + HN_1 to D_1 + HN_2 to MA. In this patient, diffuse atrophy and choroidal neovascularization progressed together. As seen in this patient, myopic choroidal neovascularization may develop in elderly highly myopic patients who are not extremely myopic and who show only slight diffuse atrophy in the fundus.

Fig. 44B. Fluorescein angiogram at the initial examination (November 1983). At 3 min after dye injection, no abnormal fluorescence is observed in the macula

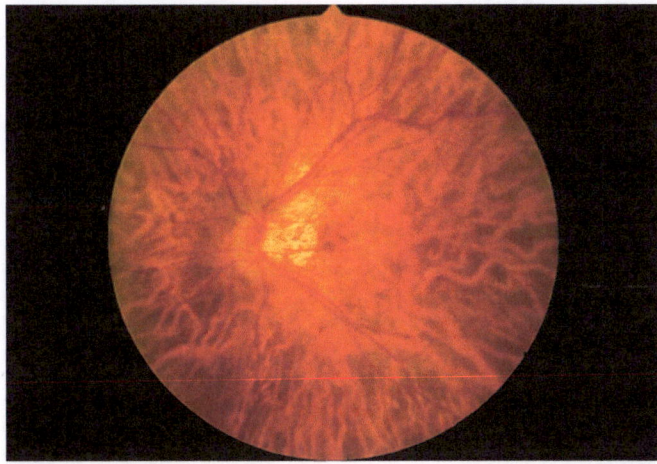

Fig. 44C. Three years later (January 1986), a linear lesion of diffuse atrophy is observed in the macula. Visual acuity is 0.8, and the refractive error is −14.00 D

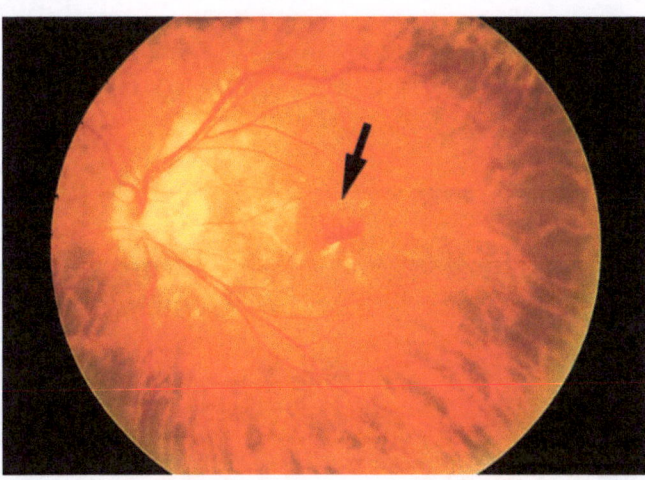

Fig. 44E. Five years after the initial examination (September 1988), choroidal neovascularization with surrounding subretinal bleeding has appeared in the foveal region (*arrow*)

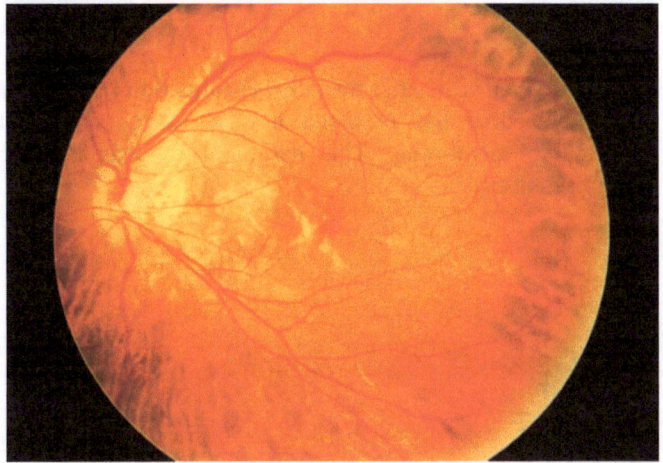

Fig. 44D. Five years after the initial examination (March 1988), linear lesions of diffuse atrophy appear obliquely across the macula. Visual acuity is 0.4, and the refractive error is −15.75 D

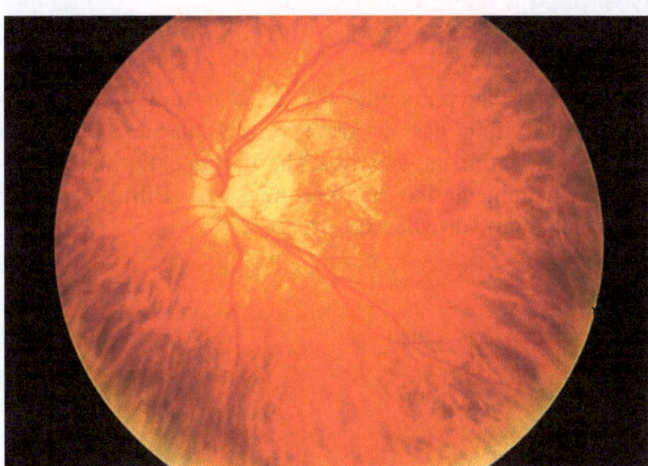

Fig. 44F. Six years after the initial examination (January 1989), subretinal bleeding caused by choroidal neovascularization has enlarged. Linear lesions of diffuse atrophy around the optic disc have also enlarged. Visual acuity is 0.1, and the refractive error is −15.5 D

Fig. 44G. Six years after the initial examination (June 1989), a half-moon-shaped atrophic lesion has appeared nasal to the neovascular membrane (*arrow*)

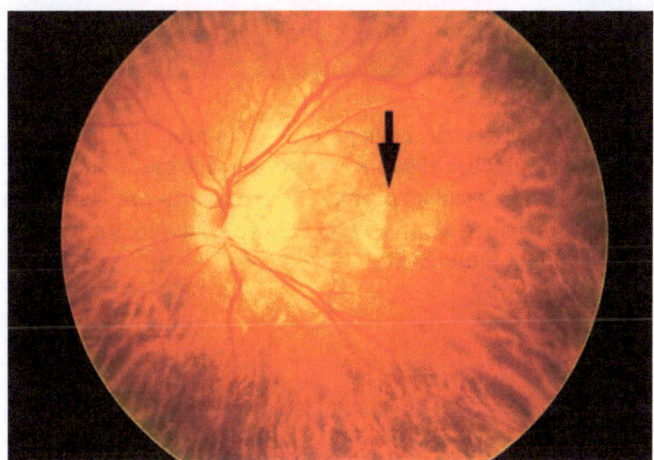

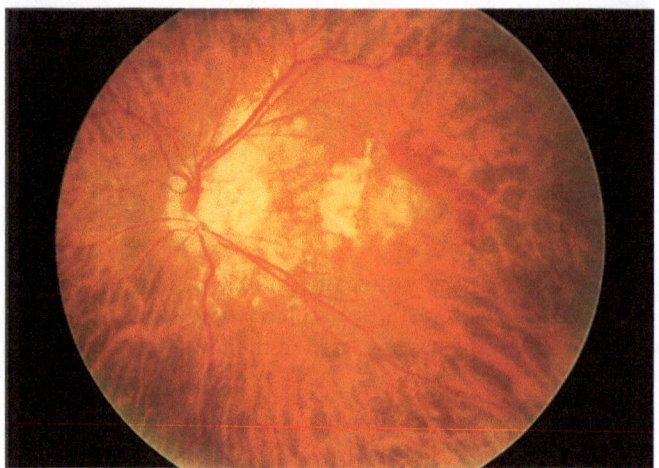

Fig. 44H. Seven years after the initial examination (March 1990), rebleeding has occurred in the macula. Choroidal neovascularization has enlarged. The margin of the half-moon-shaped atrophic lesion has become clear. Diffuse atrophy around the optic disc has also enlarged

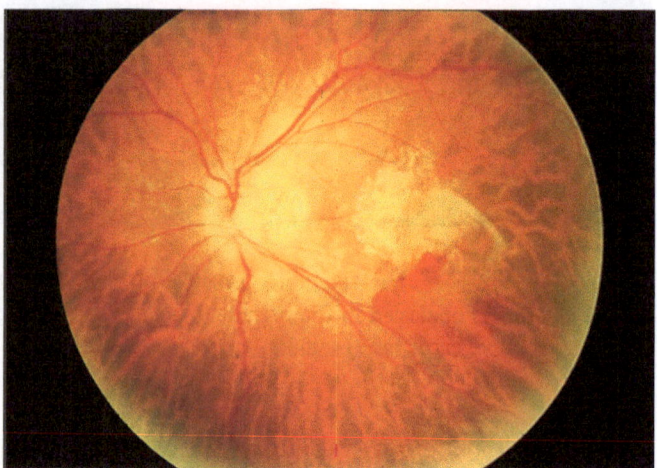

Fig. 44J. Seven years after the initial examination (November 1990), rebleeding has occurred inferior to the choroidal neovascular membrane. The half-moon-shaped atrophic lesion has enlarged

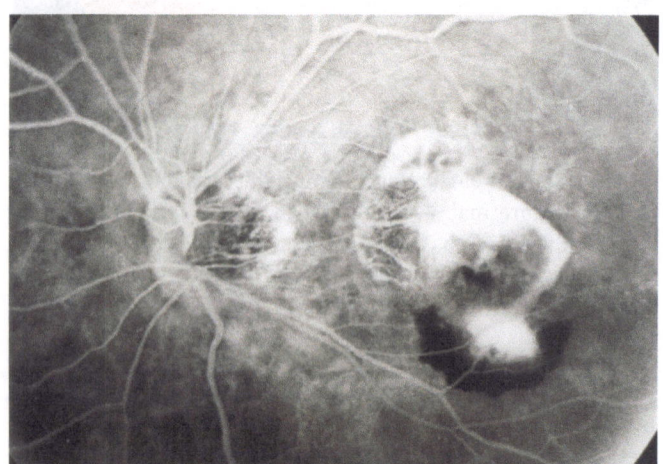

Fig. 44I. Fluorescein angiogram 7 years after the initial examination (October 1990). At 9 min after dye injection, a large choroidal neovascular membrane is hyperfluorescent. The half-moon-shaped atrophic lesion is hypofluorescent because of a choroidal filling defect

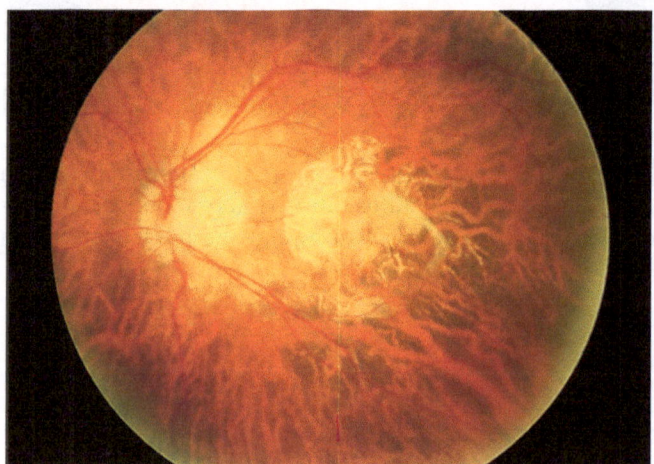

Fig. 44K. Nine years after the initial examination (May 1992), macular bleeding is completely absorbed. Fibrovascular tissue is seen in the macula. A retinochoroidal atrophic lesion is formed within the area of previous retinal edema and bleeding around the fibrovascular membrane

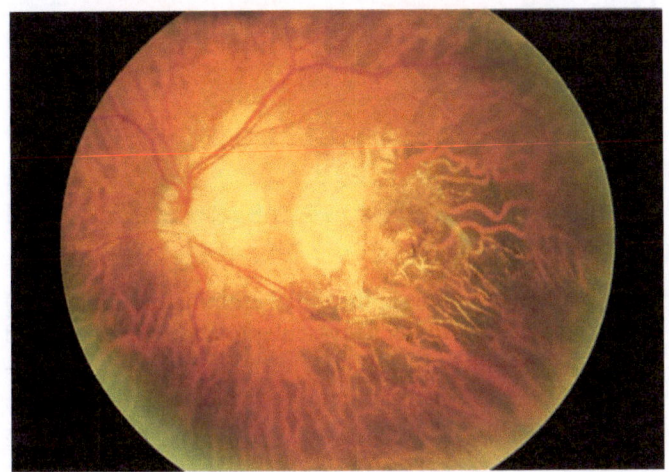

Fig. 44L. Eleven years after the initial examination (November 1994), the atrophic lesion around the fibrovascular tissue has enlarged. Pigmentation has increased within the atrophic lesion. Visual acuity is 0.08, and the refractive error is −16.0 D

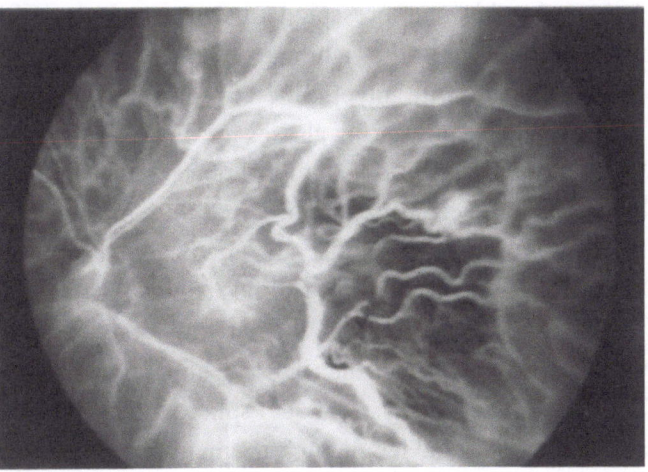

Fig. 44N. Indocyanine green angiogram 11 years after the initial examination (May 1994). The atrophic lesion is hypofluorescent in the early phase of the angiogram

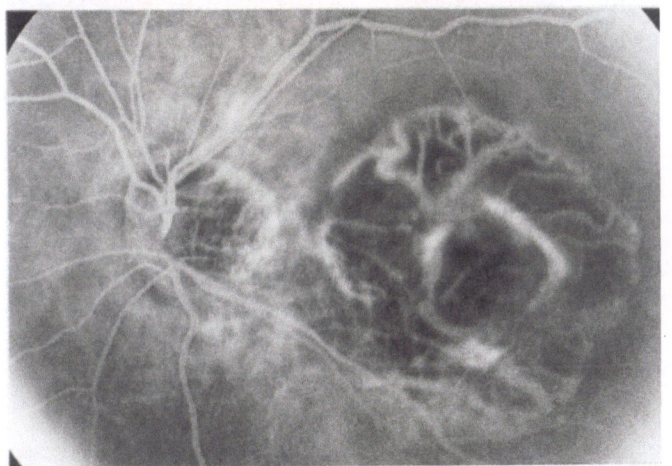

Fig. 44M. Fluorescein angiogram 11 years after the initial examination (May 1994). At 6 min after dye injection, leakage of dye from the choroidal neovascular membrane has decreased, indicating regression of the choroidal neovascularization. A large choroidal filling defect is also seen in the large atrophic lesion around the neovascular membrane

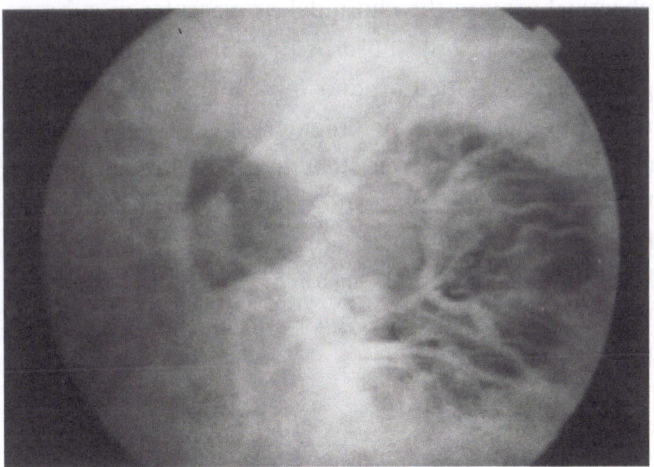

Fig. 44O. Indocyanine green angiogram 11 years after the initial examination (May 1994). The late phase of the angiogram shows consistent hypofluorescence in the atrophic lesion. Abnormal fluorescence corresponding to the choroidal neovascularization is not obvious in all the angiograms

Case 45

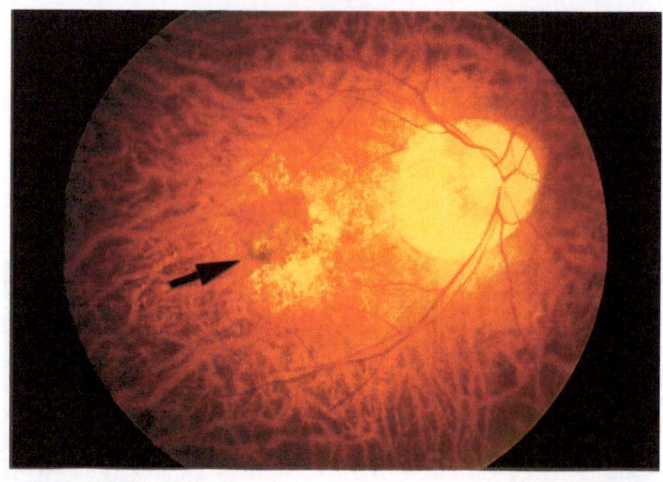

Fig. 45A. Right fundus at the initial examination (June 1991) shows a grayish choroidal neovascular membrane surrounded by bleeding in the macula (*arrow*). An enlarged lesion of diffuse atrophy is also visible around the neovascular membrane. The optic disc tilts temporally. A wide peripapillary crescent is seen temporal to the optic disc. Type I posterior staphyloma is present

A 53-year old man presented on June 1, 1991, with metamorphopsia in the right eye of 1-year duration. He was diagnosed with myopia as an elementary school student. He began wearing glasses for distance vision in high school. He noticed metamorphopsia in the right eye but received no examination for 1 year until his first visit to our high myopia clinic. His medical history was noncontributory. One of his siblings is highly myopic.

In the initial examination, the patient's best corrected visual acuity was 0.5 in the right eye and 1.0 in the left. The refractive error was −14.50 D sphere in the right eye and −15.00 D. Axial length measurements were 29.8 mm bilaterally. Intraocular pressures and anterior segments were normal in both eyes. We describe the long-term fundus changes in his right eye.

Summary

The patient has been followed up for 4 years, since 1991. At the initial examination, macular bleeding was observed around the choroidal neovascular membrane. After the bleeding absorbed, chorioretinal atrophy gradually developed around the choroidal neovascular membrane. Fluorescein angiography of chorioretinal atrophy showed a consistent hyperfluoresence during the entire angiographic examination, which is different from that seen in typical patchy atrophy. Pigmentation later appeared within the lesion of chorioretinal atrophy. His right eye showed typical progressive pattern of Fuchs' spot.

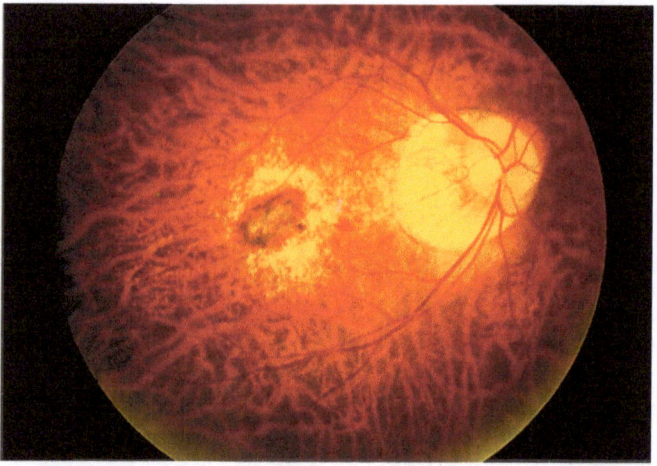

Fig. 45B. One year later (January 1992), macular bleeding is absorbed. Chorioretinal atrophy has developed around the choroidal neovascular membrane. Visual acuity is 0.3, and the refractive error is −15.00 D

Fig. 45C. Two years after the initial examination (April 1993), chorioretinal atrophy around the choroidal neovascular membrane has enlarged and its margins are clear, especially nasal to the membrane. Visual acuity is 0.1, and the refractive error is −15.00 D

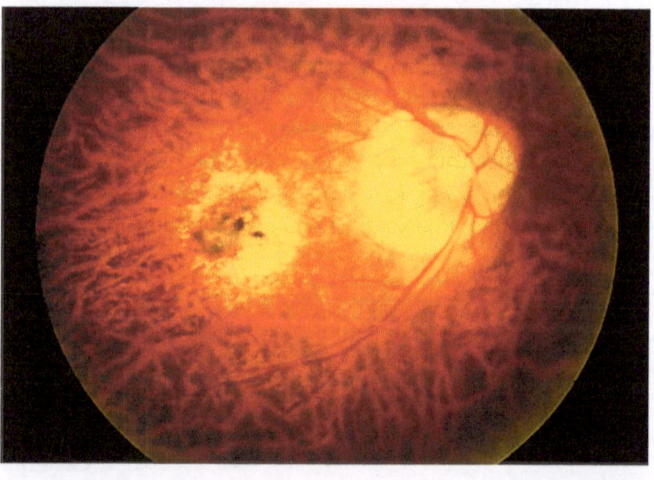

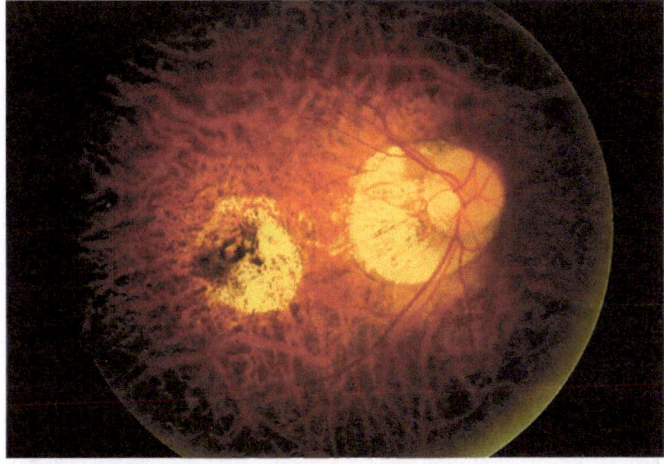

Fig. 45D. Three years after the initial examination (April 1994), chorioretinal atrophy around the neovascular membrane has enlarged. Pigmentation has increased within the area of chorioretinal atrophy

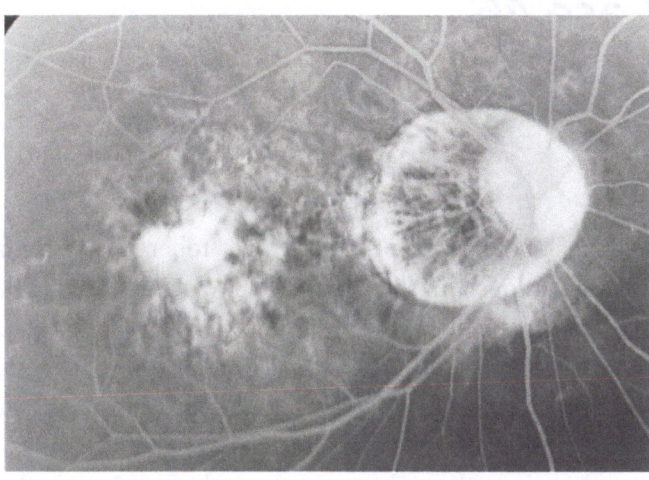

Fig. 45F. Fluorescein fundus angiogram at the initial examination (June 1991). At 9 sec after dye injection, choroidal neovascular membrane is hyperfluorescent because of tissue staining

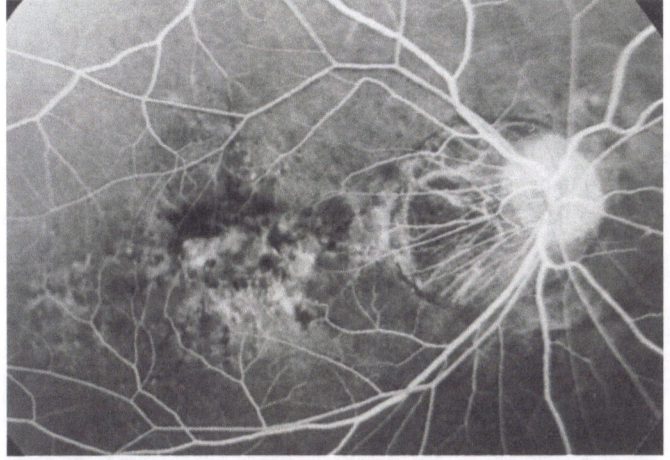

Fig. 45E. Fluorescein fundus angiogram at the initial examination (June 1991). At 14 sec after dye injection, the choroidal neovascular membrane shows irregular hyperfluorescence. Macular bleeding is visible as blocked fluorescence. Diffuse atrophy surrounding the choroidal neovascular membrane shows irregular hyperfluorescence and hypofluorescence

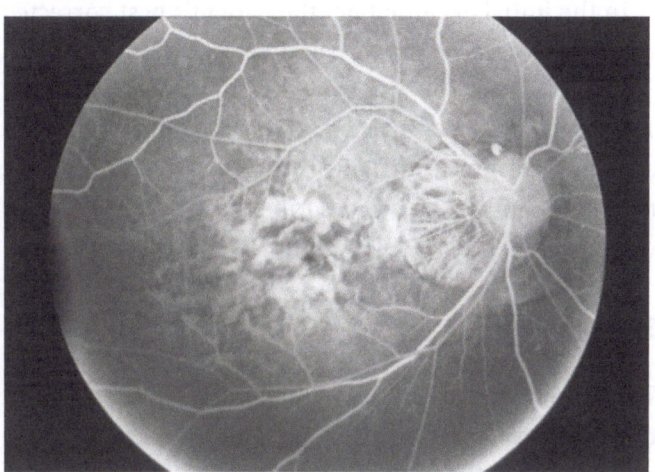

Fig. 45G. Fluorescein angiogram 1 year after the initial examination (August 1992). At 41 sec after dye injection, chorioretinal atrophy is hyperfluorescent superior to the neovascular membrane

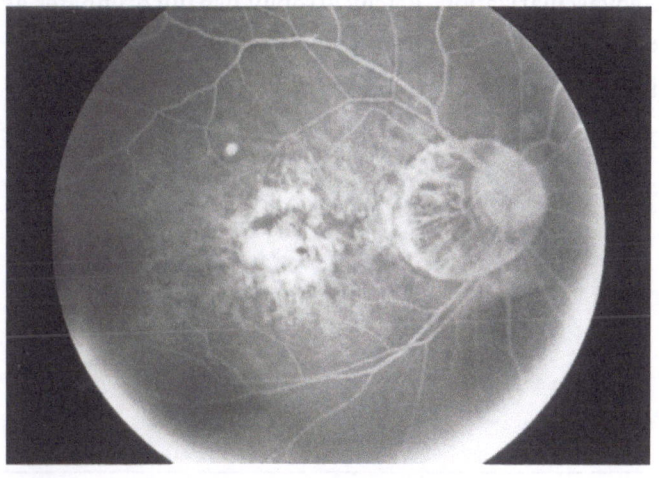

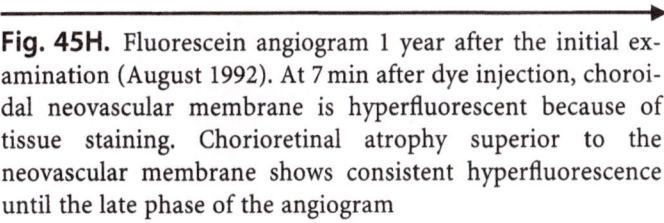

Fig. 45H. Fluorescein angiogram 1 year after the initial examination (August 1992). At 7 min after dye injection, choroidal neovascular membrane is hyperfluorescent because of tissue staining. Chorioretinal atrophy superior to the neovascular membrane shows consistent hyperfluorescence until the late phase of the angiogram

Case 46

A 39-year-old woman presented on October 5, 1983, with metamorphopsia in the left eye. She was diagnosed with myopia as an elementary school student. She began wearing contact lenses for distance vision at age 21 years. Her best corrected visual acuity at that time was 0.3 in both eyes with contact lenses. She noticed metamorphopsia in the right eye at the end of 1982, visited a general practitioner, and was referred to our high myopia clinic for macular bleeding in the left eye. Her medical history was noncontributory. No family members had severe myopia.

In the initial examination, the patient's best corrected visual acuity was 0.3 in the right eye and 0.06 in the left. The refractive error was −20.50 D sphere in both eyes. The axial length measurements were 31.7 mm in the right eye and 32.0 mm in the left. Intraocular pressures were normal in both eyes. We describe the long-term fundus changes in her left eye.

Summary

This woman was followed up for 12 years, since 1983. At the initial examination, macular bleeding with choroidal neovascularization was observed in her left eye. After that, the choroidal neovascular membrane regressed with no episodes of rebleeding. However, some areas around the neovascular membrane gradually turned yellowish white, and finally wide chorioretinal atrophy was formed around the Fuchs' spot. This pattern of development is different from that of patchy atrophy without neovascularization. Patchy atrophy usually originates as small spotty lesions that coalesce to form one large atrophic lesion.

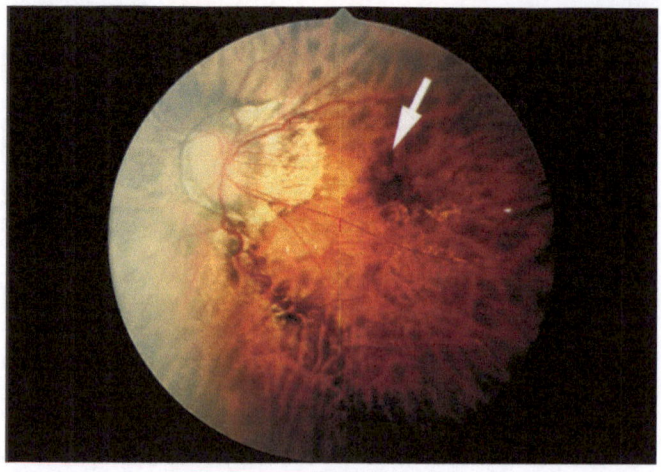

Fig. 46A. Left fundus at the initial examination (October 1983) shows a pigmented Fuchs' spot with bleeding in the macula (*arrow*). A lacquer crack lesion is also visible temporal to the Fuchs' spot. The optic disc tilts temporally. A temporal peripapillary crescent is seen. Type I posterior staphyloma is present

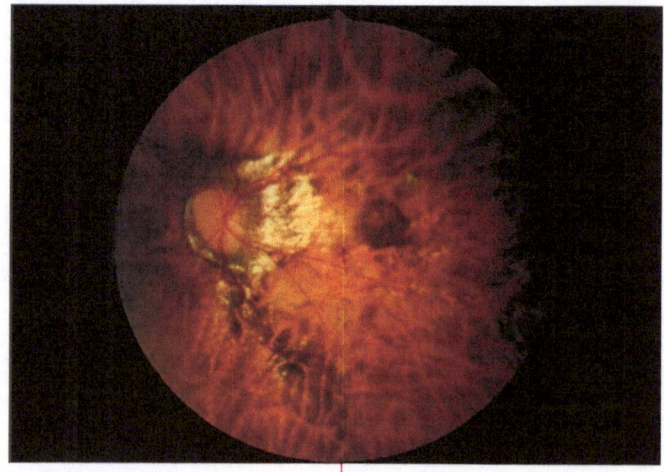

Fig. 46B. One year later (March 1984), the bleeding is absorbed. The pigmented Fuchs' spot has enlarged. Visual acuity is 0.02, and the refractive error is −20.50 D

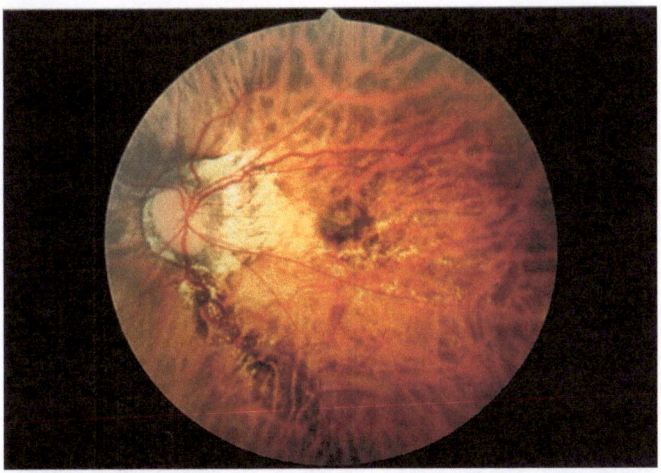

Fig. 46C. One year later (September 1984), Fuchs' spot shows no remarkable changes. Lacquer crack lesions have increased around the Fuchs' spot

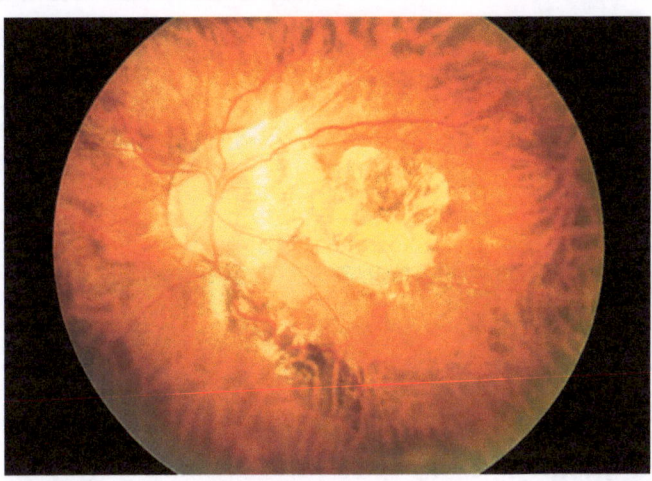

Fig. 46E. Six years after the initial examination (September 1989), chorioretinal atrophy around the Fuchs' spot has enlarged. The temporal peripapillary crescent has also enlarged

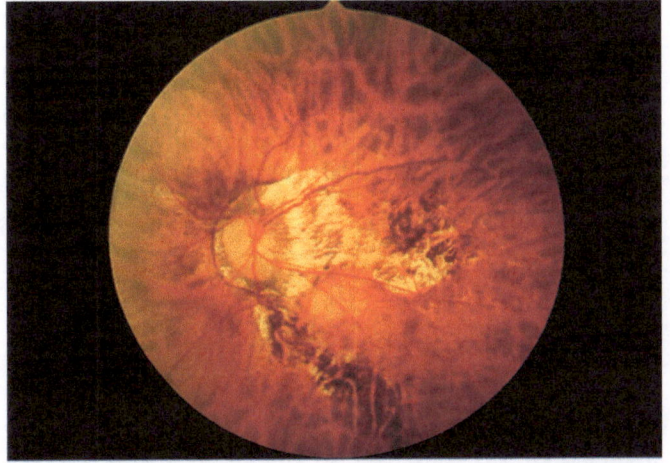

Fig. 46D. Four years after the initial examination (September 1987), chorioretinal atrophy is formed around the Fuchs' spot. Its appearance is similar to that of patchy atrophy. The Fuchs' spot has become less pigmented. Visual acuity is 0.01, and the refractive error is −20.50 D

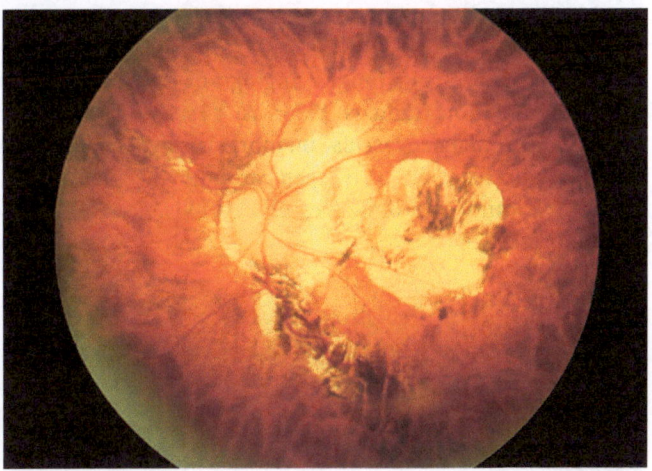

Fig. 46F. Eight years after initial examination (September 1991), chorioretinal atrophy around the Fuchs' spot has enlarged further

Fig. 46G. Ten years after the initial examination (April 1993), chorioretinal atrophy around the Fuchs' spot has continued to enlarge. Visual acuity is 0.02, and the refractive error is −19.0 D

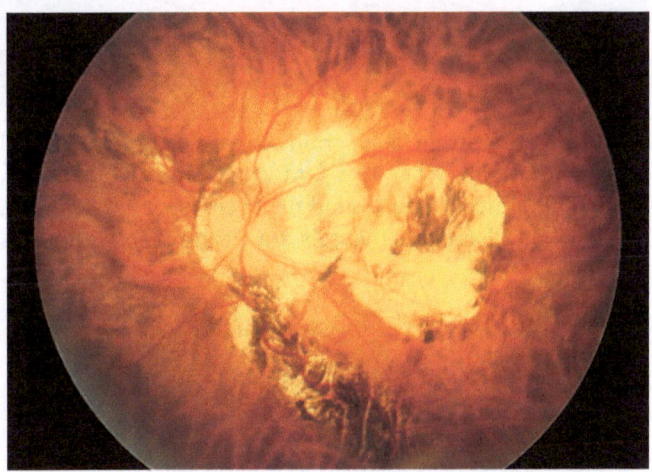

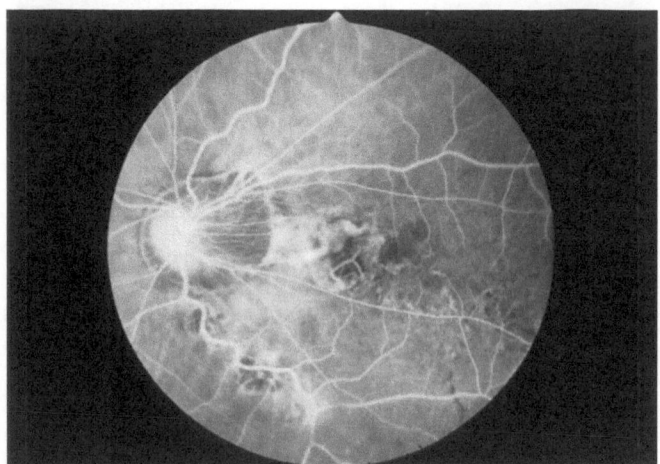

Fig. 46H. Fluorescein fundus angiogram 3 years after the initial examination (January 1986). At 42 sec after dye injection, the choroidal neovascular membrane is hyperfluorescent. A hypofluorescent area is seen around the neovascular membrane, and choroidal vessels are visible within the hypofluorescence

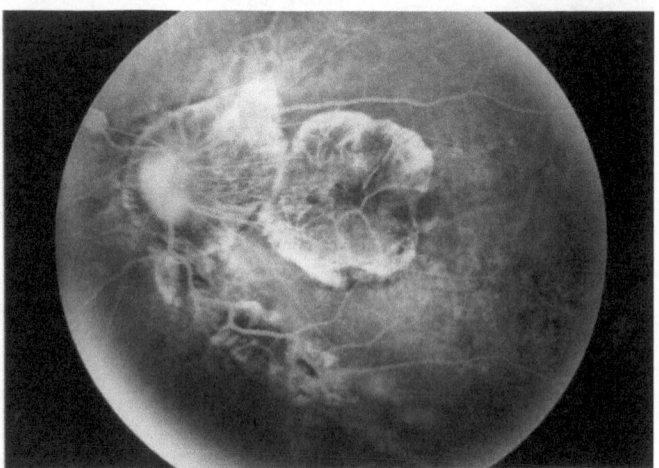

Fig. 46J. Fluorescein angiogram 12 years after the initial examination (November 1995). At 7 min after dye injection, the margin of chorioretinal atrophy around the Fuchs' spot is hyperfluorescent. The choroidal neovascular membrane shows no dye leakage

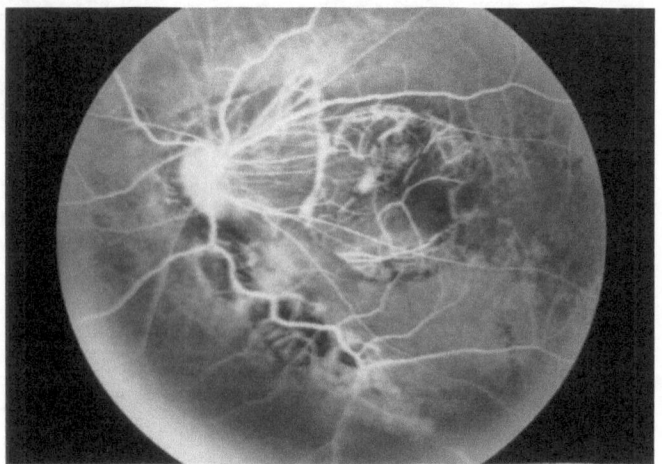

Fig. 46I. Fluorescein angiogram 12 years after the initial examination (November 1995). At 27 sec after dye injection, the hypofluorescent area around the Fuchs' spot has enlarged. Medium- and large-sized vessels are clearly seen within this lesion

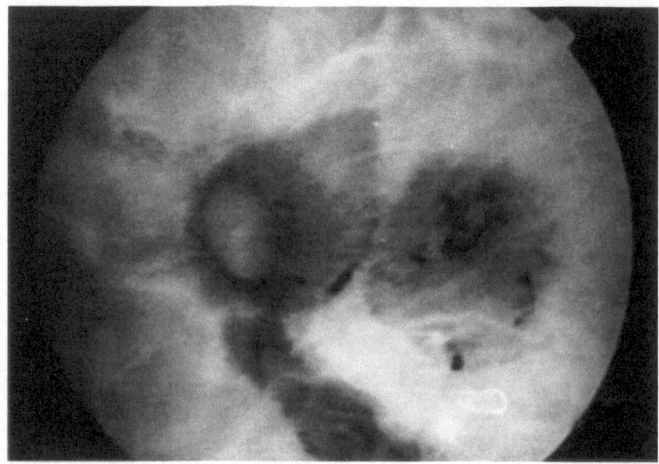

Fig. 46K. Indocyanine green fundus angiogram 12 years after the initial examination (November 1995). In the late phase of the angiogram, chorioretinal atrophy around the Fuchs' spot is hypofluorescent. Angiographic findings of chorioretinal atrophy around the Fuchs' spot are similar to patchy atrophy without neovascularization. Hyperfluorescence corresponding to the choroidal neovascular membrane is not observed

Case 47

A 65-year-old woman presented with metamorphopsia in the right eye on April 7, 1989. She was diagnosed as having myopia in elementary school. She noticed metamorphopsia in the right eye several months before the initial examination. Her medical history was noncontributory. No family members had severe myopia.

In the initial examination, the patient's best corrected visual acuity was 0.2 in the right eye and 0.6 in the left. The refractive error was −16.00 D sphere in the right eye and −9.25 D in the left. The axial length measurements were 29.3 mm in the right eye and 26.5 mm in the left. Intraocular pressures and anterior segments were normal in both eyes. We describe the long-term fundus changes in her right eye.

Summary

This woman was followed up for 6 years, since 1989. She presented with metamorphopsia caused by myopic choroidal neovascularization in the right eye. The bleeding around the choroidal neovascularization absorbed by 4 months after the initial examination. In the following 2 years, chorioretinal atrophy gradually formed around the regressed choroidal neovascular membrane. The chorioretinal atrophy developed within the lesion of diffuse atrophy but not at the site of the previous bleeding. Although the bleeding is considered one cause of chorioretinal atrophy around the neovascular membrane, the findings in this patient suggest different mechanisms of the formation of chorioretinal atrophy.

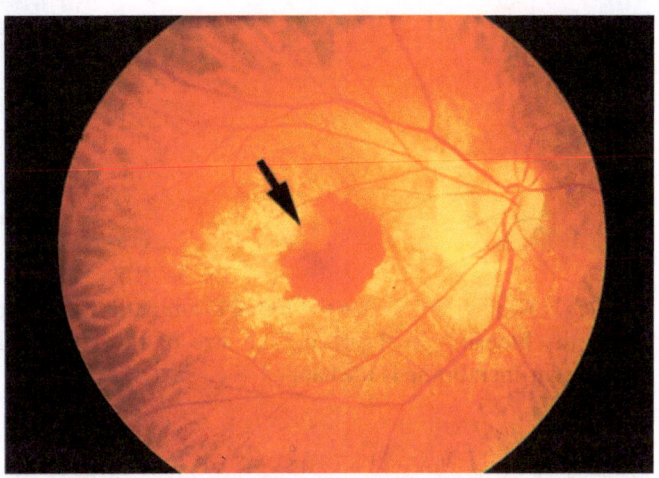

Fig. 47A. Right fundus at the initial examination (April 1989) shows macular bleeding. A grayish fibrovascular membrane of choroidal neovascularization is observed at the upper edge of the bleeding (*arrow*). The optic disc tilts temporally. A temporal peripapillary crescent is seen. Type I posterior staphyloma is present

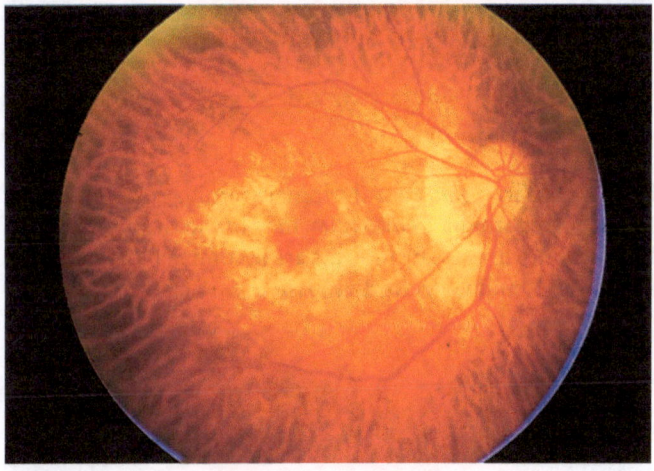

Fig. 47B. Three months later (July 1989), the bleeding is nearly absorbed. A choroidal neovascular membrane is seen within the enlarged lesion of diffuse atrophy

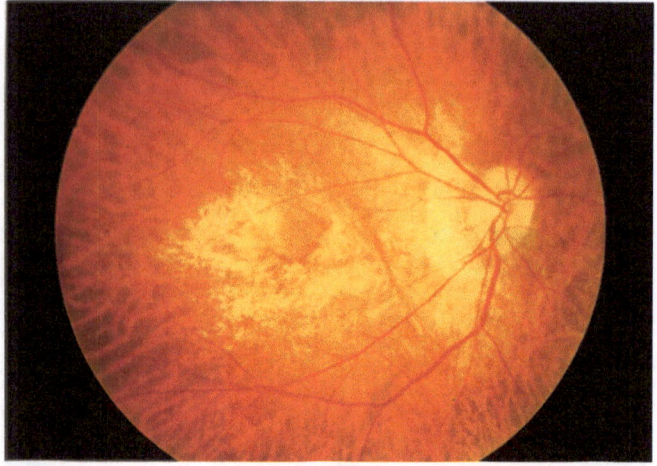

Fig. 47C. Four months after the initial examination (August 1989), the bleeding is absorbed. The size of the choroidal neovascular membrane is unchanged

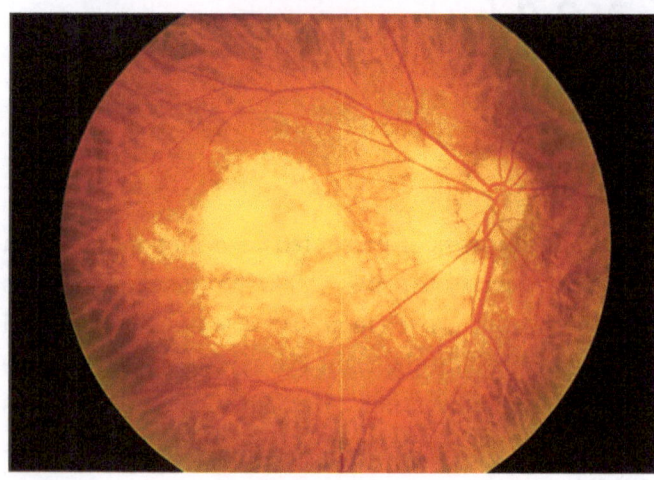

Fig. 47F. Five years after the initial examination (November 1994), the chorioretinal atrophy around the Fuchs' spot has enlarged further. Visual acuity is 0.1, and the refractive error is −14.00 D

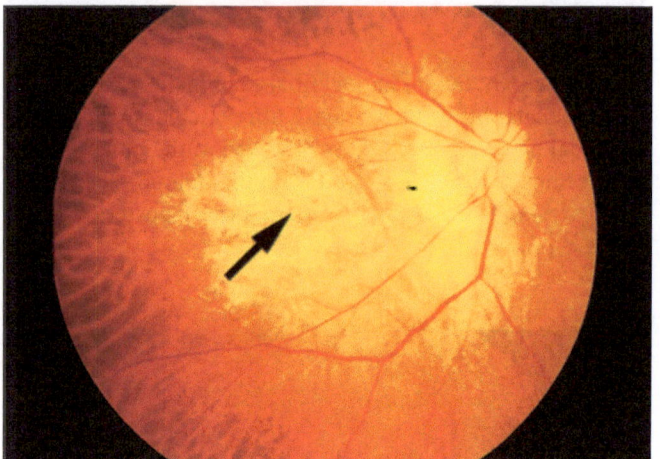

Fig. 47D. Two years after the initial examination (November 1991), the choroidal neovascular membrane has become yellowish white (*arrow*). Its margins are becoming blurred. Visual acuity is 0.3, and the refractive error is −15.00 D

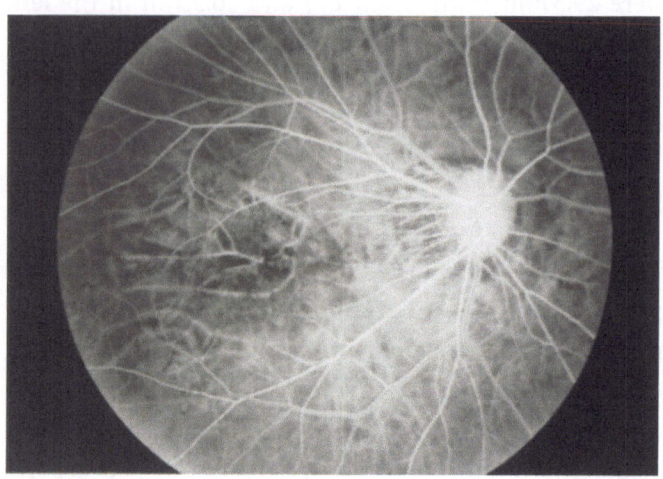

Fig. 47G. Fluorescein fundus angiogram 2 years after the initial examination (November 1991). At 19 sec after dye injection, the choroidal neovascular membrane is not obvious. The chorioretinal atrophy around the neovascular membrane also shows a filling defect. The margins of the chorioretinal atrophy are less clear

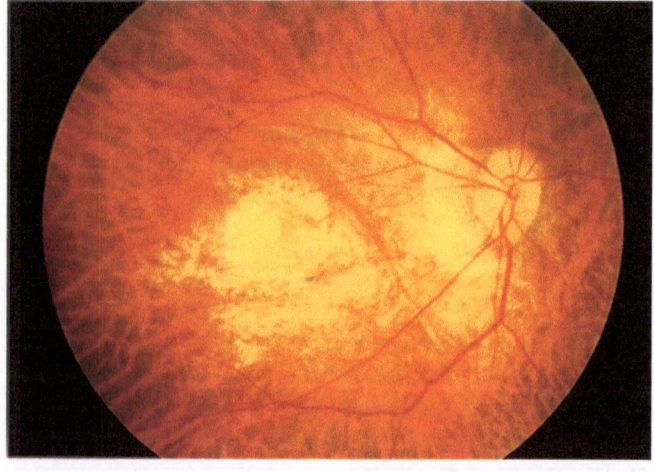

Fig. 47E. Four years after the initial examination (February 1993), the chorioretinal atrophy around the neovascular membrane has enlarged and is becoming clear. Visual acuity is 0.3, and the refractive error is −15.00 D

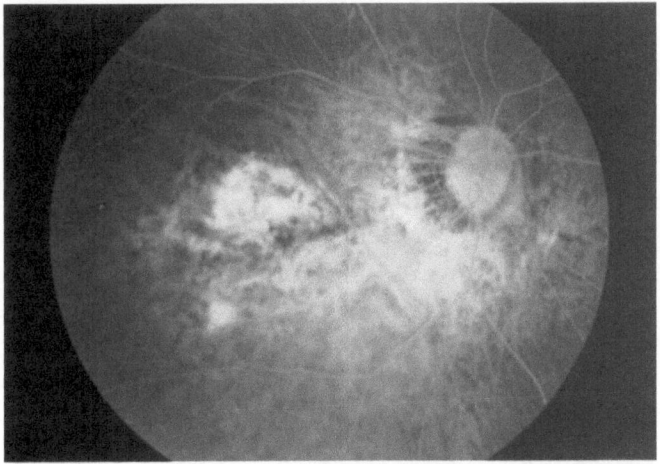

Fig. 47H. Fluorescein fundus angiogram 2 years after the initial examination (November 1991). At 8 min after dye injection, the chorioretinal atrophy around the neovascular membrane is hyperfluorescent because of tissue staining

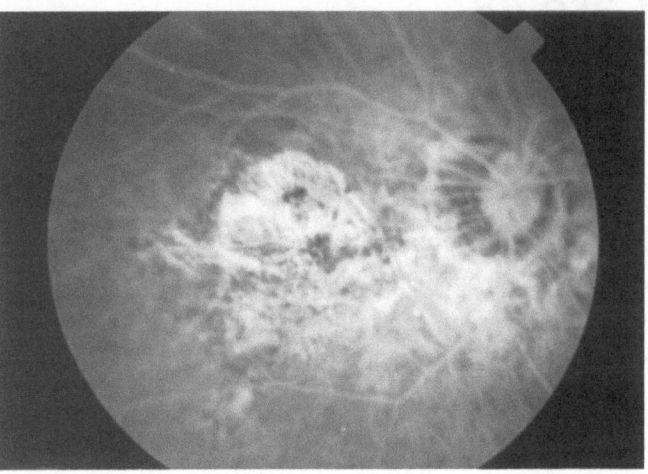

Fig. 47J. Fluorescein fundus angiogram 6 years after the initial examination (May 1995). At 6 min after dye injection, chorioretinal atrophy shows late hyperfluorescence

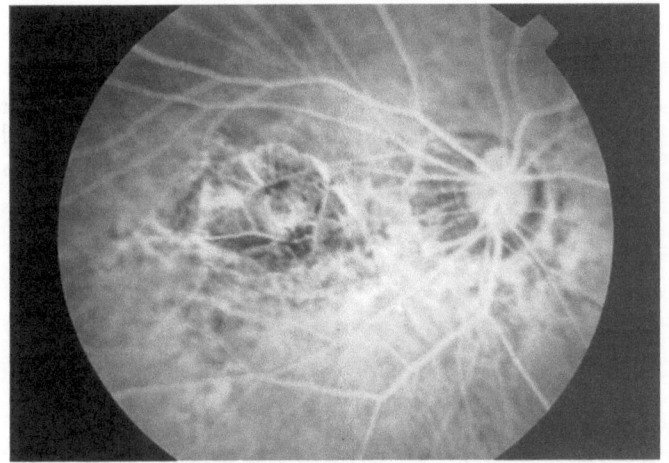

Fig. 47I. Fluorescein fundus angiogram 6 years after the initial examination (May 1995). Chorioretinal atrophy around the neovascular membrane shows a choroidal filling defect. The margins of chorioretinal atrophy are obvious

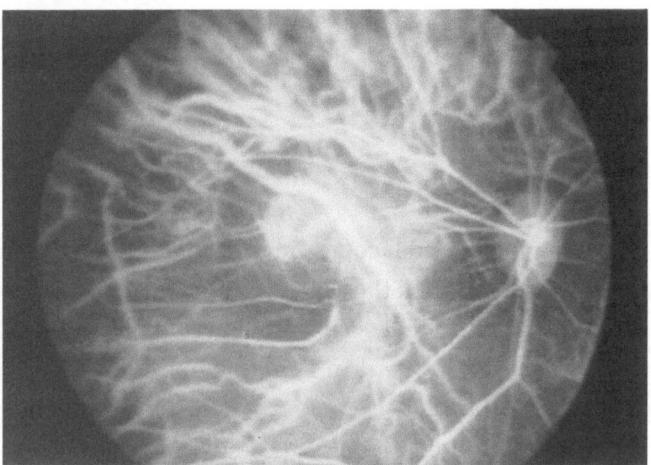

Fig. 47K. Indocyanine green fundus angiogram 6 years after the initial examination (May 1995). In the early phase of the angiogram, the chorioretinal atrophy shows slight hypofluorescence because of the filling defect. One large choroidal vein is observed to traverse the macular lesion obliquely

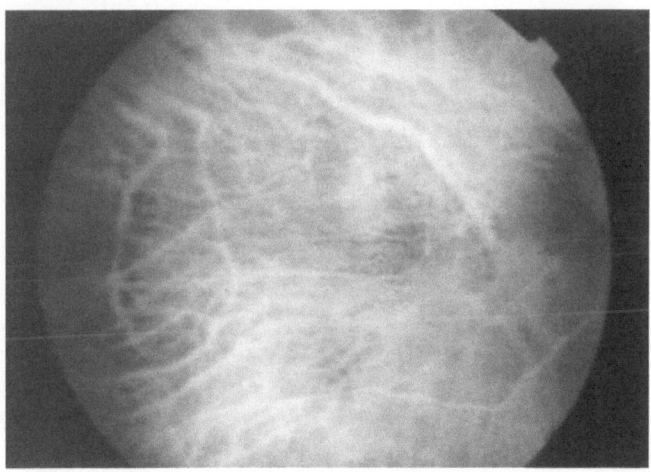

Fig. 47L. Indocyanine green fundus angiogram 6 years after the initial examination (November 1995). In the late phase of the angiogram, the chorioretinal atrophy shows slight hypofluorescence

Case 48

A 39-year-old woman was referred to our high myopia clinic on February 3, 1984, for macular bleeding in the right eye. She reported some difficulties with her distance vision in elementary school and began wearing glasses in fourth grade. She also began wearing contact lenses at age 18 years. Her medical history was noncontributory. Three of her five siblings are slightly myopic.

In the initial examination, the patient's best corrected visual acuity was 0.1 in the right and 0.5 in the left. The refractive error was −21.00 D sphere in the right eye and −15.25 D sphere in the left. The axial length measurements were 30.4 mm in the right eye and 29.1 mm in the left. Intraocular pressures and anterior segments were normal in both eyes. We describe the long-term fundus changes in her right eye.

Summary

This woman showed lacquer crack lesions and choroidal neovascularization in the right eye at the initial examination in 1984. After that, she was followed up by a general practitioner for 10 years. In 1994, she noticed a decrease in vision in the right eye and was referred to our high myopia clinic for myopic choroidal neovascularization. Wide chorioretinal atrophy had formed around the regressed Fuchs' spot. The ophthalmologic and angiographic findings of chorioretinal atrophy were similar to those of patchy atrophy. The progressive pattern of myopic fundus changes in the right eye was from HN_1 to HN_2 to MA.

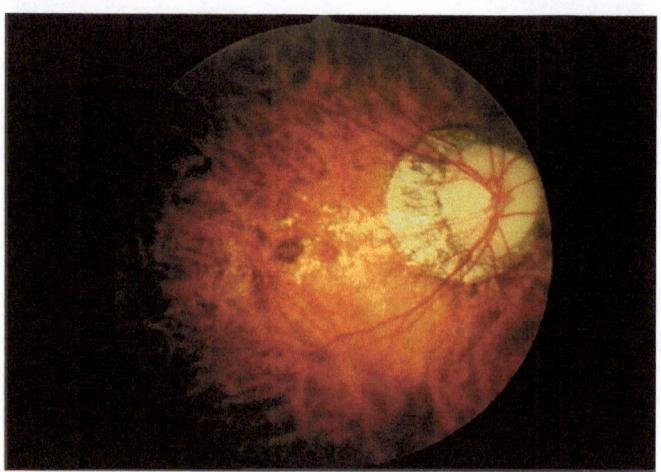

Fig. 48A. Right fundus at the initial examination (February 1984) shows a small pigmented Fuchs' spot with several lacquer crack lesions. The optic disc tilts temporally. A temporal peripapillary crescent is seen. Type II posterior staphyloma is present

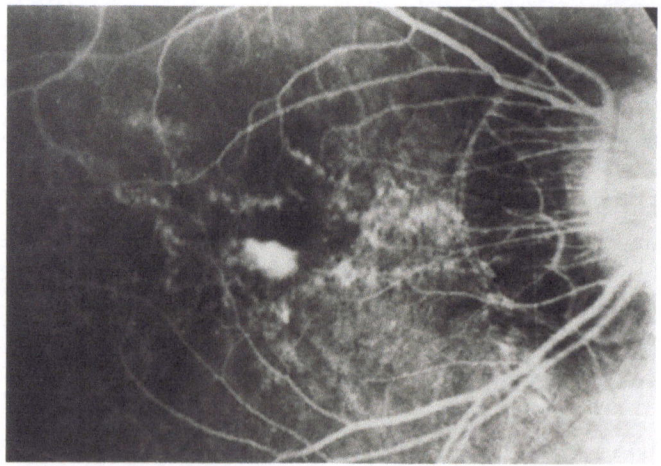

Fig. 48B. Fluorescein fundus angiogram at the initial examination. At 54 sec after dye injection, the choroidal neovascular membrane is hyperfluorescent. Lacquer crack lesions in the macula show linear hyperfluorescence

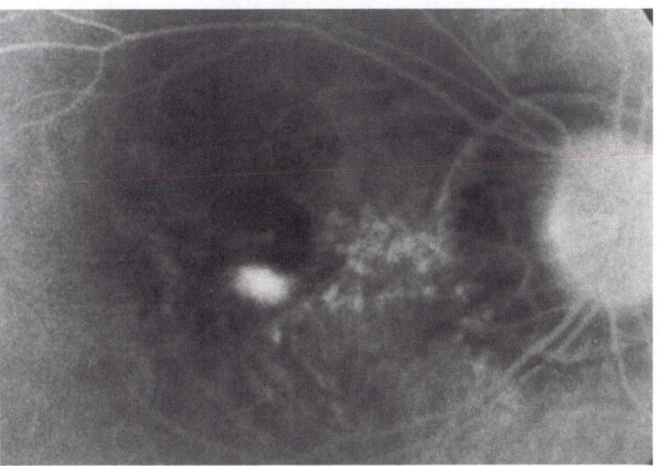

Fig. 48C. Fluorescein fundus angiogram at the initial examination. At 6 min after dye injection, slight dye leakage from the choroidal neovascular membrane is observed

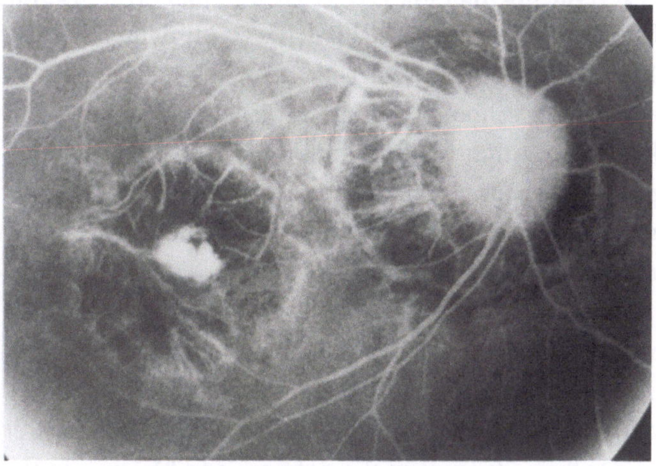

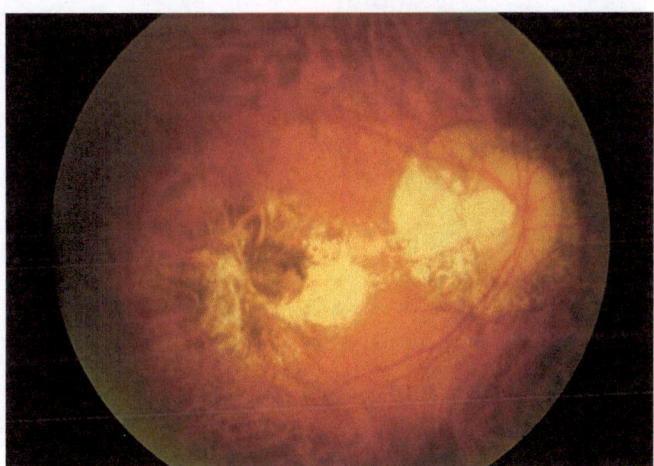

Fig. 48D. Ten years after the initial examination (March 1994), wide chorioretinal atrophy has formed around the pigmented Fuchs' spot

Fig. 48E. Fluorescein fundus angiogram 10 years after the initial examination (September 1994). At 7 min after dye injection, chorioretinal atrophy around the Fuchs' spot shows hypofluorescence caused by a choroidal filling defect. The choroidal neovascular membrane is hyperfluorescent

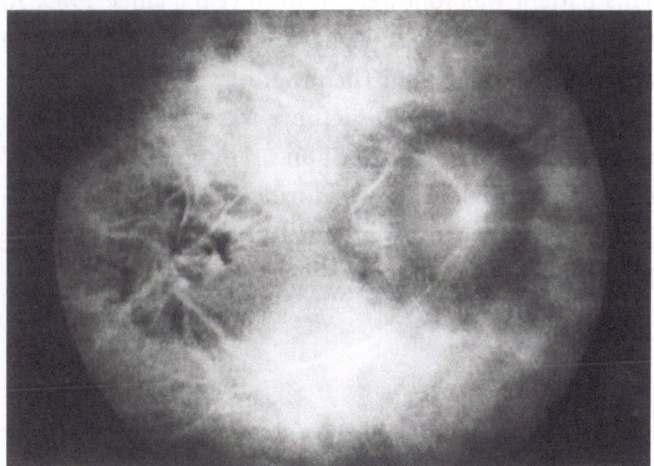

Fig. 48F. Indocyanine green fundus angiogram 11 years after the initial examination (March 1995) shows clear-margined hypofluorescence corresponding to the chorioretinal atrophy around the Fuchs' spot

Case 49

A 47-year-old man was referred to our high myopia clinic for macular bleeding in his left eye on September 27, 1985. He was diagnosed with myopia when he was an elementary school student. His visual acuity was 0.5 in both eyes at that time. In June 1985, he visited a general practitioner for visual disturbance in his left eye. Myopic macular bleeding in the left eye was found. No family members had severe myopia.

In the initial examination, the patient's best corrected visual acuity was 0.5 in the right eye and 0.15 in the left. The refractive error was −14.00 D sphere in the right eye and −17.00 D sphere in the left. Axial length measurements were 30.3 mm in the right eye and 31.1 mm in the left. Intraocular pressure and anterior segments were normal in both eyes. Slight cataractous changes were noted. We describe the long-term fundus changes in his left eye.

Summary

This patient was followed up for 8 years, since 1985. In his left fundus, a typical Fuchs' spot had formed after the absorption of bleeding. The progressive pattern of myopic fundus changes in his left eye was from HN_1 to HN_2. Chorioretinal atrophy later appeared around the Fuchs' spot and gradually enlarged during the follow-up period. Chorioretinal atrophy gradually became whitish, like patchy atrophy.

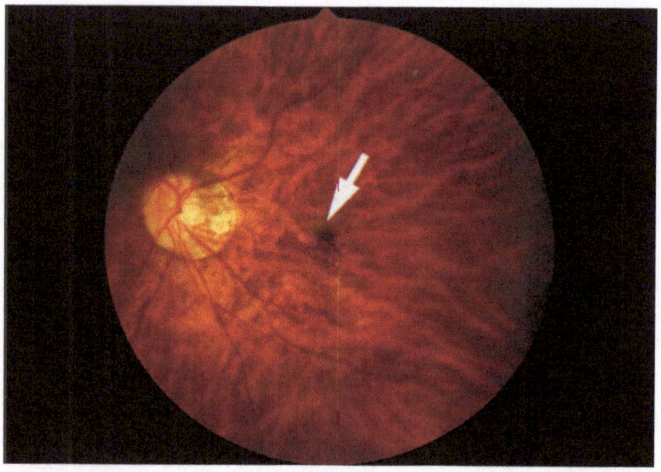

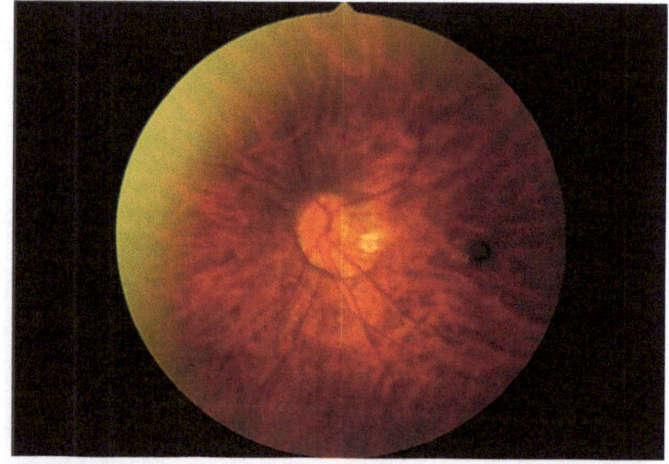

Fig. 49A. Left fundus at the initial examination (September 1985) shows a pigmented lesion (Fuchs' spot) with little bleeding in the macula (*arrow*). The optic disc tilts temporally. A temporal peripapillary crescent is seen. Slight diffuse atrophy is observed around the optic disc

Fig. 49B. One year later (April 1986), the bleeding has disappeared. Fuch's spot has slightly enlarged. Visual acuity is 0.15, and the refractive error is −16.75 D

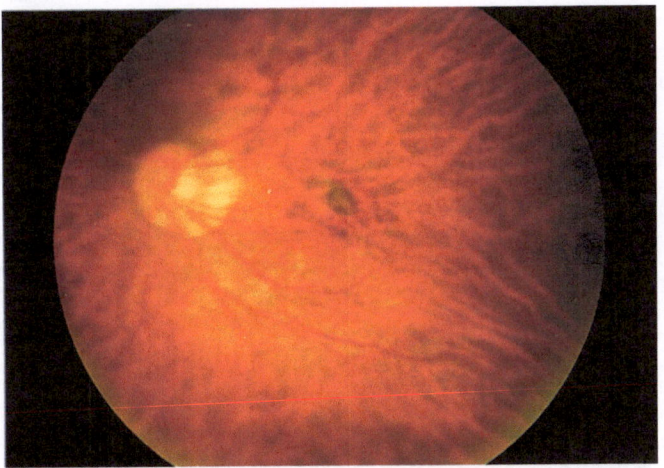

Fig. 49C. Two years after the initial examination (April 1987), new bleeding has appeared around the Fuchs' spot

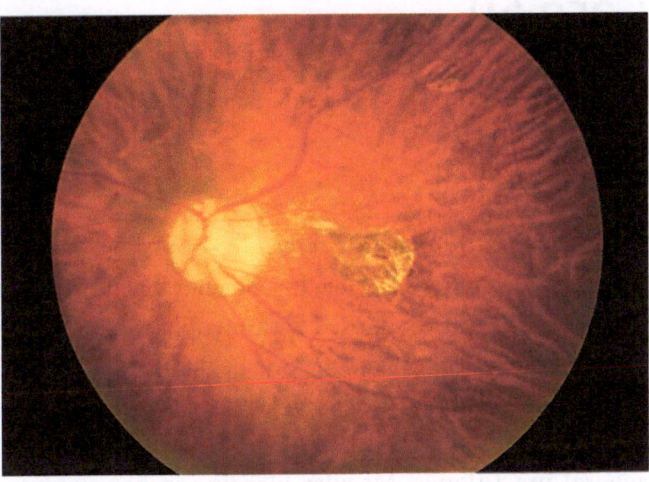

Fig. 49F. Six years after the initial examination (April 1991), chorioretinal atrophy and the Fuchs' spot have enlarged. Pigmentary change is observed within the chorioretinal atrophy

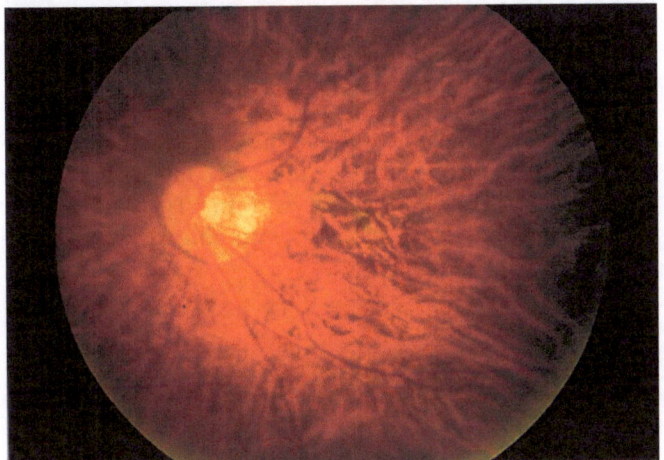

Fig. 49D. Four years after the initial examination (April 1989), bleeding is absorbed completely. Chorioretinal atrophy has formed around the Fuchs' spot. Visual acuity has dropped to 0.02 in the past 2 years

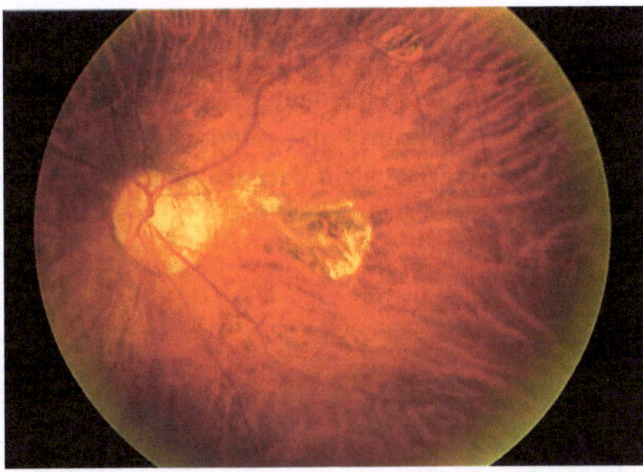

Fig. 49G. Seven years after the initial examination (March 1992), chorioretinal atrophy and Fuchs' spot have enlarged further

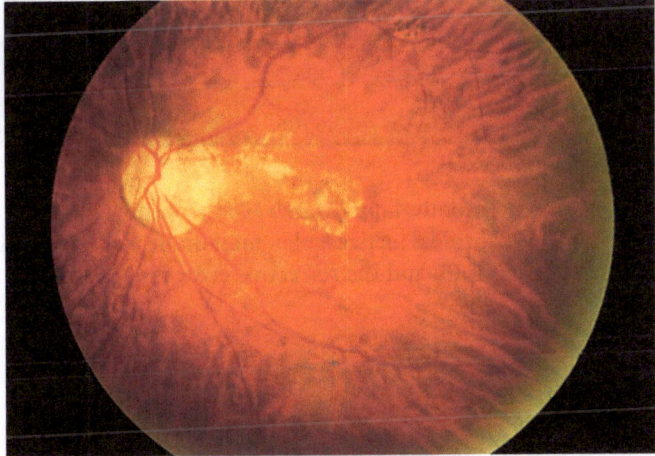

Fig. 49E. Five years after the initial examination (April 1990), Fuchs' spot and the surrounding chorioretinal atrophy have become pale and well defined

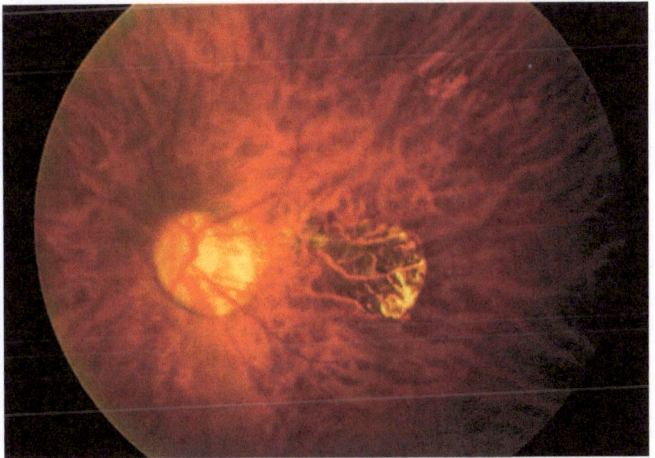

Fig. 49H. Eight years after the initial examination (March 1993), chorioretinal atrophy has continued to enlarge. Pigmentation has increased within the atrophic lesion. Visual acuity is 0.04, and the refractive error is −16.00 D

Case 50

A 56-year-old woman was referred to our high myopia clinic on November 11, 1983, for macular bleeding in her right eye. She was diagnosed with myopia when she was an elementary school student. She began wearing glasses for distance vision at age 13 years. In August 1983, she noticed a central scotoma in her right eye and visited a general practitioner. Macular bleeding in her right eye was found. Her medical history was noncontributory. All her siblings are highly myopic.

In the initial examination, the patient's best corrected visual acuity was 0.08 in the right eye and 1.0 in the left. The refractive error was $-17.00\,D$ sphere in the right eye and $-14.75\,D$ sphere in the left. Axial length measurements were 28.5 mm in the right eye and 27.1 mm in the left. Intraocular pressures and anterior segments were normal in both eyes. Slight cataractous changes were seen bilaterally. We describe the long-term fundus changes in her right eye.

Summary

This woman presented with decreased visual acuity caused by a choroidal neovascular membrane in her right eye. The course of fundus changes after the development of myopic choroidal neovascularization was typical. Chorioretinal atrophy similar to patchy atrophy formed, gradually enlarged, and finally occupied the entire macula. The progressive pattern of myopic fundus changes was from HN_1 to HN_2 to MA.

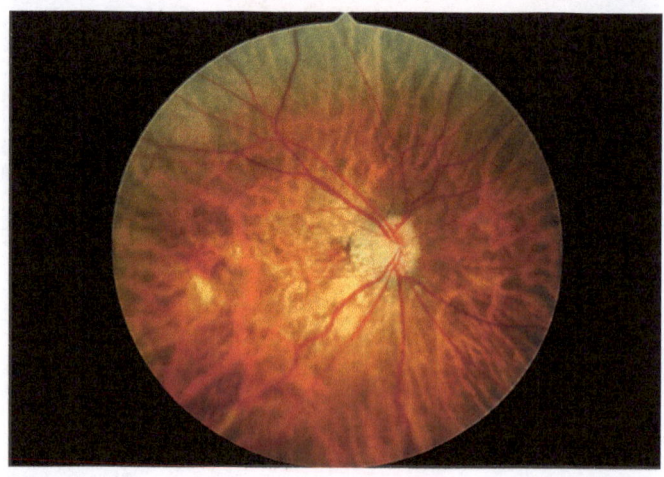

Fig. 50A. Right fundus at the initial examination (November 1983) shows choroidal neovascular membrane and surrounding bleeding in the macula. The optic disc tilts temporally. A temporal peripapillary crescent is seen. Type I posterior staphyloma is present. Diffuse atrophy is observed between the optic disc and the macula

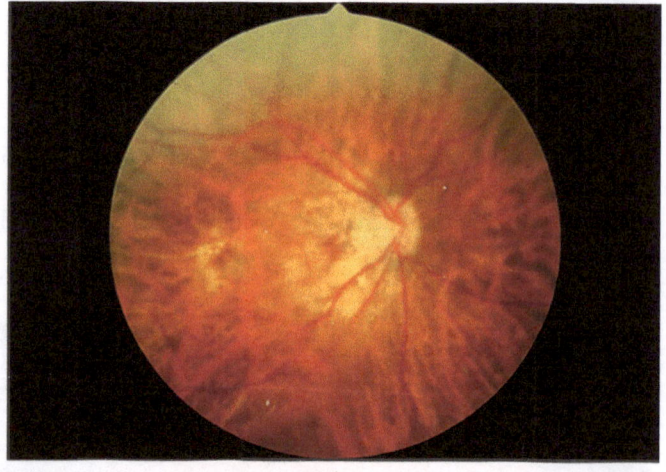

Fig. 50B. Five months later (March 1984), bleeding has disappeared. The choroidal neovascular membrane has enlarged. Visual acuity is 0.15, and the refractive error is $-17.50\,D$

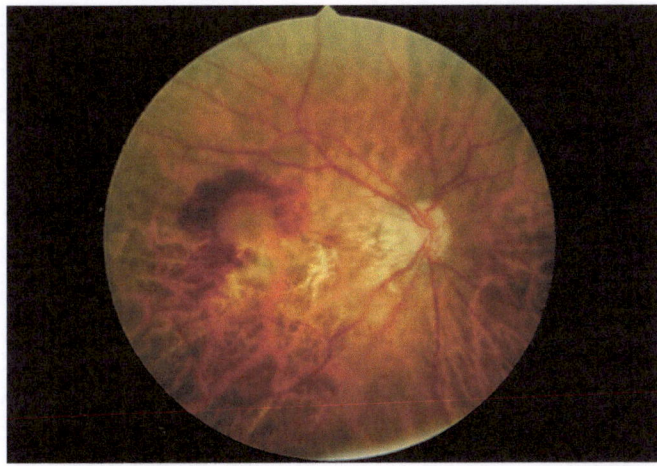

Fig. 50C. One year after the initial examination (October 1984), rebleeding has occurred. Visual acuity has decreased to 0.06

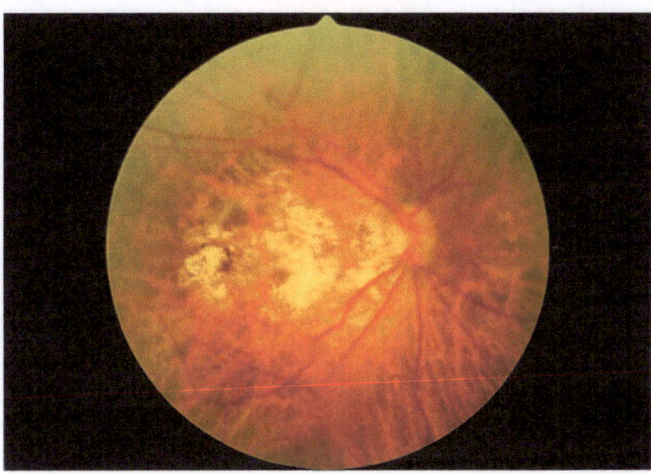

Fig. 50E. Four years after the initial examination (March 1987), chorioretinal atrophy has enlarged

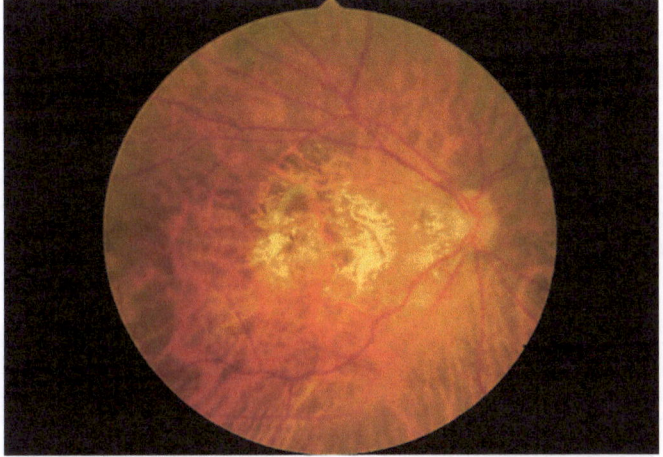

Fig. 50D. Three years after the initial examination (October 1986), chorioretinal atrophy appears around the regressed choroidal neovascular membrane. Visual acuity is 0.1, and the refractive error is −16.75 D

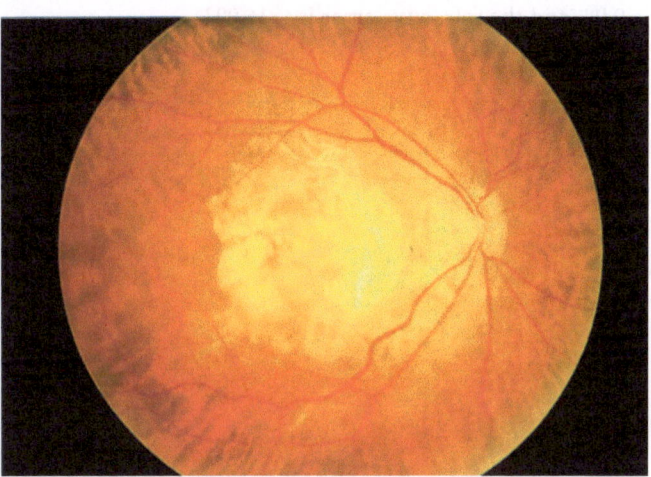

Fig. 50F. Five years after the initial examination (March 1988), the chorioretinal atrophy and choroidal neovascular membrane have enlarged further. The chorioretinal atrophy has become whitish. Visual acuity is 0.08, and the refractive error is −16.75 D

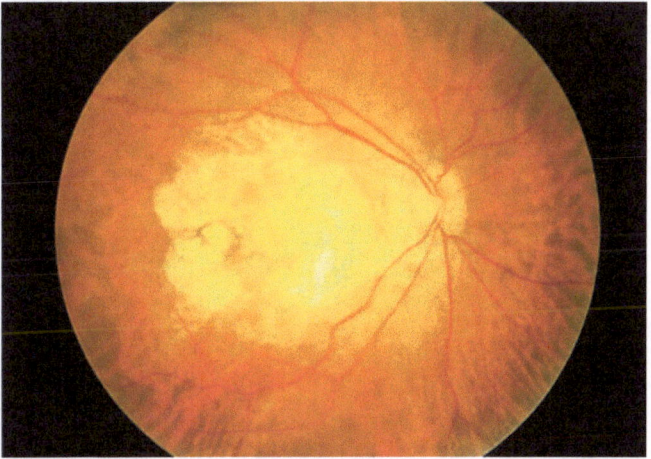

Fig. 50G. Eight years after the initial examination (January 1991), chorioretinal atrophy has enlarged, nearly covering the entire posterior fundus

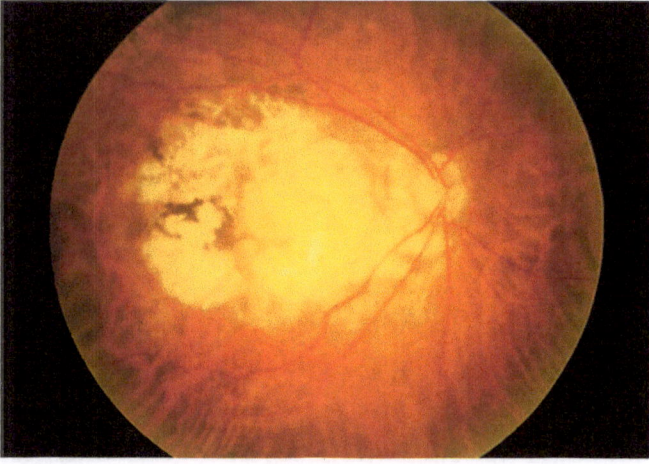

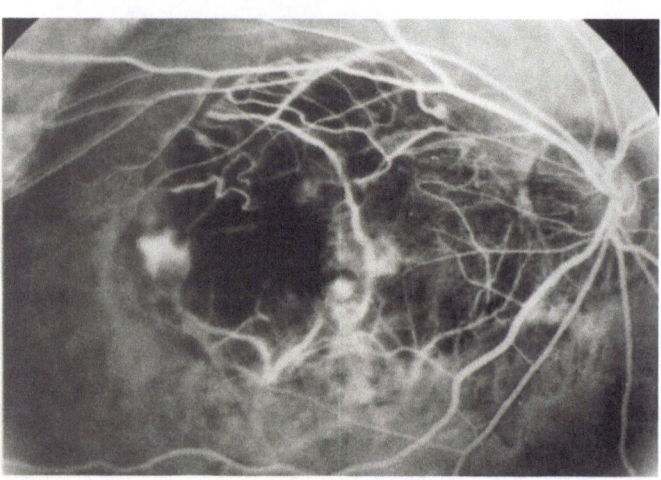

Fig. 50H. Eleven years after the initial examination (May 1994), the posterior fundus is almost entirely covered with chorioretinal atrophy. Pigmentation has increased within the chorioretinal atrophy. The choroidal neovascular membrane is obscured by surrounding chorioretinal atrophy. Visual acuity is 0.08, and the refractive error is −16.00 D

Fig. 50K. Fluorescein fundus angiogram 11 years after the initial examination (May 1994). At 1 min after dye injection, the choroidal filling defect has enlarged. The choroidal neovascular membrane has regressed and is no longer hyperfluorescent

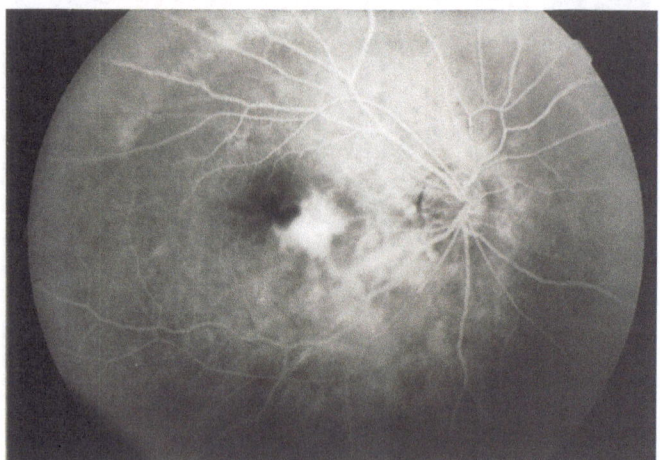

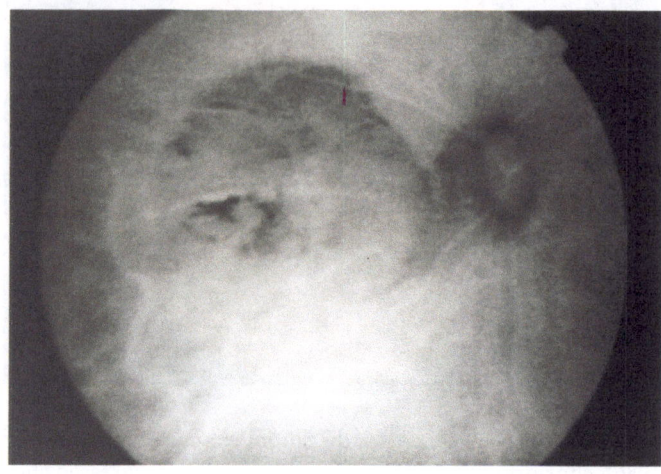

Fig. 50I. Fluorescein fundus angiogram at the initial examination. At 7 min after dye injection, the choroidal neovascular membrane shows hyperfluorescence

Fig. 50L. Indocyanine green fundus angiogram taken 11 years after the initial examination (May 1994). In the late phase of the angiogram, the chorioretinal atrophy shows hypofluorescece

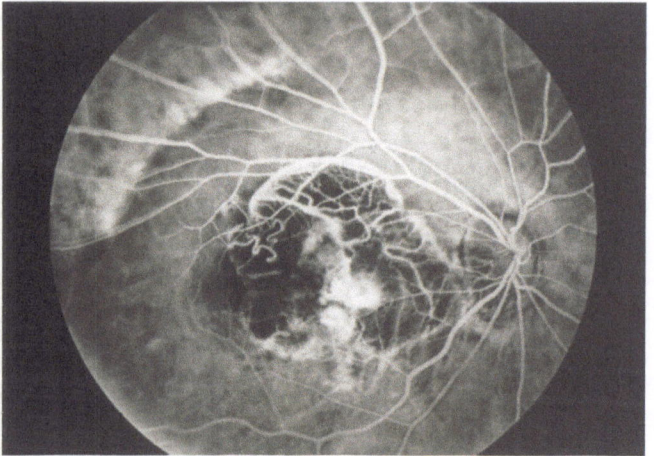

← **Fig. 50J.** Fluorescein fundus angiogram 7 years after the initial examination (October 1990). At 2 min after dye injection, the chorioretinal atrophy around the choroidal neovascular membrane shows a filling defect. Large-sized choroidal vessels are clearly seen within the chorioretinal atrophy. The choroidal neovascular membrane is still hyperfluorescent

Case 51

A 38-year-old man was referred to our high myopia clinic for macular bleeding in the right eye on August 4, 1989. He was diagnosed as having myopia when he was in elementary school. He began wearing glasses for distance vision at age 13 years. He noticed decreased visual acuity in the right eye in January 1989. Myopic choroidal neovascularization was found in that eye by a general practitioner. His medical history was noncontributory. No family members had severe myopia.

In the initial examination, the patient's best corrected visual acuity was 0.4 in the right eye and 1.2 in the left. The refractive error was −11.50 D sphere in the right eye and −9.00 D sphere in the left. Axial length measurements were 26.9 mm in the right eye and 26.2 mm in the left. Intraocular pressure and anterior segments were normal in both eyes. We show the long-term fundus changes in his right eye.

Summary

This man was followed up for 6 years, since 1989. He presented with decreased visual acuity caused by choroidal neovascular membrane. He was not extremely myopic, and no severe myopic fundus changes were observed around a Fuchs' spot. At the initial examination, a linear lesion was observed temporal to the choroidal neovascular membrane. This linear lesion was wide, and its appearance was different from a typical lacquer crack lesion. During the follow-up period, the linear lesion enlarged and progressed into chorioretinal atrophy, similar to patchy atrophy. The area of chorioretinal atrophy around the Fuchs' spot was observed beyond the area of previous bleeding.

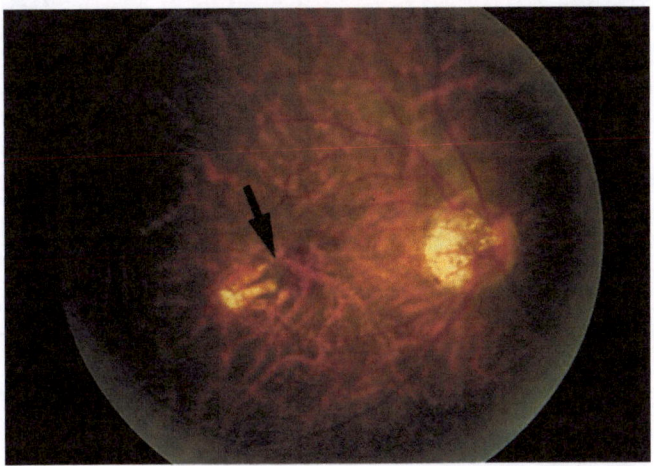

Fig. 51A. Right fundus at the initial examination (August 1989) shows choroidal neovascular membrane with pigmentation in the macula (*arrow*). Slight bleeding is present nasal to the neovascular membrane. A linear lesion is seen temporal to the choroidal neovascular membrane. The optic disc tilts temporally. A temporal peripapillary crescent is seen. No posterior staphyloma is present

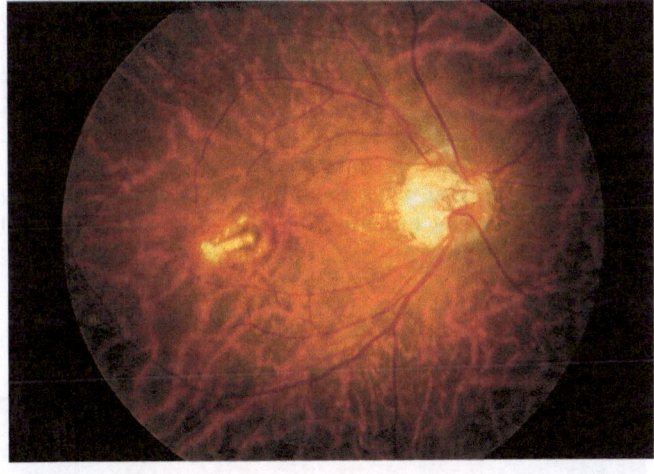

Fig. 51B. A month later (September 1989), macular bleeding is almost absorbed. Chorioretinal atrophy around the Fuchs' spot has slightly enlarged. Visual acuity is 0.4, and the refractive error is −11.00 D

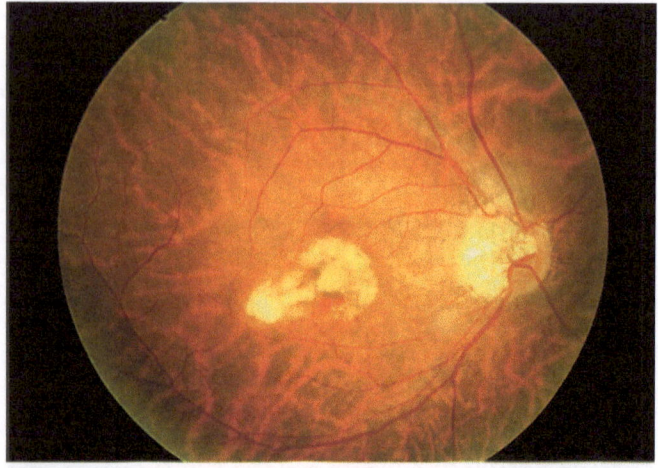

Fig. 51C. One year after the initial examination (June 1990), annular chorioretinal atrophy has developed around the choroidal neovascular membrane

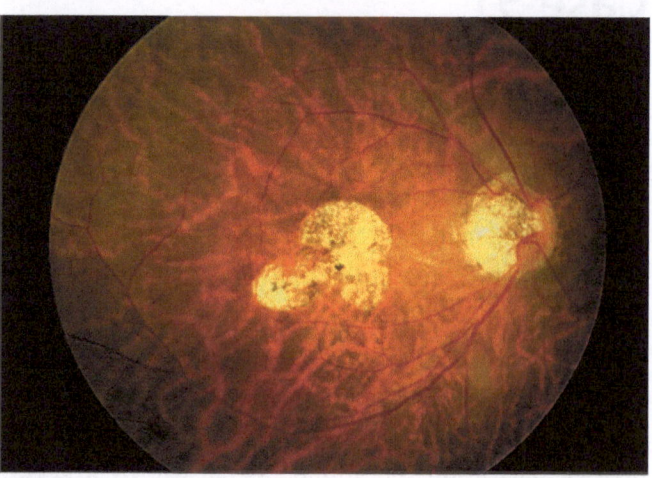

Fig. 51F. Three years after the initial examination (June 1992), chorioretinal atrophy around the choroidal neovascular membrane has enlarged. The choroidal neovascular membrane appears to have regressed

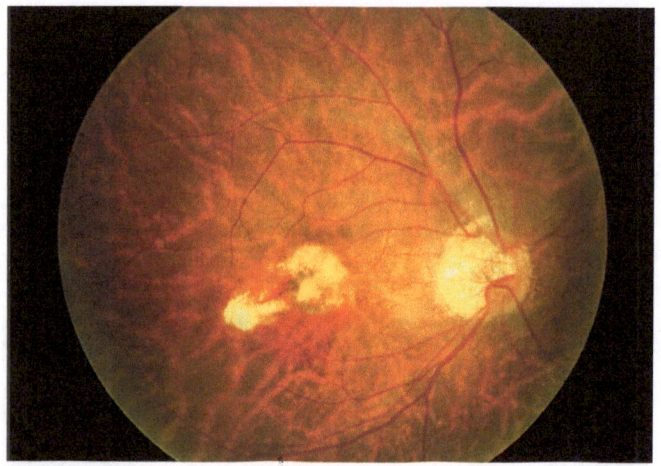

Fig. 51D. One year after the initial examination (August 1990), new bleeding has occurred inferior to the choroidal neovascular membrane. Visual acuity has decreased to 0.1, and the refractive error is −11.00 D

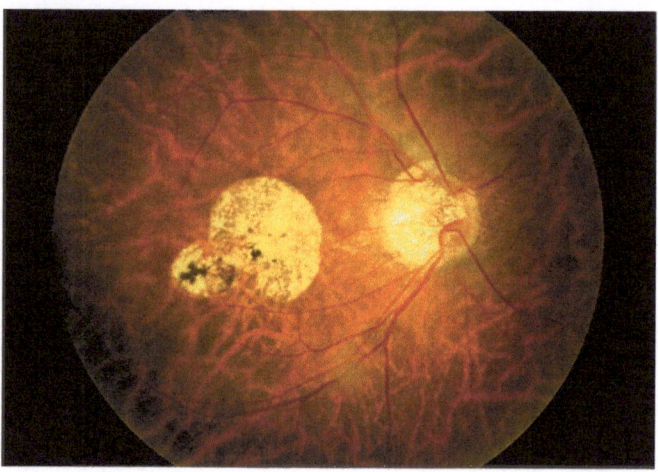

Fig. 51G. Five years after the initial examination (October 1994), chorioretinal atrophy around the neovascular membrane has enlarged further, forming one large atrophic lesion in the macula. Visual acuity is 0.1, and refractive error is −11.50 D

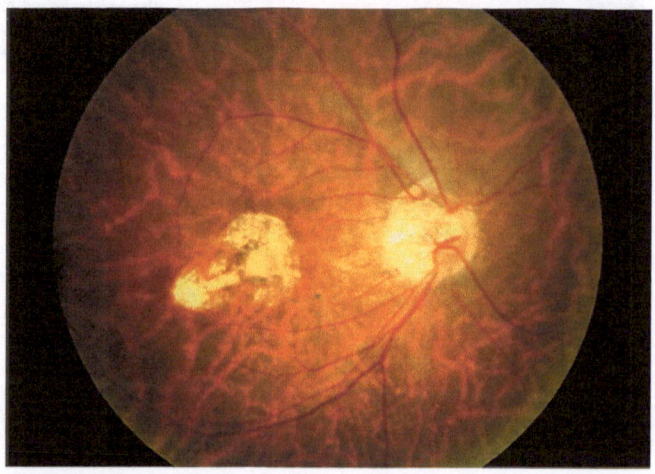

Fig. 51E. Two years after the initial examination (January 1991), chorioretinal atrophy around the choroidal neovascular membrane has enlarged

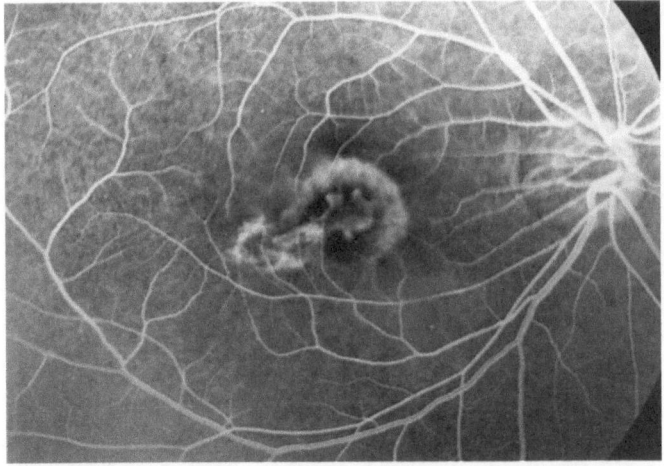

Fig. 51H. Fluorescein fundus angiogram 1 year after the initial examination (March 1990). At 23 sec after dye injection, hyperfluorescence corresponding to the choroidal neovascular membrane is seen in the macula. The chorioretinal atrophy is hyperfluorescent, especially at its margin

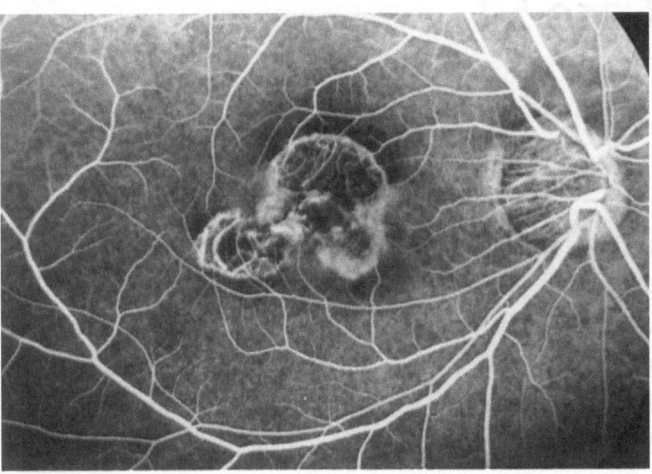

Fig. 51J. Fluorescein fundus angiogram 2 years after the initial examination (December 1991). At 22 sec after dye injection, an atrophic lesion shows a choroidal filling defect

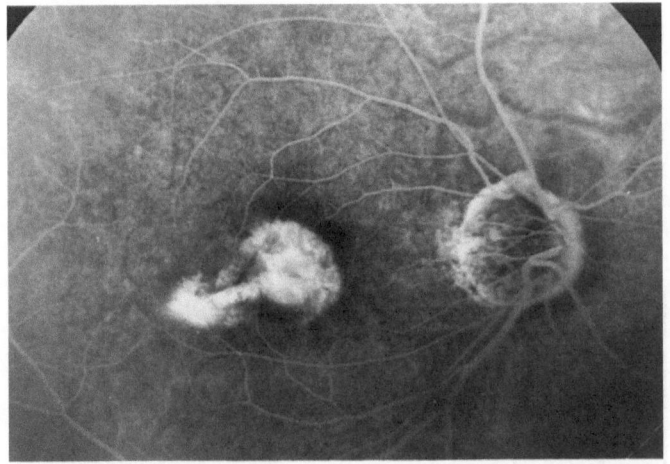

Fig. 51I. Fluorescein fundus angiogram 1 year after the initial examination (March 1990). At 8 min after dye injection, the chorioretinal atrophy and choroidal neovascular membrane are hyperfluorescent because of tissue staining

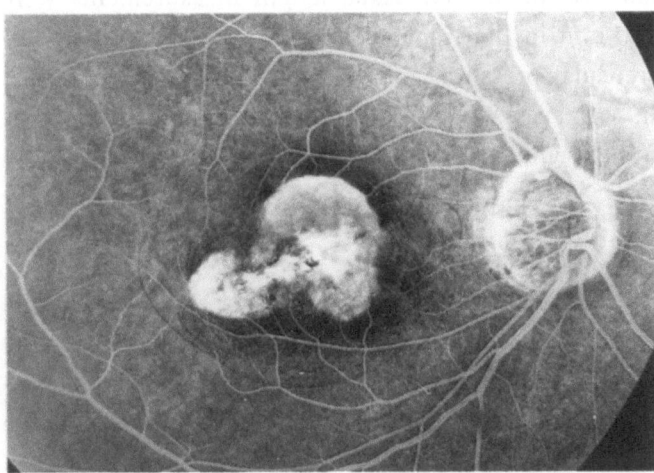

Fig. 51K. Fluorescein fundus angiogram 2 years after the initial examination (December 1991). At 8 min after dye injection, the chorioretinal atrophy shows hyperfluorescence caused by tissue staining in the late phase

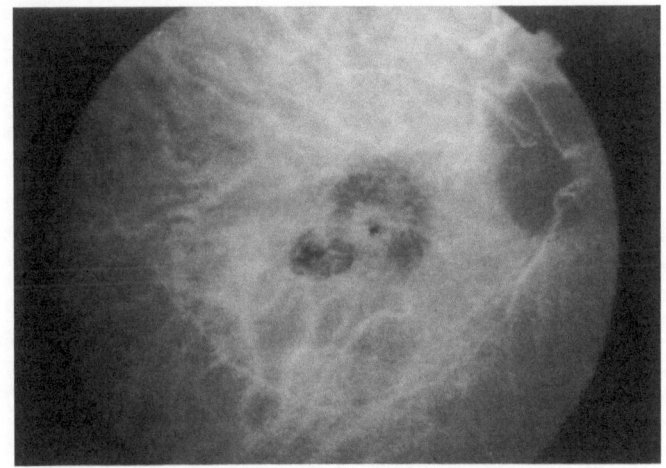

Fig. 51L. Indocyanine green fundus angiogram 4 years after the initial examination (October 1993). The chorioretinal atrophy shows hypofluorescence in the late phase of the angiogram, similar to patchy atrophy

Case 52

A 53-year-old woman presented on July 26, 1985, with decreased visual acuity in the right eye. She was diagnosed with myopia in the right eye before entering elementary school. She reported no visual disturbance because the left eye was emmetropic. She noticed a central scotoma in the right eye 2 months previous to the initial examination in our high myopia clinic. Her medical history was noncontributory. Her father and one of her three siblings are myopic.

In the initial examination, the patient's best corrected visual acuity was 0.07 in the right eye and 1.2 in the left. The refractive error was $-14.00\,D$ sphere in the right eye and $0\,D$ in the left. Axial length measurements were 28.1 mm in the right eye and 22.7 mm in the left. Intraocular pressures and anterior segments were normal in both eyes. We describe the long-term fundus changes in her right eye.

Summary

This patient was followed up for 10 years, since 1985. She was highly myopic unilaterally. After the choroidal neovascular membrane in the right eye regressed, sharp-margined chorioretinal atrophy formed around the neovascular membrane. Diffuse atrophy was also seen around the membrane before the chorioretinal atrophy developed. The progressive pattern of myopic fundus changes in this patient was from $D_2 + HN_1$ to $D_2 + HN_2$, to $D_2 + MA$.

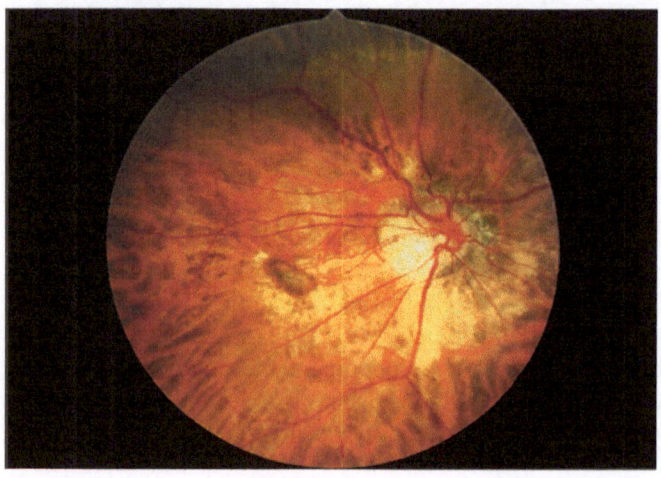

Fig. 52A. Right fundus at the initial examination (July 1985) shows a choroidal neovascular membrane surrounded by grayish pigmentation in the macula. Diffuse atrophy is also seen in the macula. The optic disc tilts temporally. A temporal peripapillary crescent is also seen. Type I posterior staphyloma is present

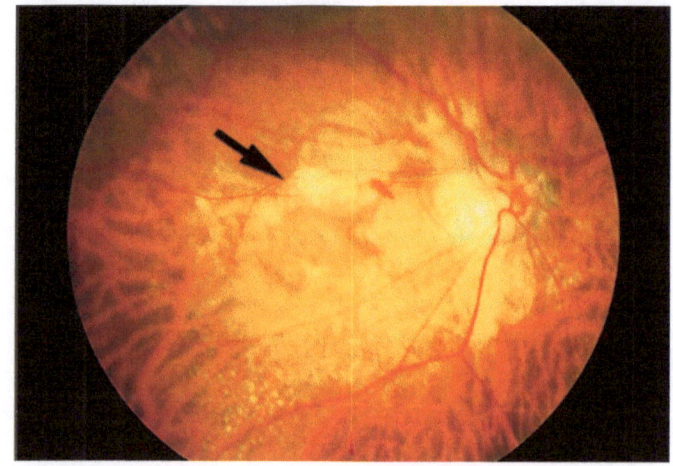

Fig. 52B. Two years later (June 1987), chorioretinal atrophy similar to patchy atrophy has appeared superior to the neovascular membrane (*arrow*). Visual acuity is 0.02, and the refractive error is $-14.00\,D$

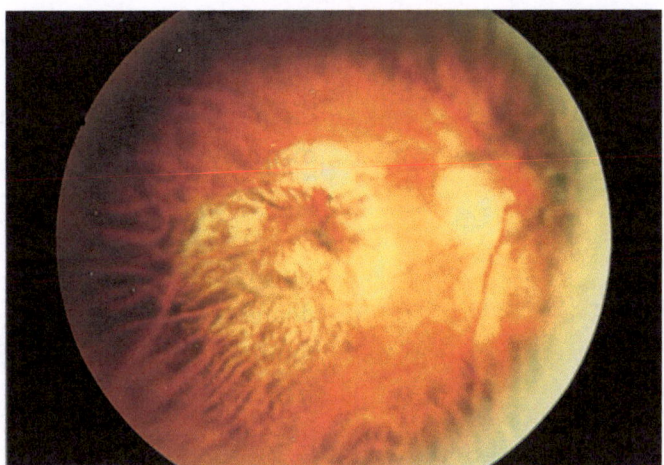

Fig. 52C. Four years after the initial examination (June 1989), the choroidal neovascular membrane has regressed. Chorioretinal atrophy around the neovascular membrane has enlarged and shows clear margins

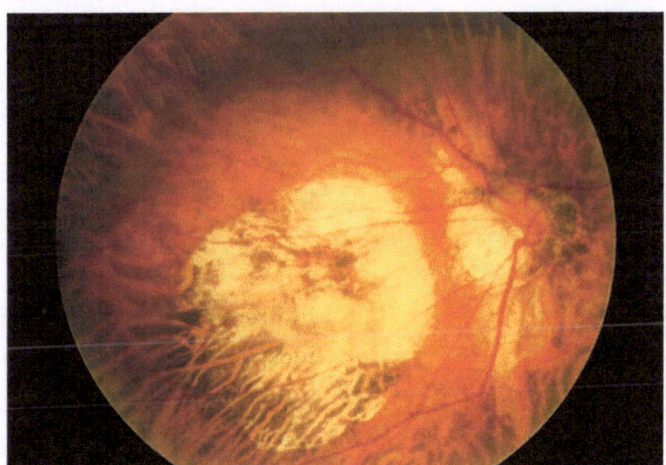

Fig. 52D. Nine years after the initial examination (May 1994), chorioretinal atrophy around the neovascular membrane has enlarged further and largely occupies the posterior fundus. Visual acuity is 0.03, and the refractive error is −14.00 D

Subject Index